The embryonic ages for Streeter's stages XII – XXII have been altered in accordance with the human data from Iffy, L. et al: Acta Anat. 66 : 178, 1967

EXTREMITIES	HEART	GUT, ABDOMEN	LUNG	UROGENITAL	OTHER
					Early blastocyst with inner cell mass and cavitation (58 cells) lying free within the uterine cavity.
					Implantation Trophoblast invasion Embryonic disc with endoblast and ectoblast
		Yolk sac			Early amnion sac Extraembryonic mesoblast, angioblast Chorionic gonadotropin
	Merging mesoblast anterior to pre-chordal plate	Stomatodeum Cloaca		Allantois	Primitive streak Hensen's node Notochord Prechordal plate Blood cells in yolk sac
	Single heart tube Propulsion	Foregut		Mesonephric ridge	Yolk sac larger than amnion sac
Arm bud	Ventric. outpouching Gelatinous reticulum	Rupture stomatodeum Evagination of thyroid, liver, and dorsal pancreas.	Lung bud	Mesonephric duct enters cloaca	Migration of myotomes from somites
Leg bud	Auric. outpouching Septum primum	Pharyngeal pouches yield parathyroids, lat. thyroid, thymus Stomach broadens	Bronchi	Ureteral evag. Urorect. sept. Germ cells Gonadal ridge Coelom, Epithelium	Rathke's pouch
Hand plate, Mesench. condens. Innervation	Fusion mid. A-V canal Muscular vent. sept.	Intestinal loop into yolk stalk Cecum Gallbladder Hepatic ducts Spleen	Main lobes	Paramesonephric duct Gonad ingrowth of coelomic epith.	Adrenal cortex (from coelomic epithelium) invaded by sympathetic cells = medulla Jugular lymph sacs
Finger rays, Elbow	Aorta Pulmonary artery Valves Membrane ventricular septum	Duodenal lumen obliterated Cecum rotates right Appendix	Tracheal cartil.	Fusion urorect. sept. Open urogen. memb., anus Epith. cords in testicle	Early muscle
Clearing, central cartil.	Septum secundum			S-shaped vesicles in in nephron blastema connect with collecting tubules from calyces	Pleuroperitoneal canals closed Superficial vascular plexus low on cranium
Shell, Tubular bone				A few large glomeruli Short secretory tubules Tunica albuginea Testicle	Superficial vascular plexus at vertex

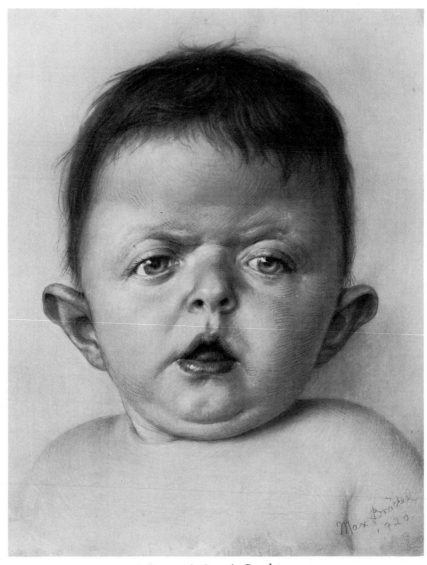

A Boy with Apert's Syndrome

Original Max Brödel drawing No. 506. Property of The Johns Hopkins
University School of Medicine, Department of Art as Applied to Medicine.

RECOGNIZABLE PATTERNS OF HUMAN MALFORMATION

Genetic, Embryologic, and Clinical Aspects

By

David W. Smith, M.D.

Professor in Pediatrics,
University of Washington School of Medicine
Seattle, Washington

Volume VII in the Series

MAJOR PROBLEMS IN CLINICAL PEDIATRICS

ALEXANDER J. SCHAFFER
Consulting Editor

W. B. Saunders Company • Philadelphia • London • Toronto • 1970

W. B. Saunders Company: West Washington Square
Philadelphia, Pa. 19105

12 Dyott Street
London W.C.1

1835 Yonge Street
Toronto 7, Ontario

Recognizable Patterns of Human Malformation

Print No.:   1   2   3   4   5   6   7   8   9

Dedication

To my wife Ann, beloved inspirational companion.

To my father William H. Smith, accomplished engineer and erstwhile physician.

To my teachers Dr. Lawson Wilkins, molder of clinicians and humanist, and Professor Dr. Gian Töndury, complete anatomist and teacher, who brings embryology into living perspective.

Foreword

We have long wanted a volume in this series on the subject of the "odd-looking baby." Proper counseling of parents faced with the birth of an infant of this nature depends entirely upon the recognition of the category into which he falls. Knowledge concerning babies with constellations of congenital defects has grown tremendously within the last few years, and not many of us have been able to keep abreast of it.

David W. Smith needs no introduction to those who have followed this literature even superficially. We have recognized the outstanding qualities which made him the logical choice to write this monograph ever since we watched his brilliant, devoted work as Resident and Fellow in Endocrinology in the Harriet Lane Home in the early 1950's. Since then he has become a Professor in Pediatrics at the University of Washington School of Medicine. He has written a book which we think no one dealing with the newborn can do without.

ALEXANDER J. SCHAFFER, M.D.

Acknowledgments

The information set forth in this book represents an amalgamation of the knowledge, contributions, and work of many individuals, some of whom are herein recognized.

TEACHERS: Dr. Lawson Wilkins, Johns Hopkins University School of Medicine, whose total clinical approach served as a guide and inspiration toward the development of this book; Dr. Klaus Patau, University of Wisconsin Medical School, from whom the author gained knowledge of cytogenetics and a critical and concise approach toward writing manuscripts; Dr. Gian Töndury, University of Zurich Medical School, from whom the author gained knowledge of embryology and the interpretation of errors in morphogenesis; and Dr. Waldo Nelson, Temple University School of Medicine, whose editorial policy toward clinical relevance and simplicity of semantics has influenced the manner in which this book was developed.

FELLOWS AND STUDENTS: The following have been especially helpful in the development of this book.

FELLOWS: Dr. Luc Lemli, Dendermonde, Belgium; Dr. John Opitz, University of Wisconsin Medical School; Dr. Robert Summitt, University of Tennessee Medical School; Dr. Arlan Rosenbloom, University of Florida Medical School; Dr. Jaime Frias, University of Concepcion Medical School, Chile, who gathered the material for and wrote up 15 of the syndromes; and Dr. Jon Aase, University of Washington Medical School, who has been an invaluable critic during the latter stages of the development of this book.

STUDENTS: Dr. Philip Marden, University of Wisconsin Medical School, whose work contributed to Chapter 5; and Dr. John Mulvihill, University of Washington Medical School, who contributed to the section on dermatoglyphics in Chapter 5 and in the appendix.

ASSOCIATES: Many individuals have contributed photos and information. Especially helpful have been the following: Dr. John Opitz, University of Wisconsin Medical School; Drs. Pierre Maroteaux and Maurice Lamy, Hospital des Enfants-Malades, Paris; Dr. Robert Gorlin, University of Minnesota Medical and Dental School; Dr. Victor McKusick, Johns Hopkins University Medical School; and my Associates at the University of Washington Medical School, Drs. Benjamin Graham, Arno Motulsky, Thomas Shepard, David Shurtleff, Pierre Ferrier, Ronald Scott, and Bruce Beckwith.

ASSISTANTS: The invaluable and dedicated secretarial assistance of Mrs. Nancy Fargo is deeply appreciated. Miss Kay Drangsveit of the University of Wisconsin Department of Pediatrics has also been of assistance, and Mrs. Nancy Laestadius deserves special mention for her assistance in the development of the tables at the end of Chapter 2 and in the preparation of photographs for many of the disorders.

RESEARCH LIBRARIAN: Mrs. Lyle Harrah is a major contributor to the development of this book. She has made available over 2200 articles, allowing for an extensive review on each syndrome, though only selected references appear in the text. Her dedication and capacity for obtaining even the most obscure references are greatly appreciated. Gerald J. Oppenheimer, Head Librarian at the University of Washington Medical School Library, has been most helpful, allowing a special room for this project.

ILLUSTRATIONS: Mrs. Phyllis Wood of the University of Washington Department of Medical Illustration prepared the illustrations in Chapter 1 as well as some of the illustrations in Chapters 3, 4 and 5. Her art work, which immeasurably augments the text itself, is greatly appreciated. Mrs. Nancy Laestadius is gratefully acknowledged for her preparation of charts in Chapters 3 and 5. Acknowledged for their assistance in photography and illustrations are the departments of medical photography at the University of Washington, University of Wisconsin, and the Children's Orthopedic Hospital of Washington. The C. V. Mosby Publishing Company of St. Louis deserves special acknowledgment for their permission to publish a large proportion of the photographs that appear in this text, many of which were previously published in the Journal of Pediatrics.

FUNDING: This work was accomplished in the Dysmorphology Unit, a unit which is dedicated to teaching, service, and research about problems of malformation and which derives its financial support from the Children's Bureau.

MEMORIAL: The Robert Gordon Schneller Memorial Fund provided funds for medical illustration and photography which greatly enhanced the educational value of this book. Mr. and Mrs. M. R. Schneller had two sons. Robert Gordon, a student at the University of Washington, was interested in problems of malformation, at least partially because his younger brother has Down's syndrome. Robert's life and his interest were cut short by a mountaineering accident at the age of 20 years. Mr. and Mrs. Schneller hope, as do I, that the contribution of his friends and relatives may assist in stimulating others to pursue the interest which Robert had in extending our knowledge about malformation problems.

DAVID W. SMITH, M.D.

Contents

Chapter Three

Chapter Four

Chapter Five

INTRODUCTION

We ought not to set them aside with idle thoughts or idle words about "curiosities" or "chances." Not one of them is without meaning; not one that might not become the beginning of excellent knowledge, if only we could answer the question—why is it rare? or being rare, why did it in this instance happen?—JAMES PAGET, Lancet, 2:1017, 1882.

The questions set forth by Paget are still applicable today. Every malformation represents an inborn error in morphogenesis. Just as the study of inborn metabolic errors has extended our understanding of normal biochemistry, so the accumulation of knowledge concerning defects in morphogenesis may assist us in further unraveling the story of structural development.

The major portion of this text is devoted to patterns of malformation, but in addition you will find relevant chapters on morphogenesis and genetics, as well as a chapter on the recognition of minor anomalies including dermatoglyphic alterations. It is hoped that the design of the book will lend itself to practical clinical application, as well as providing a basic text for the education of those interested in a better understanding of alterations in morphogenesis. Furthermore, many of the charts have been developed for direct use in the counseling of patients and parents.

Accurate diagnosis of a specific syndrome among the 0.7 per cent of babies born with multiple malformations is a necessary prerequisite to providing a prognostic evaluation and plan of management for the affected infant, as well as genetic counseling for the parents.

The following is the author's approach toward the evaluation of an individual with multiple defects:

I. Gather information. An outline of history and physical evaluation is set forth in Appendix A. Chapter Five presents some of the minor defects which are valuable diagnostic clues in patterns of malformation.

II. Interpret the patient's anomalies from the viewpoint of developmental anatomy and strive to answer the following questions:
   A. Which anomaly in the individual represents the earliest defect in morphogenesis? A table for this purpose is found in Chapter Three, Morphogenesis. From such information one can determine that the problem in development must have existed *prior to* a particular prenatal age and any environmental factor *after* that time could not be the cause of that malformation.
   B. Is a given defect primary or secondary? Morphogenesis is a timely and sequential process in which a defect of one structure may compromise the formation of subsequent structures. An attempt should be made to determine retrospectively the primary anomalies. This approach will tend to subdivide the multiple defect patients into two general categories:
      1. Those having a *single syndromic anomaly* in which the pattern of anomalies is the consequence of a single localized defect which anteceded and was the cause for the secondary anomalies. Chapter One delineates some of the single syndromic anomalies.
      2. Those having *multiple primary defects*, either within many areas of one system or involving multiple systems, as set forth in Chapter Two.

III. Attempt to arrive at a specific overall diagnosis, confirm when possible, and counsel accordingly. When possible, counsel should include the following: an understanding of how the altered structures came to be the way they are; the natural history of the condition and what measures can be utilized to assist the child; and the mode of etiology and the genetic counsel (recurrence risks).

Chapter One

SINGLE SYNDROMIC MALFORMATIONS
resulting in secondary defects

A single localized defect in morphogenesis can upset the subsequent development of other structures and result in a syndrome of multiple defects, especially when the initiating defect is one that occurs early in morphogenesis. Thus the structural consequences at birth may appear far more extensive and profound than the single early, initiating defect.

It is important to recognize such multiple defect individuals as having a single *primary* defect in morphogenesis. With the possible exception of the prechordal mesoderm defect (see Fig. 7), chromosomal studies are not presently indicated for individuals with a single primary defect. Rarely, a single mutant gene or pair of mutant genes may be implicated, and therefore a review of the family history for a similar type of defect is always indicated. With the exception of androgenic hormones causing masculinization of the external genitalia in the female fetus, quinine and possibly chloroquine causing deafness, and tetracyclines causing defective tooth development, no other environmental agent has been clearly implicated as a cause for a single malformation in an otherwise normal individual. Judging from the more common single major malformations, the predominant cause is polygenic factors with a low recurrence risk—about 5 per cent—for the same type of defect in subsequent offspring of normal parents (see Chapter Four).

For the following conditions, adequate recurrence risk data are available only for cleft lip and palate and for the meningomyelocele-anencephaly-type defect—both about 5 per cent. For the other conditions set forth in this chapter it may simply be stated that they occur sporadically in a family, with unusual exceptions.

The following are some examples of patterns of defect which appear to represent the consequences of a single initiating malformation. The unproved suppositions regarding developmental pathology, illustrated at the end of the chapter, are based on indirect evidence, much of it summarized by Willis[1] and by Gruenwald.[2-4]

1. Cleft Lip and Palate—Primary Defect in Closure of Lip (Fig. 1)

By 35 days of age the lip is normally fused. A failure of lip fusion may impair the subsequent closure of the palatal shelves, which do not completely fuse until the eighth to ninth week. Thus cleft palate is a frequent association with cleft lip.

2. Pierre Robin Anomaly—Primary Defect May Be Early Mandibular Hypoplasia (see Fig. 5)

The Pierre Robin "syndrome"[5] consists of small mandible, glossoptosis, and posterior cleft of the palate. The single initiating defect may be hypoplasia of the mandibular area prior to nine weeks, allowing the tongue to be posteriorly located and thereby impairing the closure of the posterior palatal shelves which must "grow over" the tongue to meet in the midline. The author suggests that this be termed "Pierre Robin anomaly" rather than Pierre Robin syndrome. The Pierre Robin anomaly is most commonly noted in otherwise normal individuals, whose prognosis is very good if they survive the early period of respiratory obstruction. Less commonly the anomaly may be one feature in a multiple defect syndrome such as the 18 trisomy syndrome. It is

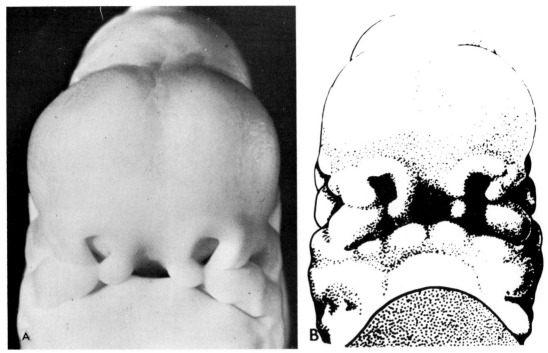

Figure 1. A, Normal face at 35 days of age, by which time the lip is fused. B, A spontaneous abortus of 35 days with unilateral hypoplasia of the lateral nasal swelling and incomplete closure of the lip on that side. (Courtesy of Prof. G. Töndury, University of Zurich.)

potentially quite misleading if all patients with the Pierre Robin anomaly are linked together under the Pierre Robin syndrome, thus including those individuals with multiple primary defects of diverse etiology and prognosis.

3. Meningomyelocele and Anencephaly — Primary Defect in Neural Tube Closure
(Figs. 2 and 6)

The initiating malformation appears to be a defect in closure of the neural groove to form an intact neural tube, which is normally completely fused by 28 days. Anencephaly[6] represents a defect in closure at the anterior portion of the neural groove. The secondary consequences are as follows: (1) the unfused forebrain develops partially and then tends to degenerate; (2) the calvarium is incompletely developed; and (3) the facial features and auricular development are secondarily altered to a variable degree, including cleft in the palate, frequent abnormality of the cervical vertebrae, and occasional incomplete development of the anterior pituitary.

Defects of closure at the mid- or caudal neural groove can give rise to meningomyelocele[7] and other secondary defects, as depicted in Figure 6. The early form of one such lesion is illustrated in Figure 2.

The recurrence risk for defects of neural tube closure, about 5 per cent for parents who have had one affected offspring, includes about an equal risk for either anencephaly or meningomyelocele. This indicates that the risk is a general one for defects of closure of the neural tube, the presumed common basis for both meningomyelocele and anencephaly.

These anomalies of neural tube closure seldom occur in patterns of multiple primary malformation. In fact, the author is not aware of any multiple defect syndrome in which anencephaly or meningomyelocele is a usual feature.

4. Holoprosencephaly, Arhinencephaly, Cebocephaly, Cyclopia — Primary Defect in Anterior Mid-line Axis Mesoderm (Prechordal Mesoderm) (see Fig. 7)

During the third week the prechordal mesoderm migrates forward into the area anterior to the notochord and is necessary in the development of the mid-face as well as having an inductive role in the morphogenesis of the forebrain. The consequences of prechordal mesoderm defect are varying degrees of deficit of midline facial development, especially the median nasal process (premaxilla), and incomplete morphogenesis of the forebrain.[1, 8] Cyclopia represents a severe

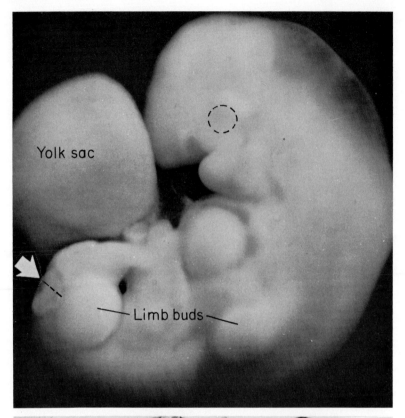

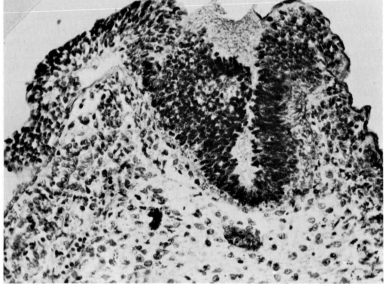

Figure 2. Otherwise normal 28 day embryo with incomplete closure of the posterior neural groove (arrow), which shows aberrant growth of cells to the side in a transverse section (lower). Had this embryo survived, it would presumably have developed a meningomyelocele. (From Lemire, R.: Anat. Record, *152*:9, 1965.

deficit in early midline facial development such that the eyes become fused, the olfactory placodes are fused into a single tube-like proboscis above the eye, and the ethmoid and other midline bony structures are missing. With cyclopia there is failure in the cleavage of the prosencephalon, with grossly incomplete morphogenesis of the forebrain. Less severe degrees of deficit result in hypotelorism and varying degrees of inade-

quate mid-facial and incomplete forebrain development that are more common than cyclopia and frequently include cleft lip and palate. The important clinical point is that incomplete midline facial development, such as hypotelorism or absence of the philtrum or nasal septum, suggests the possibility of a serious anomaly in brain development and function.

This type of anomaly has been produced by

a variety of teratogenic agents in animals[9] and has occurred in sheep as a consequence of the pregnant ewe ingesting the plant *Veratrum californicum* between the fifth and fifteenth days of gestation.[10] There is no known environmental teratogen associated with this defect in man. The anomaly has been a frequent feature of the 13 trisomy syndrome and an occasional feature of the short arm 18 deletion syndrome; for most other cases the etiology has not been determined.

The prognosis for central nervous system function in individuals with this type of defect is very poor, and the author recommends limitation of medical assistance toward survival in such patients.

5. Sirenomelia (Mermaid), Caudal Regression Anomaly — Primary Defect in Mid-posterior Axis Mesoderm[11-13] (see Fig. 8)

The most severe form of this defect, sirenomelia or sympodia, is presumably the consequence of a wedge-shaped early deficit of the posterior axis mesoderm, allowing for fusion of the early limb buds at their fibular margins with absence or incomplete development of the intervening caudal structures. The embryonic defect apparently dates back to the primitive streak stage during the third week, prior to development of the allantois, for there is usually an absence of allantoic vessels. The single umbilical artery arises directly from the aorta, rather than the usual two umbilical arteries arising from the hypogastric vessels. This defect, occurring in about one in 60,000 newborns, has a 2.7 : 1 male sex preponderance. All degrees of severity are observed, presumably dependent on the relative length and width of the early caudal deficit. The variable consequences are often called the caudal regression syndrome.[12] Conceivably, imperforate anus might represent a minor degree of this type of defect. It is important to appreciate that the following defects of the caudal axis may be present in an individual with imperforate anus: lower vertebral defects, 40 per cent; urological defects other than fistulas, 19 per cent; genital anomalies, 17 per cent; and lower limb defect, 10 per cent.

6. Potter's Syndrome[14-17] — Primary Defect of Renal Agenesis or Other Anomaly Leading to a Lack of Urine Flow into the Amniotic Space (see Fig. 9)

Renal agenesis, which must have occurred prior to 31 days, will secondarily limit the amount of amniotic fluid and thereby result in further anomalies during prenatal life. The renal agenesis may be the only primary defect, or it may be one feature of a more extensive caudal axis anomaly (see condition 5). The anomaly occurs more frequently in anatomical males, 17 of 20 in Potter's series,[14] and this might be partially explained by the observations of Schlegel et al.[17] They noted masculinization of the external genitalia in an XX female with Potter's syndrome and raised the possibility of the genital development being secondary to limited androgen excretion and degradation in this female with renal agenesis.

7. Abdominal Muscle Deficiency, Renal and Urinary Tract Dysplasia, and Cryptorchidism; the So-Called Triad Syndrome — Possibly an Early Defect of Mesoderm Contributing to Abdominal Musculature, Renal Parenchyma, Urinary Tract Musculature, and Descent of the Testicles[18-21] (see Fig. 10)

The remarkable similarity among affected individuals with abdominal muscle deficiency suggests that this "syndrome" may be the consequence of a single localized defect in early mesoderm which eventually contributes to the formation of the abdominal musculature, the urinary tract musculature, the renal parenchyma, and possibly the gubernaculum testis. The condition occurs predominantly in males who occasionally have defects of the lower limbs as well. The prognosis for these patients is mainly dependent on the degree of renal insufficiency and complications arising from poor drainage of the urinary tract. Abdominal binding will often improve respiratory exchange and assist in the patient's having bowel movements. Some improvement in abdominal muscle mass and function may occur with age; because these patients are usually of normal intelligence all supportive measures seem indicated.

8. Exstrophy of Bladder[1, 22-24] — Defect in Development of Infraumbilical Mesenchyme (Mesoderm) (see Fig. 11)

Normally the bladder portion of the cloaca and the overlying ectoderm are in direct contact (the cloacal membrane) until the infraumbilical mesenchyme migrates into the area around the sixth to seventh week, giving rise to the lower abdominal wall, genital tubercles, and pubic rami. A failure of the infraumbilical mesenchyme to invade the area allows for a breakdown in the cloacal membrane, in similar fashion to that which normally occurs at the oral, anal and urogenital areas where mesoderm does not intercede between ectoderm and endoderm. Thus the posterior bladder wall is exposed in conjunction with defects in structures derived from the infraumbilical mesenchyme.

This anomaly, six times as likely to occur in the male as in the female, continues to be a difficult one to correct, though encouraging results have followed immediate postnatal primary closure of both the bladder and the pubic rami.

9. Exstrophy of Cloaca[24-26] — Early Defect in Mesoderm Contributing to Infraumbilical Mesenchyme, Cloacal Septum, and Lumbosacral Vertebrae (see Fig. 12)

The remarkable similarity among otherwise normal individuals with this bizarre type of defect suggests a similar mode of developmental pathology having its inception as a single localized defect — theoretically in the early development of the mesoderm which will later contribute to the infraumbilical mesenchyme, cloacal septum, and caudal vertebrae. The consequences are (1) failure of cloacal septation, with the persistence of a common cloaca into which the ureters, ileum, and a rudimentary hindgut open; (2) complete breakdown of the cloacal membrane with exstrophy of the cloaca, failure of fusion of the genital tubercles and pubic rami, and often an omphalocele; and (3) incomplete development of the lumbosacral vertebrae with herniation of a grossly dilated central canal of the spinal cord (hydromyelia), yielding a soft, cystic, skin-covered mass over the sacral area — sometimes asymmetric in its positioning.

The rudimentary hindgut may contain two appendices, and there is no anal opening. The small intestine may be relatively short. Cryptorchidism is a usual finding in the male. Affected females have unfused müllerian elements with completely bifid uterine horns and short, duplicated, or atretic vagina. Most cases have a single umbilical artery, and anomalies of the lower limbs are occasionally present.

Surgical intervention has been carried out.[25, 26] However, considering the overall problem of urinary and fecal incontinence plus the incomplete genital development, the author considers that a decision toward surgical partial correction should be undertaken only after careful consideration with the family.

10. Poland's Anomaly — Possible Defect in the Mesoderm Contributing to the Pectoralis Major and Minor and the Distal Limb on the Same Side (Fig. 3)

In 1841 Poland[27] reported unilateral absence of the pectoralis minor and the sternal portion of the pectoralis major in a deceased convict who

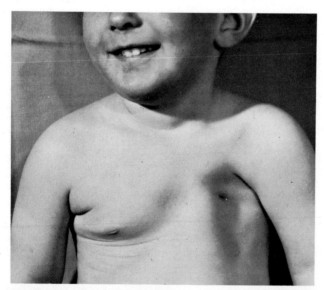
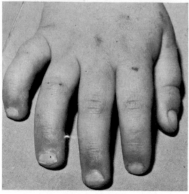
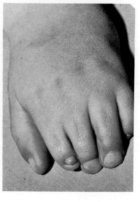

Figure 3. Poland's anomaly. The absence of the pectoralis minor and the sternal portion of the pectoralis major plus the ipsilateral syndactyly of the hand are the more usual features of this complex anomaly. The bony thoracic anomaly and the hypoplasia of the hand, as noted in this otherwise normal boy, are more severe expressions of this defect.

also had cutaneous syndactyly of the hand on the same side. This unique pattern of malformation has subsequently been noted in numerous cases, and Clarkson[28] has estimated that 10 per cent of patients with syndactyly of the hand have Poland's anomaly. It is generally a unilateral sporadic occurrence in otherwise normal individuals. This pattern of malformation may include absence of the nipple and areola, rib defects, and hypoplasia of the hand or even the whole arm on the affected side.

11. Amniotic Bands (Streeter's Bands) Causing Constriction of Developing Parts (Fig. 4)

Partial to complete ring-like constrictions occur as a rare anomaly of the limbs and very rarely involve the head. At times fibrous-appearing bands have been noted at the sites of constriction, sometimes having a broken strand connected to the amnion proper. These bands, when present, become necrotic after birth. There has been much controversy over their origin. Streeter[29] considered the primary lesion to be within the developing limb mesenchyme, the outer bands being a secondary phenomena. The author agrees with the older interpretation of Ballantyne[30] which ascribes the primary abnormality to the amnion, with amniotic strands encircling fetal parts, especially the distal limbs. These bands become constrictive with growth, even to the point of amputation. Torpin[31] has summarized and extended the evidence which indicates that the primary defect is an early rupture of the amnion, with the chorion remaining intact and amniotic bands occurring as a secondary phenomenon. This anomaly is usually a sporadic one in families and generally occurs in an otherwise normal individual. A surgical procedure, Z-plasty, may occasionally be indicated for a constrictive "ring."

12. Athyrotic Hypothyroidism – Primary Defect in Development of Thyroid Gland[32] (see Fig. 13)

Severe hypothyroidism is seldom clinically evident at the time of birth, indicating at least partial prenatal protection of the fetus by maternal thyroid hormone. Postnatally, morphogenesis and function are grossly impaired as a metabolic consequence of the lack of thyroid hormone. Adequate thyroid hormone replacement therapy, at least 3/4 grain of U.S.P. desiccated thyroid for the affected infant, will allow for a complete return to physical normality for age. However, the detrimental effect of the hypothyroid state on morphogenesis and function of the brain is irreparable. Therefore the earlier a diagnosis is made and adequate thyroid hormone therapy instituted, the better is the prognosis for mental function.

Athyrotic hypothyroidism is usually a sporadic occurrence in an otherwise normal child.

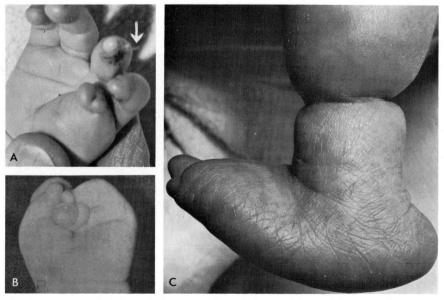

Figure 4. Amniotic bands. Three different newborn infants with partial to complete amputations considered to be due to amniotic bands. *A,* Note the strand extending from the ring-like constricting band on the third finger. *B,* Several fingers were surrounded by one band, resulting in this aberrant appearance by the time of birth. *C,* Partial constriction of the ankle with altered form of the foot as a presumed secondary consequence. Note the toe amputations as well.

PIERRE ROBIN SYNDROME
A Primary Anomaly in Mandibular Development
Hypoplasia of Mandible Prior to 9 Weeks

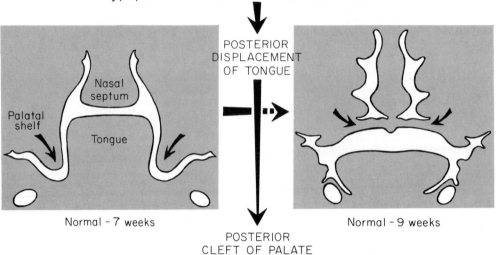

POSTERIOR DISPLACEMENT OF TONGUE

Nasal septum

Palatal shelf

Tongue

Normal – 7 weeks

Normal – 9 weeks

POSTERIOR CLEFT OF PALATE

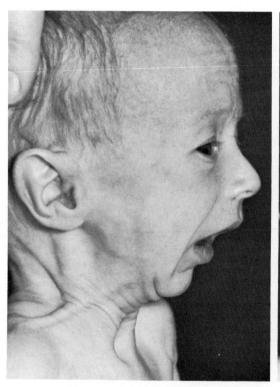

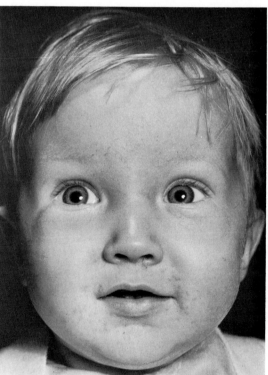

Pierre Robin anomaly with upper respiratory obstruction and failure to thrive in 3 week old (weight, 4.9 lbs.).

Same patient at 13 months showing catch-up in mandibular growth. Patient thriving with normal growth (weight, 14.8 lbs.).

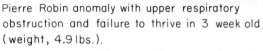

Figure 5. (Photographs from Dennison, W. M.: Pediatrics, *36*:336, 1965.)

DEFECTS IN CLOSURE OF NEURAL TUBE

DORSAL VIEW OF NORMAL EMBRYO OF 23 DAYS

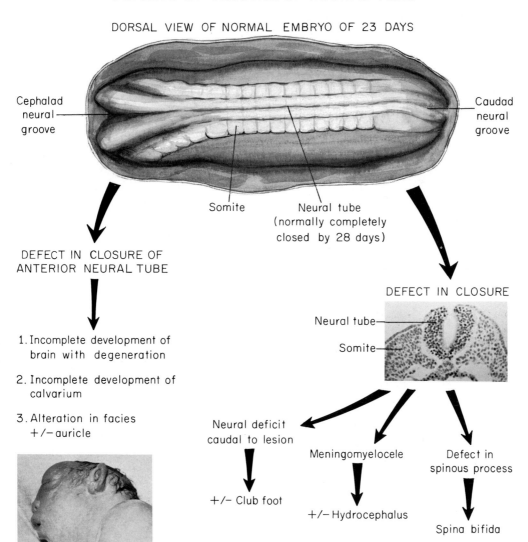

Cephalad neural groove

Caudad neural groove

Somite

Neural tube (normally completely closed by 28 days)

DEFECT IN CLOSURE OF ANTERIOR NEURAL TUBE

1. Incomplete development of brain with degeneration

2. Incomplete development of calvarium

3. Alteration in facies +/−auricle

DEFECT IN CLOSURE

Neural tube

Somite

Neural deficit caudal to lesion

+/− Club foot

Meningomyelocele

+/−Hydrocephalus

Defect in spinous process

Spina bifida

Anencephaly

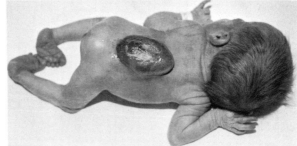

Meningomyelocele with partially epithelialized sac

Figure 6.

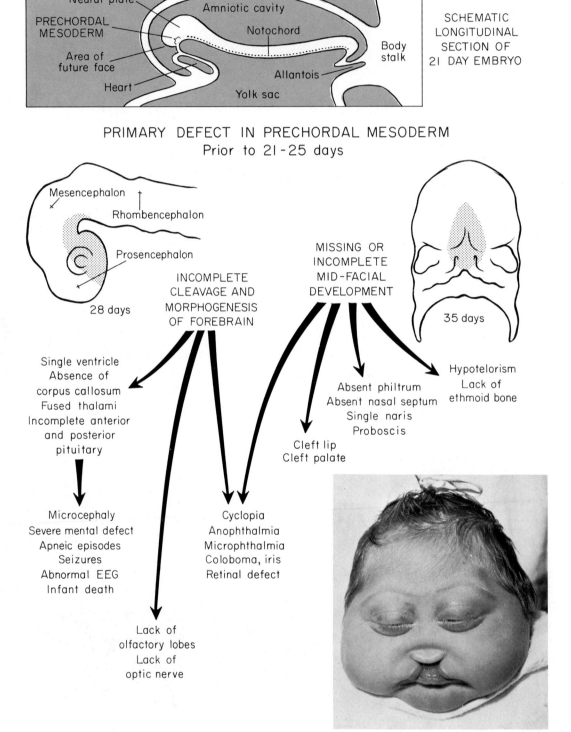

Figure 7.

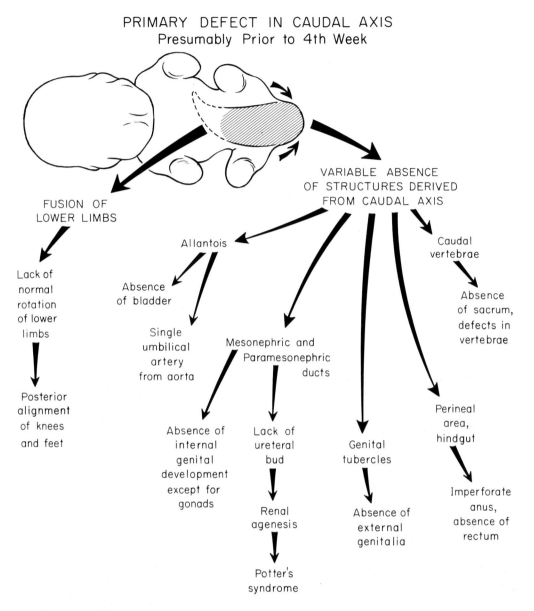

PRIMARY DEFECT IN CAUDAL AXIS
Presumably Prior to 4th Week

FUSION OF
LOWER LIMBS

VARIABLE ABSENCE
OF STRUCTURES DERIVED
FROM CAUDAL AXIS

Allantois

Caudal
vertebrae

Lack of
normal
rotation
of lower
limbs

Absence
of bladder

Absence
of sacrum,
defects in
vertebrae

Single
umbilical
artery
from aorta

Mesonephric and
Paramesonephric
ducts

Posterior
alignment
of knees
and feet

Absence of
internal
genital
development
except for
gonads

Lack of
ureteral
bud

Genital
tubercles

Perineal
area,
hindgut

Renal
agenesis

Absence of
external
genitalia

Imperforate
anus,
absence of
rectum

Potter's
syndrome

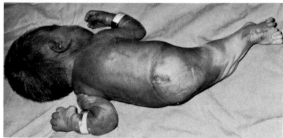

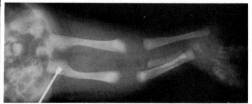

Newborn with sirenomelia, a severe caudal axis deficit

Figure 8.

POTTER'S SYNDROME
The Consequences of Renal Agenesis

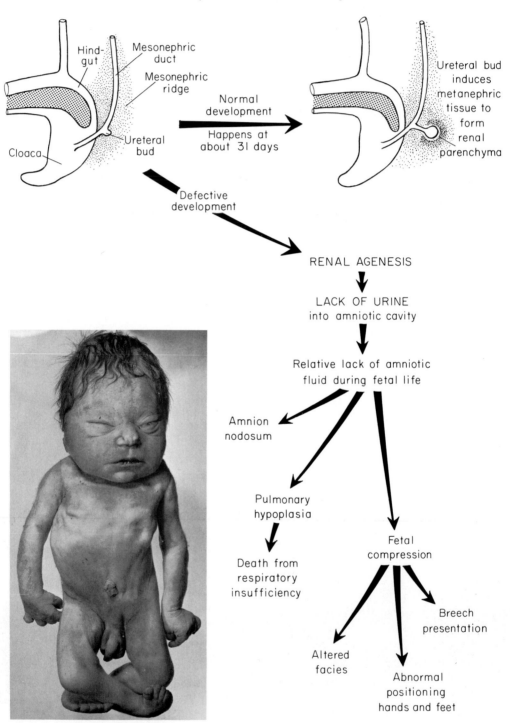

Figure 9.

THE TRIAD SYNDROME
Abdominal Muscle Deficiency, Renal and Urinary Tract Anomalies, and Cryptorchidism

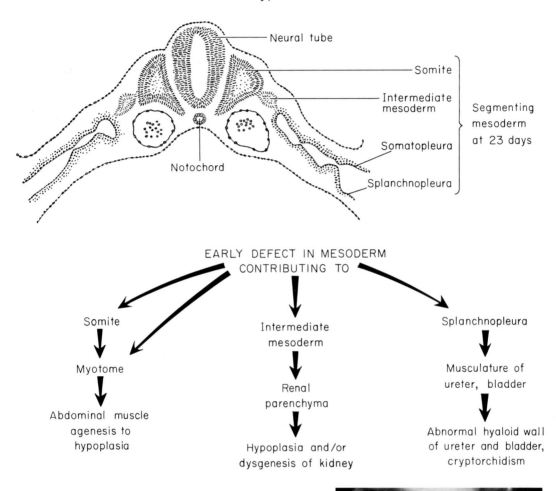

EARLY DEFECT IN MESODERM
CONTRIBUTING TO

Somite	Intermediate mesoderm	Splanchnopleura
Myotome	Renal parenchyma	Musculature of ureter, bladder
Abdominal muscle agenesis to hypoplasia	Hypoplasia and/or dysgenesis of kidney	Abnormal hyaloid wall of ureter and bladder, cryptorchidism

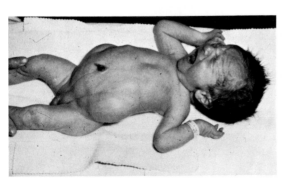

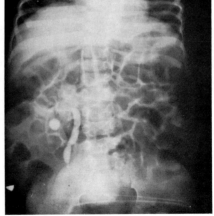

Figure 10.

EXSTROPHY OF BLADDER

Urorectal
septum   Gut

Body stalk

Urachus

Tail gut

Cloaca

29 days

Genital
tubercle   Cloacal
membrane

Infraumbilical
mesenchyme

Genital
tubercle

40 days

Infraumbilical mesoderm
fills in all of cloacal membrane
except urogenital floor.
Genital tubercles fuse

Failure of
infraumbilical mesoderm
to invade cloacal membrane

Breakdown of cloacal
membrane exposing
posterior wall of bladder

Incomplete fusion
of genital tubercles,
often with epispadias

Separated pubic rami,
short lower abdominal wall,
+/− inguinal herniae

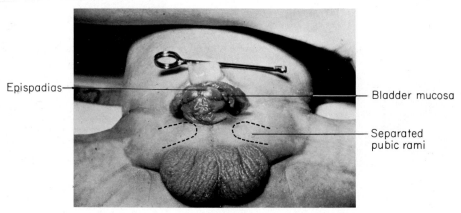

Epispadias

Bladder mucosa

Separated
pubic rami

Figure 11.

EXSTROPHY OF CLOACA
Defect in early mesoderm which will contribute to:

1. Urorectal septum
2. Infraumbilical mesenchyme
3. Lumbosacral somites

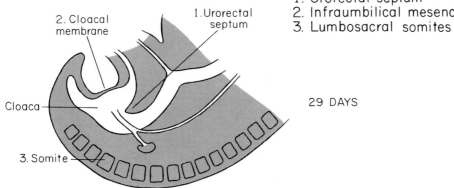

2. Cloacal membrane

1. Urorectal septum

Cloaca

29 DAYS

3. Somite

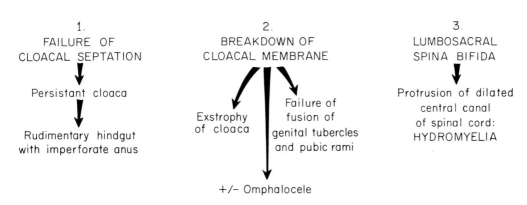

1.
FAILURE OF CLOACAL SEPTATION

↓

Persistant cloaca

↓

Rudimentary hindgut with imperforate anus

2.
BREAKDOWN OF CLOACAL MEMBRANE

Exstrophy of cloaca

Failure of fusion of genital tubercles and pubic rami

+/− Omphalocele

3.
LUMBOSACRAL SPINA BIFIDA

↓

Protrusion of dilated central canal of spinal cord: HYDROMYELIA

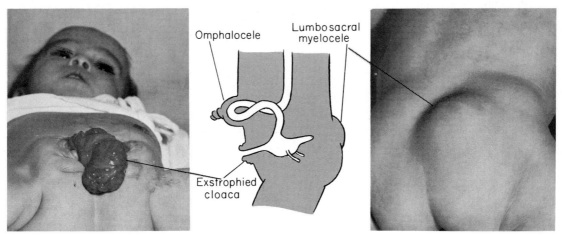

Omphalocele

Lumbosacral myelocele

Exstrophied cloaca

Infant with exstrophy of the cloaca (prolapsed intestine). Note separation of scrotal folds and genital tubercle.

Figure 12.

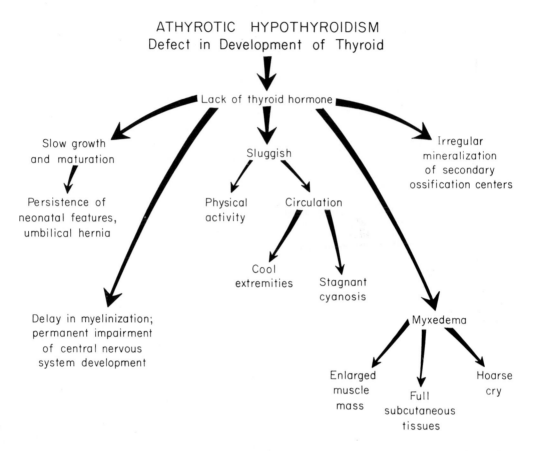

ATHYROTIC HYPOTHYROIDISM
Defect in Development of Thyroid

Lack of thyroid hormone

Slow growth
and maturation

Persistence of
neonatal features,
umbilical hernia

Sluggish

Physical
activity

Circulation

Irregular
mineralization
of secondary
ossification centers

Cool
extremities

Stagnant
cyanosis

Delay in myelinization;
permanent impairment
of central nervous
system development

Myxedema

Enlarged
muscle
mass

Full
subcutaneous
tissues

Hoarse
cry

Athyrotic Patients

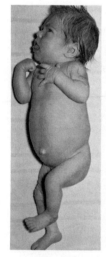 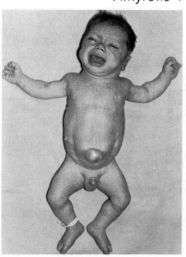 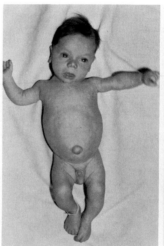 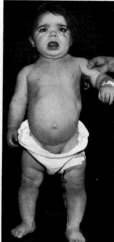

Age - 2 months
Height age - 1 mo.
Bone age - birth

Age - 9 months
Height age - 2 months
Bone age - birth

⟶ After 3 weeks of thyroid
replacement

Age - 3 years, untreated
Height age - 12 mo.
Bone age - 3 months

Figure 13.

REFERENCES

1. Willis, R. A.: The Borderland of Embryology and Pathology. Washington, D.C., Butterworth, 1962.
2. Gruenwald, P.: Mechanisms of abnormal development. I. Causes of abnormal development in the embryo. Arch. Path., *44*:398, 1947.
3. Gruenwald, P.: Mechanisms of abnormal development. II. Embryonic development of malformations. Arch. Path., *44*:495, 1947.
4. Gruenwald, P.: Mechanisms of abnormal development. III. Postnatal developmental abnormalities. Arch. Path., *44*:648, 1947.
5. Dennison, W. M.: The Pierre Robin syndrome. Pediatrics, *36*:336, 1965.
6. Giroud, A.: Causes and morphogenesis of anencephaly. Ciba Foundation Symposium on Congenital Malformations, 1960, pp. 199-218.
7. Lemire, R. J., Shepard, T. H., and Alvord, E. C., Jr.: Caudal myeloschisis (lumbo-sacral spina bifida cystica) in a five millimeter (horizon XIV) human embryo. Anat. Record, *152*:9, 1965.
8. DeMyer, W., Zeman, W., and Palmer, C. G.: The face predicts the brain: diagnostic significance of median facial anomalies for holoprosencephaly (arhinencephaly). Pediatrics, *34*:256, 1964.
9. Adelmann, H. B.: The problem of cyclopia. Part II. Quart. Rev. Biol., *11*:284, 1936.
10. Babbott, F. L., Binns, W., and Ingalls, T. H.: Field studies of cyclopian malformations in sheep. Arch. Environ. Health, *5*:109, 1962.
11. Wolff, E.: Les bases de la tératogénèse expérimentale des vértebrés amniotes, d'après les résultats de méthodes directes. Arch. d'Anat., d'Histol. et d'Embryol., *22*:1, 1936.
12. Duhamel, B.: From the mermaid to anal imperforation: the syndrome of caudal regression. Arch. Dis. Childhood, *36*:152, 1961.
13. Crawfurd, M. d'A., Ismail, S. R., and Wigglesworth, J. S.: A monopodal sireniform monster with dermatoglyphic and cytogenetic studies. J. Med. Genet., *3*:212, 1966.
14. Potter, E. L.: Bilateral renal agenesis. J. Pediat., *29*:68, 1946.
15. Bain, A. D., and Scott, J. S.: Renal agenesis and severe urinary tract dysplasia. A review of 50 cases with particular reference to the associated anomalies. Brit. Med. J., *1*:841, 1960.
16. Passarge, E., and Sutherland, J. M.: Potter's syndrome. Chromosome analysis of three cases with Potter's syndrome or related syndromes. Am. J. Dis. Children, *109*:80, 1965.
17. Schlegel, R. J., Aspillaga, M. J., Nev, R. L., Carneiro-Leano, J., and Gardner, L. I.: An XX sex chromosome complement in an infant having male-type external genitals, renal agenesis, and other anomalies. J. Pediat., *69*:812, 1966.
18. Parker, R. W.: Case of an infant in whom some of the abdominal muscles were absent. Clin. Soc. Trans., *28*:201, 1895.
19. Silverman, F. N., and Huang, N.: Congenital absence of the abdominal muscles. Am. J. Dis. Children, *80*:91, 1950.
20. Lattimer, J. K.: Congenital deficiency of abdominal musculature and associated genitourinary anomalies. J. Urol., *79*:343, 1958.
21. Miller, R. M., Kind, R. E., and Rich, R. W.: Congenital anomalies of the abdominal musculature and urogenital tract in a foal. Vet. Med., *61*:652, 1966.
22. Wyburn, G. M.: The development of the infra-umbilical portion of the abdominal wall, with remarks on the aetiology of ectopia vesicae. J. Anat., *71*:201, 1937.
23. Muecke, E. C.: The role of the cloacal membrane in exstrophy: the first successful experimental study. J. Urol., *92*:659, 1964.
24. Beckwith, J. B.: The congenitally malformed. VII. Exstrophy of the bladder and cloacal exstrophy. Northwest Med., *65*:407, 1966.
25. Zwiren, G. T., and Patterson, J. H.: Exstrophy of the cloaca: report of a case treated surgically. Pediatrics, *35*:687, 1965.
26. Spencer, R.: Exstrophia splanchnica (exstrophy of the cloaca). Surgery, *57*:751, 1965.
27. Poland, A.: Deficiency of the pectoral muscles. Guy's Hosp. Rep., *6*:191, 1841.
28. Clarkson, P.: Poland's syndactyly. Guy's Hosp. Rep., *111*:335, 1962.
29. Streeter, G. L.: Focal deficiencies in fetal tissues and their relation to intra-uterine amputation. Contribs. Embryol., No. 126. Washington, D.C., Carnegie Institute of Washington, 1930.
30. Ballantyne, J. W.: Manual of Antenatal Pathology and Hygiene. The Foetus. Edinburgh, W. Greene and Sons, 1902.
31. Torpin, R.: Fetal Malformations Caused by Amnion Rupture During Gestation. Springfield, Ill., Charles C Thomas, 1965.
32. Wilkins, L.: The Diagnosis and Treatment of Endocrine Disorders in Childhood and Adolescence. Springfield, Ill., Charles C Thomas, 1965.

DYSMORPHIC SYNDROMES
of multiple primary defects

Once it has been determined that an individual has multiple *primary* areas of faulty morphogenesis, the question is no longer an anatomical one; rather, the question becomes that of an overall diagnosis. Aside from Down's syndrome, the recognized syndromes of multiple primary defect are individually rare, but collectively they are numerous and new ones are continuing to be reported. It is quite difficult for a clinician to become personally acquainted with many of them, and hence this chapter was developed to assist in the recognition of such syndromes, as well as to provide a nucleus of information about the natural history and etiology of each disorder. References to other texts which may be of further assistance regarding such syndromes are listed at the end of this chapter.

GENERAL COMMENTS CONCERNING SPECIFIC DEFECTS AND PATTERNS OF ANOMALY

Growth. The same etiology which results in multiple defects in morphogenesis often has an adverse effect on skeletal development and may lead to hypoplasia of the whole individual. Therefore shortness of stature is a frequent feature in many of these syndromes. When the small size in a patient with multiple defects has been of prenatal onset the clinician can be reassured that it is not due to an endocrine abnormality, and he can usually anticipate a continuation of the slow rate of linear growth.

Central Nervous System Dysfunction. Because the development of the nervous system is so prolonged and complex, it is not surprising that mental deficiency, behavioral aberrations, and neurological abnormalities are frequent features in these syndromes. The overall pattern of central nervous system function tends to be similar in individuals with the same multiple defect syndrome. Hence one of the values in a specific diagnosis is the enhanced ability to anticipate future performance.

Nonspecificity of Individual Defects. With rare exceptions a clinical diagnosis of one of these syndromes cannot be made on the basis of a single defect, as is evident in the tables at the end of this chapter. Even a rare defect may be a feature in several syndromes of variant etiology. A specific diagnosis is usually dependent on recognition of the overall *pattern of anomalies,* and the detection of minor defects may be as helpful as major anomalies in this regard. (See Chapter Five.)

Variance in Expression. Variance in extent of abnormality (expression) among individuals with the same etiological syndrome is a usual phenomenon. Except for such nonspecific general features as mental deficiency and small stature, it is unusual to find a given anomaly in 100 per cent of patients with the same etiological syndrome. For example, in full 21 trisomy Down's syndrome only mental deficiency is ubiquitous; hypotonia is a frequent feature, but most of the other individual clinical features are found in less than 80 per cent of such patients. However, a specific diagnosis of Down's syndrome can generally be rendered, based on the *total pattern of anomalies.*

Intraindividual variability in expression is also frequent, with variance in the degree of abnormality on the left versus the right side of the individual.

Heterogeneity. Similar phenotypes (overall physical similarity) may result from *different* etiologies. Only by finer discrimination of the phenotype or mode of etiology can such similar entities be distinguished. For example, Marfan's syndrome and homocystinuria were initially discriminated on the basis of homocystinuria, next by a difference in mode of etiology (autosomal dominant for Marfan's syndrome and autosomal recessive in homocystinuria), and finally by closer scrutiny of the phenotype. As another example, achondroplasia is frequently misdiagnosed among individuals who have chondrodystrophies which only superficially resemble true achondroplasia. A diagnosis should be rendered only when there is close resemblance in the overall pattern of malformation between the patient and the disorder under consideration.

Etiology. Most of the syndromes herein set forth have a genetic basis. Chapter Four provides the background information relative to genetic counseling for these conditions. Only three disorders, the rubella syndrome, the thalidomide syndrome (not included), and the aminopterin syndrome, are known to be caused by environmental teratogens.

Besides the following established syndromes, roughly half the individuals with multiple defects have conditions which have not yet been recognized as a specific syndrome. A small percentage of such patients (8 per cent in Summitt's study)[1] have a structural chromosomal abnormality. In such cases genetic counsel should be withheld until it has been determined whether either parent is a balanced translocation carrier of the chromosomal abnormality. In the absence of an evident chromosomal abnormality or familial data suggesting a particular mode of etiology, it is generally impossible to state any accurate risk of recurrence for unknown patterns of multiple malformation. It is presumptuous to inform the parents that "this is a rare condition and therefore unlikely to recur in your future children." Under these circumstances the author's present approach is to inform the parents that the lowest recurrence risk is zero and the highest risk with each pregnancy would be 25 per cent. The latter figure is predicated on the possibility of recessive inheritance or a nondetectable chromosomal abnormality from a balanced translocation carrier parent.

METHOD AND UTILITY OF PRESENTATION OF THE SYNDROMES

Each syndrome has a listing of anomalies. The main list consists of defects which occur in at least 25 per cent and usually more than 50 per cent of patients. Sometimes the actual percentage or number is stated for each anomaly. Below these are listed the occasional defects that occur with a frequency of from 1 to 25 per cent, most commonly 5 to 10 per cent. The occurrence of these "occasional abnormalities" is of interest and has been loosely ascribed to "developmental noise." In other words, an adverse influence that usually causes a particular pattern of malformation may occasionally cause other anomalies as well. Possibly it is differences of genetic background, environment, or both that allow some individuals to express these "occasional" anomalies. The important feature is that they are not random for a particular syndrome. For example, clinicians who have seen a large number of children with Down's syndrome are not surprised to see "another" Down's syndrome baby with duodenal atresia, web neck, or tetralogy of Fallot.

The references listed for each syndrome have been selected as those that give the best account of that disorder, provide recent additional knowledge, or represent the initial description.

A word of caution is indicated. This book does not contain a number of syndromes, especially those reported after April, 1968. Furthermore, the conditions have been limited to those which appear to be a concise entity, omitting such questionable disease entities as Klippel-Feil syndrome, Grieg's syndrome, and the lissencephaly syndrome.

All the syndromes, including alternative designations, are alphabetically listed with the number for that disorder. This is done to facilitate the finding of a particular disorder. Following the alphabetical listing are summary tables that include the several "diagnostic manifestations," which together are highly indicative of a particular diagnosis; whether mental deficiency, shortness of stature, or both are usual features; and the genetic mode of etiology. These tables are set forth for perspective and differential diagnosis. The numbers listed in parentheses for some syndromes are the numbers for other listed conditions that merit special consideration in the differential diagnosis for that syndrome; the numbers following some subcategories refer to other listed syndromes that may also have the feature of that subcategory. The order of presentation of the syndromes is based on physical similarities, system or area involved, and – in the case of chromosomal abnormalities – by mode of etiology. These are summarized as follows:

A. Chromosomal abnormality syndromes

This is followed by a miscellaneous group which has been arbitrarily subcategorized on the basis of single features or groups of features that are major components of the respective syndromes:

B. Unusually small stature with associated defects
C. Senile-like appearance with associated defects
D. Joint dysplasia with associated defects
E. Muscular disorders with associated defects
F. Neurological disorders other than mental deficiency with associated defects
G. Facial defects as predominant features
H. Oral-facial-digital associations of defects
I. Hematopoietic disorders with associated defects

J. Genital anomalies with associated defects
K. Deafness with associated defects
L. Presumed metabolic aberrations affecting morphogenesis; basic pathogenesis unknown
M. Hamartoses: abnormal admixture of tissue components as a feature
N. Ectodermal dysplasias: abnormal tissues derived predominantly from embryonic ectoderm

These are followed by the skeletal dysplasias.

O. Osteochondrodysplasias
P. Osteopetroses
Q. Craniosynostoses
R. Other skeletal dysplasias, including some with short metacarpal bones
S. Mucopolysaccharidoses
T. Connective tissue disorders

Lastly there are a group of miscellaneous syndromes which, although they have features of altered morphogenesis, are not generally thought of as patterns of altered morphogenesis. They are included here because they may enter into the differential diagnostic consideration of syndromes of malformation. This group could be deleted or vastly extended to include such entities as the lipidoses.

U. Other miscellaneous syndromes

Certain of the syndromes have been placed out of context to a particular category. This was done because of similarities to an adjacent syndrome, and these conditions have been labeled *(Insert)* in the tables.

The tables at the end of this chapter list individual anomalies and the syndromes in which that defect is a usual or occasional feature. These tables may assist the reader in finding the appropriate syndromes with which to compare a given patient with multiple defects.

ALPHABETICAL LISTING OF SYNDROMES

SUMMARY TABLES

A. Chromosomal Abnormality Syndromes. The following *chromosomal abnormalities* give rise to particular patterns of multiple defect which allow for clinical recognition. They are grouped together to aid the clinician in deciding which multiple malformation patients clearly merit chromosomal study for confirmatory diagnosis and genetic counsel.

SYNDROME	DIAGNOSTIC MANIFESTATIONS			MENTAL DEFICIENCY	SHORT STATURE	CHROMOSOME
	Craniofacial	*Limbs*	*Other*			
1. Down's syndrome (mongolism) (2,10,28)	Upward slant to palpebral fissures, flat facies	Short hands with clinodactyly of fifth finger	Hypotonia	+	+/-	21 Trisomy
2. XXXXY syndrome (1,25,26)	Inner epicanthic fold and/or upslanting of palpebral fissures	Limited elbow pronation, low dermal ridge count on fingertips (arches)	Hypogenitalism	+	+	XXXXY
3. 18 Trisomy syndrome (4,52)	Microstomia, short palpebral fissure	Clenched hand, second finger over third; low arches on fingertips	Short sternum	+	+	18 Trisomy
4. 13 (D₁) Trisomy syndrome (3,5,14)	Defects of eye, nose, lip, and forebrain of holoprosencephaly type	Polydactyly, narrow hyperconvex fingernails	Skin defects, posterior scalp	+	+	13 Trisomy
5. Chromosome No. 4 short arm deletion (4)	Ocular hypertelorism +/- prominent glabella; low set simple ear with preauricular dimple +/- cleft lip and palate		+/- Mid-line scalp defects	+	+	No. 4 p—
6. Cri-du-chat syndrome	Epicanthic folds and/or slanting palpebral fissures, microcephaly with round facial contour		Cat-like cry in infancy	+	+	No. 5 p—
7. Chromosome No. 18 long arm deletion	Mid-facial hypoplasia, atretic or narrow ear canal	High frequency of whorl digital pattern		+	+	No. 18 q—
8. Chromosome No. 21 long arm deletion	Downslanting palpebral fissures, large malformed external ears, micrognathia			+	+	No. 21 q—
9. Coloboma of iris–anal atresia–extra chromosome syndrome	Hypertelorism with slight downslanting palpebral fissures, coloboma of iris and/or pre-auricular sinus		Anal atresia	+/-		Small extra chromosome
10. Penta-X syndrome (1,2,28)	Upward slant to palpebral fissures	Small hands with clinodactyly of fifth finger	Patent ductus arteriosus	+	+	XXXXX
11. XO (Turner's) syndrome (12)	Heart shaped facies, prominent ears, webbing of posterior neck	Congenital lymphedema or its residua	Broad chest with widely spaced nipples, low posterior hairline	+/-	+	XO
(Insert)						
12. Turner-like syndrome (male Turner's, Noonan's syndrome) (11)	Webbing of posterior neck		Pectus excavatum, cryptorchidism, pulmonic stenosis	+/-	+	?

Numbers in parentheses indicate numbers of other listed syndromes which merit special consideration in the differential diagnosis.

B. Unusually Small Stature with Associated Defects. (3,5-8,11,12,52,56,57,88,89,93,94,109,112,114,115-119,122)

	CRANIOFACIAL	LIMBS	OTHER	MENTAL DEFICIENCY	SHORT STATURE	GENETICS
13. Cornelia de Lange syndrome	Synophrys (continuous eyebrows), thin downturning upper lip	Small or malformed hands and feet, proximal thumb	Hirsutism	+	+	?
14. Rubinstein-Taybi syndrome (4,23,48)	Microcephaly, slanting palpebral fissures, maxillary hypoplasia	Broad thumbs and toes		+	+	?
15. Silver's syndrome	Triangular hypoplastic facies with downturning mouth	Skeletal asymmetry, clinodactyly of fifth finger			+	?
16. Bloom's syndrome	Photosensitivity with telangiectatic erythema, malar hypoplasia		In vitro chromosomal breakage		+	Aut. rec.
17. Seckel's syndrome	Facial hypoplasia with prominent nose, microcephaly	Multiple joint and skeletal abnormalities		+	+	Aut. rec.
18. Hallerman-Streiff syndrome (19)	Microphthalmia and cataracts, micrognathia, small pinched nose		Hypotrichosis		+	?Aut. dom.

C. Senile-Like Appearance with Associated Defects. (18,75)

	FACIAL	CUTANEOUS	OTHER	MENTAL DEFICIENCY	SHORT STATURE	GENETICS
19. Progeria (18,21)	Facial bone hypoplasia	Alopecia, thin skin with atrophy of subcutaneous fat	Straight femoral neck, short distal phalanges, premature atherosclerosis		+	?
20. Werner's syndrome	Cataract	Thin skin, thick fibrous subcutaneous tissues	Gray, sparse hair		+	Aut. rec.
21. Cockayne's syndrome (19)	Retinal degeneration	Hypotrichosis, photosensitive thin skin, diminished subcutaneous fat	Impaired hearing	+	+	Aut. rec.

Numbers in parentheses indicate numbers of other listed syndromes which merit special consideration in the differential diagnosis.

D. Joint Dysplasia with Associated Defects.   (2,3,17,27,32,33,46,47,52,85,86,89,90,92,94,98,116–122)

	CRANIOFACIAL	LIMBS	OTHER	MENTAL DEFICIENCY	SHORT STATURE	GENETICS
22. Familial dwarfism with stiff joints (24)	Hyperopia	Stiff joints			+	Aut. dom.
23. Leri's pleonosteosis (14,48)	Upward slant to palpebral fissures	Broad valgus thumb, joint limitation, flexion of fingers				Aut. dom.
24. Stickler's progressive arthro-ophthalmopathy (22)	Progressive myopia with retinal detachment	Degenerative joint limitation from childhood	Sensorineural deafness			Aut. dom.
(Insert)						
25. Laurence-Moon-Biedl syndrome (2,26,107)	Retinal pigmentation	Polydactyly	Obesity	+	+/–	Aut. rec.

E. Muscular Disorders with Associated Defects.   (1–3,127)

	CRANIOFACIAL	LIMB AND OTHER	MUSCLE DYSFUNCTION	MENTAL DEFICIENCY	SHORT STATURE	GENETICS
26. Prader-Willi syndrome (2,25)	+/– Upward slant to palpebral fissures	Obesity from latter infancy, hypogenitalism, diabetes mellitus	Hypotonia, especially in early infancy	+	+	?
(Insert)						
27. Larsen's syndrome	Flat facies	Multiple joint dislocation, short fingernails				?
28. Cerebro-hepato-renal syndrome (1,29)	High forehead, flat facies	Hepatomegaly, death in early infancy	Hypotonia	? +	+	? Aut. rec.
29. Lowe's syndrome (Oculo-cerebro-renal syndrome (28)	Cataract	Renal tubular dysfunction	Hypotonia	+	+	X-linked rec.
30. Rieger's syndrome (31)	Hypodontia, iris dysplasia		Myotonic dystrophy	+/–		Aut. dom.
31. Myotonic dystrophy of Steinert (30)	Cataract	Hypogonadism	Myotonia with muscle atrophy	+/–		Aut. dom.
32. Freeman-Sheldon "whistling face" syndrome (33)	Hypoplastic alae nasi	Club feet	Mask-like "whistling face"		+/–	? Aut. dom.
33. Schwartz's syndrome (32)	Blepharophimosis	Joint limitation	Myotonia		+/–	? Aut. rec.

Numbers in parentheses indicate numbers of other listed syndromes which merit special consideration in the differential diagnosis.

F. Neurological Disorders Other Than Mental Deficiency, with Associated Defects. (1-3,62,63,66,67,73,127)

	NEUROLOGICAL	OTHER	MENTAL DEFICIENCY	SHORT STATURE	GENETICS
34. Marinesco-Sjögren syndrome	Cerebellar ataxia, hypotonia	Cataract, sparse hair	+	+	Aut. rec.
35. Biemond syndrome	Ataxia	Short fourth metacarpal			Aut. dom.
36. Ataxia telangiectasia	Development of ataxia	Telangiectasia, frequent upper respiratory infections		+	Aut. rec.
37. Sjögren-Larsson syndrome	Spasticity, especially legs	Ichthyosis	+	+	Aut. rec.
38. Menkes' syndrome	Progressive cerebral deterioration with seizures	Twisted, fractured stubby hair	+	+	X-linked rec.

G. Facial Defects as Predominant Features. (108)

	DIAGNOSTIC MANIFESTATIONS		OTHER	MENTAL DEFICIENCY	SHORT STATURE	GENETICS
39. Treacher Collins syndrome (mandibulofacial dysostosis) (40)	Malar and mandibular hypoplasia	Defect of lower eyelid, downslanting palpebral fissures	Malformation of external ear			Aut. dom.
40. Goldenhar's syndrome (39)	Malar hypoplasia	Epibulbar dermoid and/or lipodermoid +/- other eye defect	Malformed ear with preauricular tags			Unknown; ? aut. rec.
41. Familial blepharophimosis	Lateral displacement of inner canthi	Inverted inner canthal fold	Ptosis of eyelids			Aut. dom.
42. Lower lip fistula and cleft lip (43) (Insert)	Lower lip fistulas (pits)	Cleft lip and/or cleft palate				Aut. dom.
43. Popliteal web syndrome (42)	Lower lip pits, cleft palate	Popliteal web				? Aut. rec. or aut. dom.

H. Oral-Facial-Digital Associations of Defects.

	CRANIOFACIAL	LIMBS	OTHER	MENTAL DEFICIENCY	SHORT STATURE	GENETICS
44. Oral-facial-digital syndrome (46)	Hypoplasia of alae nasi, oral frenula and clefts	Digital asymmetry		+/-		Dom. ? lethal in male
45. Mohr syndrome	Cleft tongue	Partial duplication of hallux	Deafness, conductive		+/-	? Aut. rec.

Numbers in parentheses indicate numbers of other listed syndromes which merit special consideration in the differential diagnosis.

(Table continued on following page.)

H. Oral-Facial-Digital Associations of Defects. (Continued)

	CRANIOFACIAL	LIMBS	OTHER	MENTAL DEFICIENCY	SHORT STATURE	GENETICS
46. Mietens' syndrome (44)	Narrow nose, corneal opacity	Flexion contracture at elbow		+	+	? Aut. rec.
47. Oculo-dento-digital syndrome	Narrow nose, microphthalmos, +/– glaucoma	Camptodactyly of fifth fingers	Enamel hypoplasia		+	? Aut. rec.
48. Taybi's oto-palato-digital syndrome (14,23)	Cleft soft palate, microstomia	Broad distal digits, "tree-frog-like"	Deafness, conductive	+/–	+	? X-linked

I. Hematopoietic Disorders with Associated Defects. (16,56,74,102)

	LIMBS	OTHER	MENTAL DEFICIENCY	SHORT STATURE	GENETICS
49. Fanconi's syndrome of pancytopenia and multiple defects (50,74)	Hypoplastic thumb and/or radius	Hyperpigmentation, development of pancytopenia	+/–	+	? Aut. rec.
50. Radial aplasia-thrombocytopenia syndrome (49)	Radial aplasia	Thrombocytopenia with megalokarycytopenia +/– cardiac defect			Aut. rec.
(Insert)					
51. Holt-Oram syndrome (cardiac-limb syndrome)	Upper limb defect, especially thumb and radius	Cardiac septal defect, narrow shoulders			Aut. dom.

J. Genital Anomalies with Associated Defects. (2–4,25,26,60)

	CRANIOFACIAL	LIMBS	OTHER	MENTAL DEFICIENCY	SHORT STATURE	GENETICS
52. Smith-Lemli-Opitz syndrome (3)	Anteverted nostrils and/or ptosis of eyelid	Syndactyly of second and third toes	Hypospadias and cryptorchidism	+	+	? Aut. rec.
53. Fraser syndrome	Cryptophthalmos (fused eyelids) defect of auricle		Genital anomaly			? Aut. rec.
54. Hypertelorism-hypospadias syndrome	Hypertelorism		Hypospadias	+/–		? Aut. dom.

K. Deafness with Associated Defects. (4,39,40,48,77–80,101,102,117,118)

	CRANIOFACIAL	LIMBS	OTHER	MENTAL DEFICIENCY	SHORT STATURE	GENETICS
55. Rubella syndrome	Cataract		Deafness, patent ductus arteriosus			
56. Waardenburg's syndrome	Lateral displacement of inner canthi and puncta		+/– Deafness; partial albinism; white forelock, heterochromia of iris, vitelligo	+/–	+/–	Aut. dom.

Numbers in parentheses indicate numbers of other listed syndromes which merit special consideration in the differential diagnosis.

L. Presumed Metabolic Aberrations Affecting Morphogenesis; Basic Pathogenesis Unknown.

SYNDROME	FACIAL	OTHER	MENTAL DEFICIENCY	SHORT STATURE	GENETICS
57. Leprechaunism (Donohue's syndrome)	Full lips, facial hirsutism	Adipose deficiency, enlarged phallus, extreme growth deficiency with relatively large hands and feet	?	+	Aut. rec.
58. Berardinelli's lipodystrophy syndrome		Tall stature and muscle hypertrophy, phallic hypertrophy, lipoatrophy, hepatomegaly and hyperlipemia	+/-		Aut. rec.
59. Hypercalcemia, peculiar facies, supravalvular aortic stenosis	Full lips, small nose with anteverted nostrils	+/- Hypercalcemia in infancy, supravalvular aortic stenosis	+	+	?
60. Wiedemann-Beckwith syndrome	Macroglossia	Omphalocele, macrosomia, cytomegaly of fetal adrenal cortex, +/- hypoglycemia	+/-		? Aut. rec.
61. Cerebral gigantism		Large size in early life, poor coordination	+/-		?

M. Hamartoses. The hamartoses are a group of diseases in which there is an organizational defect leading to abnormal admixture of tissues, often with a tumor-like excess of one or more tissues. Included are hemangiomata, melanomata including altered skin pigmentation, fibromata, lipomata, adenomata, and some strange admixtures which create nosological confusion such as the "adenoma sebaceum"—which are not derived from sebaceous glands—in tuberous sclerosis. Certain hamartomatous lesions are liable to grow locally or metastasize, a low risk phenomenon in some of these diseases such as the Peutz-Jeghers syndrome but a major risk in others such as Gardner's syndrome. Altered morphogenesis other than hamartomata occurs in some of these conditions, notably the altered facies of the basal cell nevus syndrome and syndactyly in Goltz's syndrome.

SYNDROME	CRANIOFACIAL	SKELETAL	OTHER	MENTAL DEFICIENCY	SHORT STATURE	GENETICS
62. Sturge-Weber syndrome	Flat hemangiomata of face, most commonly in trigeminal region		Hemangiomata of meninges with seizures	+/-		?
63. Von Hippel-Lindau syndrome	Retinal angiomata		Cerebellar hemangioblastoma			Aut. dom.
64. Riley's syndrome	Macrocephaly, pseudopapilledema		Cutaneous hemangiomata			? Aut. dom.
65. Maffucci's syndrome		Enchondromatosis	Cavernous hemangiomata			?
66. Tuberous sclerosis (adenoma sebaceum)	Hamartomatous pink to brownish facial skin nodules	+/- Bone lesions	Seizures	+/-		Aut. dom.
67. Neurofibromatosis		+/- Bone lesions	Neurofibromata, cafe au lait spots			Aut. dom.
68. McCune-Albright syndrome		Polyostotic fibrous dysplasia	Irregular skin pigmentation, sexual precocity in female			?

Numbers in parentheses indicate numbers of other listed syndromes which merit special consideration in the differential diagnosis.

(Table continued on following page.)

M. Hamartoses. (Continued)

SYNDROME	CRANIOFACIAL	SKELETAL	OTHER	MENTAL DEFICIENCY	SHORT STATURE	GENETICS
69. Peutz-Jeghers syndrome	Mucocutaneous spotty pigmentation, especially lips		Intestinal polyposis, benign			Aut. dom.
70. Gardner's syndrome (110)		Osteomas	Intestinal polyposis, fibromatous growths in scars, epidermal cysts			Aut. dom.
71. Basal cell nevus syndrome	Broad facies	Rib anomalies	Basal cell cutaneous nevi	+		Aut. dom.
72. Goltz's syndrome (focal dermal hypoplasia) (75); mainly female	Dental anomalies	Cutaneous syndactyly	Poikiloderma with focal dermal hypoplasia		+/-	Dom.
73. Incontinentia pigmenti; mainly female	+/- Dental defect	Irregular skin pigmentation in fleck, whorl, or spidery form, +/- patchy alopecia		+/-		Dom.
74. Dyskeratosis congenita syndrome (49)		Nail dystrophy, hyperpigmentation, leukoplakia, development of pancytopenia, +/- hemangiomata			+/-	? Aut. rec.
75. Rothmund-Thomson syndrome (poikiloderma congenita) (72)	Development of cataracts	Development of poikiloderma, other features of ectodermal dysplasia			+/-	Aut. rec.

N. Ectodermal Dysplasias. The ectodermal dysplasias, so categorized because the abnormal tissues were predominantly derived from embryonic ectoderm, include hypoplasis of skin and its derivatives, plus defects of nails, teeth, lens, and /or sensorineural deafness. The most common type is the anhidrotic ectodermal dysplasia. The other types are called hidrotic ectodermal dysplasias because no serious problem in terms of sweating is involved.

SYNDROME	FACIAL	NAILS	OTHER	MENTAL DEFICIENCY	SHORT STATURE	GENETICS
76. Anhidrotic ectodermal dysplasia	Peg-shaped teeth, partial anodontia, mid-facial hypoplasia		Hypoplasia to aplasia of sweat glands, hyperthermia, alopecia			X-linked
HIDROTIC ECTODERMAL DYSPLASIAS:						
77. Marshall type	Cataract, mid-facial hypoplasia		Deafness			Aut. dom.
78. Robinson type (79)	Peg-shaped teeth	Hypoplastic nails	Deafness			Aut. dom.
79. Feinmesser type (78)		Rudimentary nails	Deafness			? Aut. rec.
80. Pili torti and deafness			Deafness; hair twisted, fine, and short			? Aut. rec.
81. Clouson type		Nail dystrophy	Dyskeratotic thick palms and soles		+/-	Aut. dom.
82. Basan type		Thin, fragile nails	Smooth palms and soles			Aut. dom.
83. Enamel hypoplasia and curly hair (*Insert*)	Enamel hypoplasia	+/- Nail dystrophy	Hair thick and curly			Aut. dom.
84. Pachyonychia congenita		Thick nails	Hyperkeratosis, foot blisters			Aut. dom.

Numbers in parentheses indicate numbers of other listed syndromes which merit special consideration in the differential diagnosis.

O. Osteochondrodysplasias

SYNDROME	CRANIOFACIAL	LIMBS	OTHER	MENTAL DEFICIENCY	SHORT STATURE	GENETICS
85. Achondroplasia (86–90,92)	Low nasal bridge, +/- macrocephaly	Short limbs, short hands and feet, limited elbow extension	Caudal narrowing of spinal canal, short ilium		+	Aut. dom.
86. Metatropic dwarfism (85,90,92)	Normal facies	Short limb, small epiphyses, metaphyseal flare	Severe early kyphoscoliosis, flattened vertebrae		+	? Aut. rec.
87. Thoracic asphyxiant dystrophy (85,88,90)	Normal facies	Short limbs, short hands, +/- polydactyly	Constricted small thorax +/- renal disease		+	Aut. rec.
88. Ellis-van Creveld syndrome (chondroectodermal dysplasia) (87)	Neonatal teeth, hypoplasia of teeth	Short distal limbs, polydactyly, nail hypoplasia	Small thorax, cardiac defect		+	Aut. rec.
89. Diastrophic dwarfism (85,86,92)	Hypertrophied or cystic auricular cartilage	Short limbs, short first metacarpal, joint limitations, club foot			+	Aut. rec.
90. Pseudoachondroplastic type spondyloepiphyseal dysplasia (85–87,89,92)	Normal facies	Postnatal onset of short limbs, irregular epiphyses and metaphyses, limited elbow extension			+	Aut. dom.
91. X-linked spondyloepiphyseal dysplasia (119)	Normal facies	Onset at 5-10 years of epiphyseal irregularity	Short trunk, flattening of vertebrae		+ (late)	X-linked rec.
92. Multiple epiphyseal dysplasia	Normal facies	Short fingers, epiphyseal hypoplasia, metaphyseal flaring	Joint limitation, eventual osteoarthritis of hip		+	Aut. dom.
93. Metaphyseal dysostosis, Jansen type (94–96)	Small face, prominent eyes	Wide irregular metaphyses, flexion deformities of joints	Small thorax		+	
94. Metaphyseal dystostosis, Schmid type (93,95,96)	Normal facies	Bow legs, irregular wide metaphyses	Variable limitation in full extension of fingers		+	Aut. dom.
95. Cartilage-hair hypoplasia (94)	Fine, sparse hair; normal facies	Mild bowing of legs, wide slightly irregular metaphyses	+/- Intestinal malabsorption		+	Aut. rec.
96. X-linked hypophosphatemic rickets (93–95)	Normal facies	Bowed lower limbs	Hypophosphatemia		+	X-linked
97. Multiple exostoses	Normal facies	Diaphyseal outgrowths leading to limb deformity	+/- Short metacarpals		+/-	Aut. dom.
98. Conradi's disease; chondrodystrophia calcificans congenita	Flattened nasal bridge, cataracts	Short proximal long bones, joint contractures	Calcific stippling in developing cartilage	+/-	+	Aut. rec.
99. Hypophosphatasia	Delayed closure of fontanels, early loss of deciduous teeth, craniosynostosis	Bowing of legs, poor irregular mineralization, especially at metaphyses			+	Aut. rec.
100. Kenny's syndrome	Myopia	Slim medullary cavity	Transient hypocalcemia		+	? Aut. dom.

Numbers in parentheses indicate numbers of other listed syndromes which merit special consideration in the differential diagnosis.

P. Osteopetroses

No. Syndrome	Feature 1	Feature 2	Feature 3			Inheritance
101. Pyle's syndrome of cranio-metaphyseal dysplasia	Broad flat nasal bridge, thick calvarium with cranial nerve compression	Enlarging splayed metaphyseal ends of long bones, knock knee			+/−	Aut. rec.
102. Osteopetrosis, severe (Albers-Schönberg disease)	Thick calvarium with cranial nerve compression, +/− macrocephaly	Dense, thick, fragile bones	Secondary pancytopenia, splenomegaly		+/−	Aut. rec.
103. Pyknodysostosis of Maroteaux and Lamy (104,105)	Tooth anomalies, delayed closure of fontanels, facial bone hypoplasia	Osteosclerosis, shortening of distal phalanges			+	Aut. rec.
104. Cleidocranial dysostosis (103)	Delayed closure of fontanels, late eruption of teeth		Defect of outer clavicle		+	Aut. dom.
105. Stanesco's syndrome (103)	Brachycephaly with thin cranium, facial bone hypoplasia	Mild osteosclerosis, relatively short upper arms			+	Aut. dom.

Q. Craniosynostoses

No. Syndrome	Feature 1	Feature 2	Feature 3			Inheritance
106. Apert's syndrome (acrocephalosyndactyly) (107)	Craniosynostosis, irregular mid-facial hypoplasia and hypertelorism	Syndactyly, broad distal thumb and toe		+		Aut. dom.
107. Carpenter's syndrome (25,106)	Craniosynostosis, lateral displacement of inner canthi	Polydactyly, syndactyly	Obesity	+	+/−	Aut. rec.
108. Crouzon's disease (craniofacial dysostosis)		Shallow orbits, maxillary hypoplasia, craniosynostosis				Aut. dom.

R. Other Skeletal Dysplasias. Including some with short metacarpal bones.

No. Syndrome	Feature 1	Feature 2	Feature 3			Inheritance
109. Aminopterin-induced syndrome	Cranial dysplasia with low nasal bridge, low set ears			?	+	
110. Nail-patella syndrome		Patella hypoplasia, nail hypoplasia	Iliac horns, scoliosis			Aut. dom.
111. Dyschondrosteosis of Leri-Weill		Short forearms with Madelung deformity	+/− Short lower leg		+	Aut. dom.
WITH SHORT METACARPALS:						
112. Albright's hereditary osteodystrophy (113,114)	Rounded facies	Short metacarpals, especially fourth	Obesity, hypocalcemia, extra-skeletal mineralization	+	+	?X-linked dom.
113. Brachydactyly, type E (112,114)		Brachydactyly, short third and fifth metacarpals			+	Aut. dom.
114. Weill-Marchesani syndrome (112,113)	Small spherical lens	Brachydactyly			+	Aut. rec.

Numbers in parentheses indicate numbers of other listed syndromes which merit special consideration in the differential diagnosis.

S. *Mucopolysaccharidoses.* The mucopolysaccharidoses are categorized together on the basis of finding excess tissue storage and/or urinary excretion of mucopolysaccharide. Clinically, all tend to produce some coarsening of the facial features. Other manifestations found in this group are broadening and altered configuration of bone, joint limitation, corneal opacity, hepatosplenomegaly, mental deterioration, and cardiovascular changes—all features of the prototype, Hurler's syndrome. The age of onset may be a helpful clinical clue in these disorders. With the exception of generalized gangliosidosis, these disorders become clinically manifest *after* birth.

SYNDROME	FACIAL	SKELETAL	OTHER	MENTAL DEFICIENCY	SHORT STATURE	GENETICS
115. Generalized gangliosidosis	Coarse facies, hypertrophy of alveolar ridges at birth	Kyphosis in early infancy	Renal dysfunction	? +	+	? Aut. rec.
116. Hurler's syndrome (MPS type I) (117,118)	Coarse facies, cloudy cornea, early	Stiff joints by one year, kyphosis by one-two years	Valvular heart disease	+	+ Onset 6-18 mo.	Aut. rec.
117. Maroteaux-Lamy syndrome (MPS type VI) (116,118)	Mild coarse facies, cloudy cornea	Stiff joints, kyphosis			+ Onset 1-3 yr.	Aut. rec.
118. Hunter's syndrome (MPS type II) (116,117)	Coarse facies, clear cornea	Stiff Joints, seldom develop kyphosis	Deafness develops	+	+ Onset 2-4 yr.	X-linked rec.
119. Morquio's disease (MPS type IV) (86,90,91)	Mild coarse facies, cloudy cornea, late	Mildly stiff joints, development of flattened vertebrae and severe kyphosis			+ Onset 1-3 yr.	Aut. rec.
120. Sanfilippo syndrome (MPS type III) (121)	Mild coarse facies, clear cornea	Mildly stiff joints, no kyphosis		+		Aut. rec.
121. Scheie syndrome (MPS type V) (120)	Broad mouth, cloudy cornea	Stiff joints by 5-8 yr., no kyphosis				Aut. rec.
(Insert) 122. Leroy's syndrome 'I' cell disease (116–118)	Early hypertrophy of alveolar ridges	Limited extension of joints	Thick "tight" skin	+	+	Aut. rec.

T. *Connective Tissue Disorders.* The connective tissue disorders, so categorized because the basic problem appears to be in fibrous tissue and its derivatives, include defects in development and support within connective tissue. Relative laxity of joints, bluish sclerae, and inguinal hernias are rather nonspecific and may be found as features of syndromes 123-126. Abnormality in blood vessels may lead to serious vascular disease in conditions 123-125 and 128.

SYNDROME	FACIAL	LIMBS	OTHER	MENTAL DEFICIENCY	SHORT STATURE	GENETICS
123. Marfan's syndrome (124)	Lens subluxation	Arachnodactyly	Aortic dilatation			Aut. dom.
124. Homocystinuria (113)	Lens subluxation malar flush	Osteoporosis	Venous thromboses	+/−		Aut. rec.

Numbers in parentheses indicate numbers of other listed syndromes which merit special consideration in the differential diagnosis.

(Table continued on following page.)

T. Connective Tissue Disorders. (Continued)

SYNDROME	FACIAL	LIMBS	OTHER	MENTAL DEFICIENCY	SHORT STATURE	GENETICS
125. Ehlers-Danlos syndrome		Hyperextensible joints	Hyperextensible skin, poor wound healing with thin scar, subcutaneous nodules			Aut. dom.
126. Osteogenesis imperfecta	Bluish sclerae, odontogenesis imperfecta	Fragile bone	+/− deafness		+/−	Aut. dom.
127. Fibrodysplasia ossificans progressiva (myositis ossificans)		Short hallux +/− short thumb	Fibrous dysplasia in muscle and subcutaneous fat, leading to mineralization		+/−	Aut. dom.
128. Pseudoxanthoma elasticum	Angioid retinal streaks	Thickened yellowish skin in flexural areas	Artery medial degeneration with hemorrhagic tendency			Aut. rec.

U. Other Miscellaneous Syndromes

SYNDROME	FACIAL	DIAGNOSTIC MANIFESTATIONS	OTHER	MENTAL DEFICIENCY	SHORT STATURE	GENETICS
129. X-linked hydrocephalus	Hydrocephalus	Short flexed thumbs		+		X-linked rec.
130. Fabry's syndrome	Dark nodular angiectases	Attacks of burning pain	Renal insufficiency			X-linked rec.
131. Osler's disease	Multiple telangiectases	Epistaxes				Aut. dom.
132. Riley-Day syndrome	Dysautonomia	Poor coordination	Lack of tearing	+/−	+/−	Aut. rec.
133. Schwachman's syndrome		Lack of exocrine pancreas, failure to thrive	Neutropenia +/− anemia and thrombocytopenia			Aut. rec.
134. Wiskott-Aldrich syndrome	Eczema	Immunological deficit of IgM and lymphocytes	Thrombocytopenia			X-linked rec.
135. Chediak-Higashi syndrome	Partial albinism	Photophobia, nystagmus	Neutropenia, leukocyte inclusions, infection, lymphoma			Aut. rec.

Numbers in parentheses indicate numbers of other listed syndromes which merit special consideration in the differential diagnosis.

1. DOWN'S SYNDROME

(21 Trisomy Syndrome)

Hypotonia, Flat Facies, Slanted Palpebral Fissures

Down's[1] report of 1866 on the ethnic classification of idiots stated that a "large number of congenital idiots are typical Mongols," and he set forth the clinical description of Down's syndrome. The textbook by Penrose and Smith[2] provides an excellent overall appraisal of this disease which has an incidence of 1 : 660 newborns, making it the most common pattern of malformation in man.

ABNORMALITIES

General. Hypotonia with tendency to keep mouth open and protrude the tongue; diastasis recti.

Hyperflexibility of joints.

Relatively small stature with awkward gait.

Central Nervous System. Mental deficiency (100 per cent).

Craniofacial. Brachycephaly with relatively flat occiput.

Thin cranium with late closure of fontanels.

Hypoplasia to aplasia of frontal sinuses.

Small nose with low nasal bridge.

Ears. Small, overfolding of angulated upper helix; sometimes prominent; small or absent earlobes.

Eyes. Upward slant to palpebral fissures.

Inner epicanthic folds.

Speckling of iris (Brushfield's spots) with peripheral hypoplasia of iris.

Fine lens opacities by slit lamp examination (59 per cent).

Refractive error.

Dentition. Hypoplasia, irregular placement.

Neck. Appears short.

Hands. Relatively short metacarpals and phalanges.

Fifth finger: hypoplasia of mid-phalanx of fifth finger (60 per cent) with clinodactyly (50 per cent), a single crease (40 per cent), or both.

Simian crease (45 per cent).

Distal position of palmar axial triradius (84 per cent).

Ulnar loop dermal ridge pattern on all digits (35 per cent).

Feet. Wide gap between first and second toes.

Plantar crease between first and second toes.

Open field dermal ridge patterning in hallucal area of sole (50 per cent).

Pelvis. Hypoplasia with outward lateral flare of iliac wings and shallow acetabular angle.

Heart. Anomaly in about 40 per cent; atrioventricular communis, ventricular septal defect, patent ductus arteriosus, auricular septal defect, and aberrant subclavian artery, in decreasing order of frequency.

Skin. Loose folds in posterior neck (infancy).

Cutis marmorata, especially in extremities (43 per cent).

Dry hyperkeratotic skin (with time) in 75 per cent.

Hair. Fine, soft, and often sparse; straight pubic hair at adolescence.

Genitalia. Male: relatively small penis. Infertile (100 per cent).

OCCASIONAL ABNORMALITIES. Seizures (less than 5 per cent); strabismus (33 per cent), nystagmus (15 per cent), keratoconus (6 per cent), cataract (1.3 per cent); low placement of ears; web neck; two ossification centers in manubrium sterni; funnel or pigeon breast; tracheoesophageal fistula, duodenal atresia; tetralogy of Fallot; incomplete fusion of vertebral arches of lower spine (37 per cent); only 11 ribs; cryptorchidism (27 per cent from birth to nine years and 14 per cent after 15 years); syndactyly of second and third toes. The incidence of leukemia is about 1 : 95, or close to 1 per cent.

PRINCIPAL FEATURES IN NEWBORN. The diagnosis can generally be made shortly after birth, and therefore the following ten features of Down's syndrome in the newborn are presented as set forth by Hall,[3] who found at least four of these abnormalities in all of 48 newborns with Down's syndrome, and six or more in 89 per cent of them.

Hypotonia	80%
Poor Moro reflex	85%
Hyperflexibility of joints	80%
Excess skin on back of neck	80%
Flat facial profile	90%
Slanted palpebral fissures	80%
Anomalous auricles	60%
Dysplasia of pelvis	70%
Dysplasia of mid-phalanx of fifth finger	60%
Simian crease	45%

NATURAL HISTORY. Muscle tone tends to improve with age, whereas the rate of develop-

(Text continued)

mental progress slows with age. For example 23 per cent of a group of Down's syndrome children under three years had a developmental quotient above 50, whereas none of those in the three to nine year group had intelligence quotients above 50. Though the I.Q. range is generally said to be 25 to 50 with an occasional individual above 50, the mean I.Q. for older patients is 24. Fortunately, social performance is usually beyond that expected for mental age, averaging three and one third years above mental age for the older individuals. Generally "good babies" and happy children, they tend toward mimicry, are friendly, have a good sense of rhythm, and enjoy music. Mischievousness and obstinacy may also be characteristics, and 13 per cent have serious emotional problems. Coordination is often poor, and the voice tends to be raucous.

Growth is relatively slow, and during the first eight years secondary centers of ossification are often late in development. However, during later childhood the osseous maturation is more "normal," and final height is usually attained around 15 years of age. Adolescent sexual development is usually somewhat less complete than normal. The girls may menstruate and can be fertile, whereas the males are considered infertile.

The major cause for early mortality is congenital heart defects, and 44 per cent of those with cardiac anomalies die in infancy. Lower respiratory infections may pose a serious problem; however, between infancy and 40 years of age the mortality rate is not much greater than the normal. Low grade frequent problems are chronic rhinitis, conjunctivitis, and periodontal disease, none of which are easy to "cure."

ETIOLOGY. Trisomy for all or a large part of chromosome 21. The combined results of 11 unselected surveys totaling 784 cases showed the following relative frequencies of particular types of chromosomal alteration for Down's syndrome:[3]

Full 21 trisomy	94%
21 Trisomy/normal mosaicism	2.4%
Translocation cases (with about equal occurrence of D/G and G/G translocations)	3.3%

Faulty chromosome distribution leading to Down's syndrome is more likely to occur at older maternal age, as shown in the following figures of incidence for Down's syndrome for particular maternal ages: 15 to 29 years, 1 : 1500; 30 to 34 years, 1 : 800; 35 to 39 years, 1 : 270; 40 to 44 years, 1 : 100, and over 45 years, 1 : 50.

Though the general likelihood for *recurrence* of Down's syndrome is 1 per cent, the principal problem in giving recurrence risk figures to parents is first to determine whether the Down's syndrome child is a translocation case with a parent who is a translocation carrier and thereby a relatively high risk for recurrence. The likelihood of finding a translocation in the Down's syndrome child of a mother under 30 years of age is 6 per cent, and of such cases only one out of three will be found to have a translocation carrier parent. Therefore the estimated probability that either parent of a Down's syndrome patient born of a mother under 30 years is a G/D or G/G translocation carrier is 2 per cent versus 0.3 per cent when the Down's syndrome patient is born of a mother over 30 years of age. Having excluded a translocation carrier parent, the risk for recurrence may be stated as less than 1 per cent. The recurrence risk for the rare translocation carrier parent will depend on the type of translocation and the sex of the parent.

REFERENCES

1. Down, J. L. H.: Observations on an ethnic classification of idiots. Clinical Lecture Reports, London Hospital, *3*:259, 1866.
2. Penrose, L. S., and Smith, G. F.: Down's Anomaly. Boston, Little, Brown & Company, 1966.
3. Hall, B.: Mongolism in newborn infants. Clin. Pediat., *5*:4, 1966.
4. Richards, B. W., Stewart, A., Sylvester, P. E., and Jasiewicz, V.: Cytogenetic survey of 225 patients diagnosed clinically as mongols. J. Ment. Defic. Res., *9*:245, 1965.

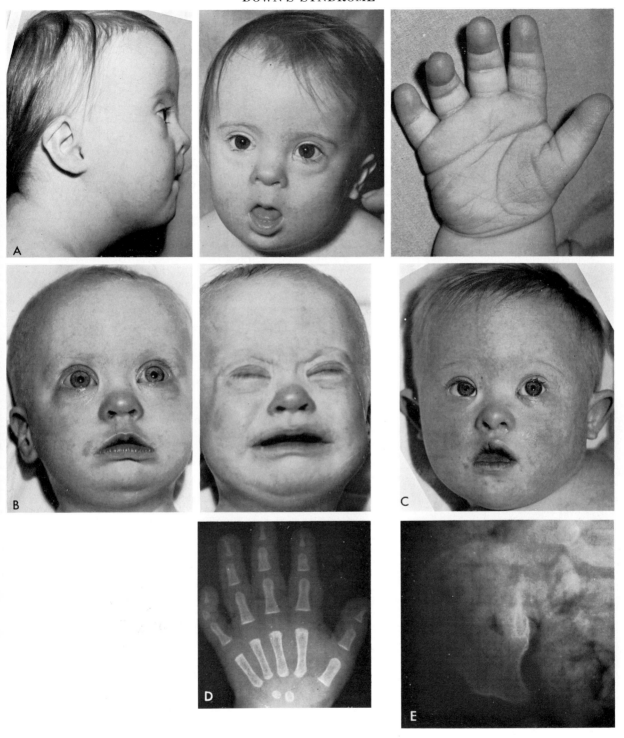

A, Young infant. Flat facies, straight hair; protrusion of tongue; single crease on inturned fifth finger.

B and *C*, Inner canthal folds. Speckling of iris with lack of peripheral patterning. Small auricles, prominent at right. "Pouting" expression when crying. (From Smith, D. W.: J. Pediat., *70*:474, 1967.)

D, Hypoplasia, mid-phalanx of fifth finger.

E, Shallow acetabular angle with small iliac wings having the shape of elephant ears.

2. XXXXY SYNDROME

Hypogenitalism, Limited Elbow Pronation, Low Dermal Ridge Count on Fingertips

Since the initial report of Fraccaro et al.[1] in 1960, at least 40 cases of the XXXXY aneuploidy syndrome have been reported.

ABNORMALITIES. Frequencies based on from 17 to 32 cases for each anomaly:[2]

Performance. Mental deficiency, intelligence quotient of 19 to 57, mean I.Q. of 34 — 100%

Hypotonia, joint laxity, or both — about one third of cases

Growth. Tendency to low birth weight, shortness of stature, retarded osseous maturation — 53%

Craniofacial. Sclerotic cranial sutures — 57%

Wide set eyes — 80%

Upward slant, palpebral fissures — 79%

Inner epicanthic folds — 82%

Strabismus — 59%

Low nasal bridge; wide or upturned nasal tip — 95%

Mandibular prognathism — 50%

Auricular anomaly (large, low set, malformed) — 70%

Neck. Short neck — 72%

Thorax. Thick sternum — 75%

Extremities. Limited pronation at elbow — 95%

Radioulnar synostosis — 42%

Clinodactyly of fifth finger — 90%

Coxa valga — 25%

Genu valga — 50%

Pes planus — 73%

Dermal ridge patterns.[3] High frequency of low arch pattern on fingertips, with mean total ridge count of only 50, versus the average male total ridge count of 144.

Genitalia. Small penis — 80%

Small testes, hypoplastic tubules, diminished Leydig cells — 94%

Cryptorchidism — 28%

Hypoplastic scrotum — 80%

OCCASIONAL ABNORMALITIES. Obesity, flat occiput, microcephaly, antimongoloid slant to palpebral fissures, Brushfield speckled iris, myopia, cleft palate, small peg-shaped teeth, web neck (12 per cent), pectus excavatum, congenital heart defect (especially patent ductus arteriosus), umbilical hernia, scoliosis, simian creases, club foot, abnormal toes, wide gap between first and second toes, hypospadias, bifid scrotum.

NATURAL HISTORY. Perinatal problems in adaptation have been frequent; linear growth is generally slow with moderately short final height attainment. Infertility and inadequate virilization may be anticipated.

ETIOLOGY. The XXXXY diagnosis may be confirmed by the finding of as many as three sex chromatin masses in interphase nuclei (buccal smear) in a male who is found to have 49 chromosomes with three extra C group chromosomes.

COMMENT. Although some of the features may initially suggest Down's syndrome, the total pattern of anomalies is usually at variance with this diagnosis.

REFERENCES

1. Fraccaro, M., Kaijser, K., and Lindsten, J.: A child with 49 chromosomes. Lancet, *2*:899, 1960.
2. Zaleski, W. A., Houston, C. S., Pozsonyi, J., and Ying, K. L.: The XXXXY chromosome anomaly: report of three new cases and review of 30 cases from the literature. Canad. Med. Ass. J., *94*:1143, 1966.
3. Penrose, L. S.: Finger-print pattern and the sex chromosomes. Lancet, *1*:298, 1967.

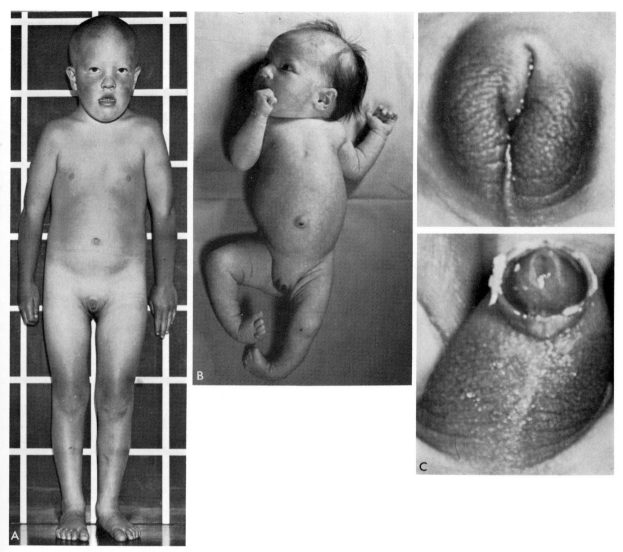

A, Six year old with height age of five years. (From Smith, D. W.: J. Pediat., *70*:476, 1967.)
B, Neonate. Note club feet and small genitalia. He had delayed tooth eruption and also had eczema.
C, Genitalia of patient shown in B. The small penis was revealed by pushing back the tissues.

3. 18 TRISOMY SYNDROME

Clenched Hand, Short Sternum, Low Arch Dermal Ridge Patterning on Fingertips

This condition was first recognized as a specific entity in 1960 by discovery of the extra 18 chromosome in babies with a particular pattern of malformation (Edwards et al.,[1] Patau et al.,[2] and Smith et al.[3]). It is the second most common multiple malformation syndrome, with an incidence of about 0.3 per 1000 newborn babies. There has been a 3 : 1 preponderance of females to males. Several good reviews set forth a full appraisal of this syndrome.[4-7]

More than 130 different abnormalities have been noted in the literature on patients with the 18 trisomy syndrome, and therefore the listing of abnormalities has been divided into those which occur in 50 per cent or more of patients, in 10 to 50 per cent of patients, and less than 10 per cent of patients.

ABNORMALITIES FOUND IN 50 PER CENT OR MORE OF PATIENTS

General. Feeble fetal activity, weak cry.
Altered gestational timing; one third premature, one third postmature.
Polyhydramnios, small placenta, single umbilical artery.
Growth deficiency; mean birth weight, 2340 gm.
Hypoplasia of skeletal muscle, subcutaneous and adipose tissue.
Mental deficiency, hypertonicity (after neonatal period).
Diminished response to sound.
Craniofacial. Prominent occiput, narrow bifrontal diameter.
Low set, malformed auricles.
Short palpebral fissures.
Small oral opening, narrow palatal arch.
Micrognathia.
Hands and Feet. Clenched hand, tendency for overlapping of index finger over third, fifth finger over fourth.
Absence of distal crease on fifth finger with or without third and fourth fingers.
Low arch dermal ridge pattern on six or more fingertips.
Hypoplasia of nails, especially on fifth finger and toes.
Short hallux, frequently dorsiflexed.
Thorax. Sternum short, with reduced number of ossification centers.
Small nipples.
Abdominal Wall. Inguinal or umbilical hernia and/or diastasis recti.

Pelvis and Hips. Small pelvis, limited hip abduction.
Genitalia. Cryptorchidism (male).
Skin. Redundancy, mild hirsutism of forehead and back, prominent cutis marmoratum.
Cardiac. Ventricular septal defect, patent ductus arteriosus.

ABNORMALITIES OCCURRING IN 10 TO 50 PER CENT OF CASES

Craniofacial. Wide fontanels, microcephaly, hypoplasia of orbital ridges.
Inner epicanthic folds, ptosis of eyelid, corneal opacity.
Cleft lip, cleft palate, or both.
Hands and Feet. Ulnar or radial deviation of hand, hypoplastic to absent thumb, simiam crease.
Equinovarus, rocker-bottom feet, syndactyly of second and third toes.
Thorax. Relatively broad, with or without widespread nipples.
Genitalia. Female: hypoplasia of labia major with prominent clitoris.
Anus. Malposed or funnel-shaped anus.
Cardiac. Auricular septal defect, bicuspid aortic and/or pulmonic valves, nodularity of vale leaflets, pulmonic stenosis.
Lung. Malsegmentation to absence of right lung.
Diaphragm. Muscle hypoplasia with or without eventration.
Abdomen. Meckel's diverticulum, heterotopic pancreatic and/or splenic tissue.
Incomplete rotation of colon.
Renal. Horseshoe defect, ectopic kidney, double ureter.

ABNORMALITIES FOUND IN LESS THAN 10 PER CENT OF CASES

Central Nervous System. Facial palsy, paucity of myelination, microgyria, cerebellar hypoplasia, defect of corpus callosum, hydrocephalus, meningomyelocele.
Craniofacial. Wormian cranial bones, shallow elongated sella. Slanted palpebral fissures, hypertelorism, colobomata of iris, cataract, microphthalmos, choanal atresia.
Hands. Syndactyly of third and fourth fingers, polydactyly, short fifth metacarpals, ectodactyly.
Other Skeletal. Radial aplasia. Incomplete ossification of clavicle. Hemivertebrae, fused

vertebrae, short neck, scoliosis, rib anomaly, pectus, dislocated hip.

Genitalia. Male: hypospadias, bifid scrotum.
Female: bifid uterus, ovarian hypoplasia.

Cardiovascular. Anomalous coronary artery, transposition, tetralogy of Fallot, coarctation of aorta, dextrocardia, aberrant subclavian artery, and intimal proliferation in arteries with arteriosclerotic change and medial calcification.

Abdominal. Pyloric stenosis, omphalocele, extrahepatic biliary atresia, hypoplastic gallbladder, gallstones, imperforate anus.

Renal. Hydronephrosis, polycystic (small cysts).

Endocrine. Thyroid or adrenal hypoplasia.

Other. Hemangiomata, thymic hypoplasia, tracheoesophageal fistula, thrombocytopenia.

NATURAL HISTORY. Babies with the 18 trisomy syndrome are usually feeble and have limited capacity for survival. Resuscitation is often performed at birth, and they may have apneic episodes in the neonatal period. Poor sucking capability may necessitate nasogastric tube feeding, but even with optimal management they fail to thrive. Thirty per cent die within the first month and 50 per cent by two months; only 10 per cent survive the first year[8] as severely mentally defective individuals. Once the diagnosis has been established, the author recommends limitation of all medical means for prolongation of life.

ETIOLOGY. Trisomy for all or a large part of the number 18 chromosome. The great majority of cases have full 18 trisomy, the result of faulty chromosomal distribution, which is most likely to occur at older maternal age; the mean maternal age at birth of babies with this syndrome is 32 years. Translocation cases, the result of chromosomal breakage, can only be excluded by chromosomal studies, and when such a case is found the parents should also have chromosomal studies to determine whether one of them is a balanced translocation carrier with high risk for recurrence in future offspring. Though no adequate studies or recurrence risk exist for full 18 trisomy cases, it seems safe to presume that the recurrence risk would be even lower than the 1 per cent for full 21 trisomy syndrome cases. This latter statement is predicated on the indication that most 18 trisomic individuals die in embryonic or fetal life, as suggested by the chromosomal findings in spontaneous abortuses.

REFERENCES

1. Edwards, J. H., Harnden, D. G., Cameron, A. H., Crosse, V. M., and Wolff, O. H.: A new trisomic syndrome. Lancet, *1*:787, 1960.
2. Patau, K., Smith, D. W., Therman, E., Inhorn, S. L., and Wagnes, H. P.: Multiple congenital anomaly caused by an extra autosome. Lancet, *1*:790, 1960.
3. Smith, D. W., Patau, K., Therman, E., and Inhorn, S. L.: A new autosomal trisomy syndrome. J. Pediat., *57*:338, 1960.
4. Smith, D. W.: Autosomal abnormalities. Am. J. Obstet. & Gynec., *90*:1055, 1964.
5. Taylor, A., and Polani, P. E.: Autosomal trisomy syndromes, excluding Down's. Guy's Hosp. Rep., *13*:231, 1964.
6. Butler, L. J., Snodgrass, A. J. A. I., France, N. E., Sinclair, L., and Russell, A.: No. E (16-18) trisomy syndrome: analysis of 13 cases. Arch. Dis. Childhood, *40*:600, 1965.
7. Warkany, J., Passarge, E., and Smith, L. B.: Congenital malformations in autosomal trisomy syndromes. Am. J. Dis. Children, *112*:502, 1966.
8. Weber, W. W.: Survival and the sex ratio in trisomy 17-18. Am. J. Human Genet., *19*:369, 1967.

18 TRISOMY SYNDROME
Some Pathological Features

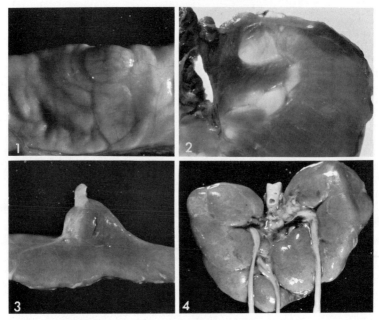

1. Ectopic pancreatic tissue in duodenum.
2. Meckel's diverticulum.
3. Defects of muscle development in diaphragm.
4. Horseshoe fused kidneys with extra ureter.

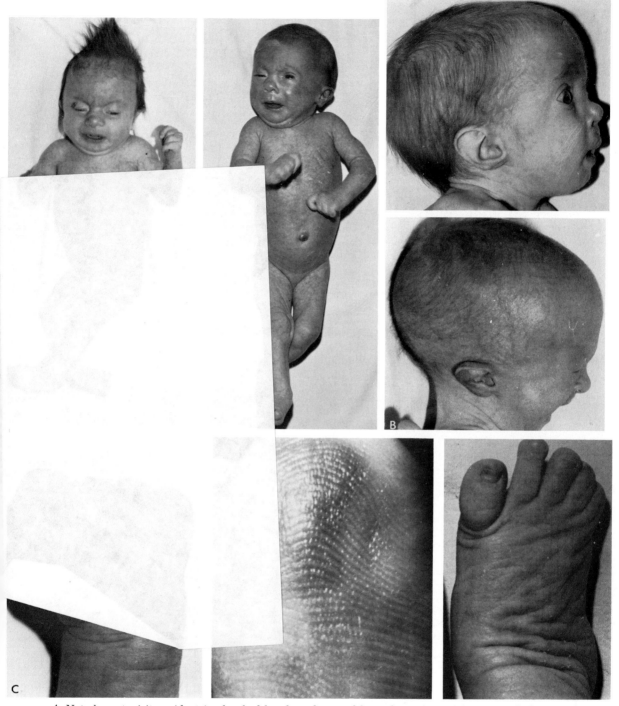

A, Note hypertonicity evident in clenched hands and crossed legs; short sternum (arrow marks lower end); narrow pelvis.

B, Prominent occiput; low-set, slanted auricle.

C, Clenched hand with index finger overlying third, hypoplasia of fifth fingernail, low arch dermal ridge configuration on fingertip, and dorsiflexed short hallux.

(From Smith, D. W.: Am. J. Obstet. & Gynec., *90*:1055, 1964.)

4. 13 TRISOMY SYNDROME

(D₁ Trisomy Syndrome)

Defects of Eye, Nose, Lip, and Forebrain of Holoprosencephaly Type; Polydactyly;
Narrow Hyperconvex Fingernails; Skin Defects, Posterior Scalp

Apparently described by Bartholin in 1657,[1] this syndrome was not generally recognized until its trisomic etiology was discovered by Patau et al.[2] in 1960. The incidence is about one per 5000 births.

ABNORMALITIES FOUND IN 50 PER CENT OR MORE OF PATIENTS

Central Nervous System. Holoprosencephaly type defect with varying degrees of incomplete development of forebrain and olfactory and optic nerves.

Minor motor seizures, often with hypsarrhythmic EEG pattern.

Apneic spells in early infancy.

Severe mental defect.

Hearing. Apparent deafness (defects of organ of Corti in the two cases studied).

Cranium. Moderate microcephaly with sloping forehead.

Wide sagittal suture and fontanels.

Eyes. Microphthalmia, colobomata of iris, or both.

Retinal dysplasia, often including islands of cartilage.

Mouth. Cleft lip, cleft palate, or both.

Auricles. Abnormal helices with or without low set ears.

Skin. Capillary hemangiomata, especially forehead.

Localized scalp defects in parieto-occipital area.

Loose skin, posterior neck.

Hands and Feet. Distal palmar axial triradii.

Simian crease.

Hyperconvex narrow fingernails.

Flexion of fingers with or without overlapping and camptodactyly.

Polydactyly of hands and sometimes feet.

Posterior prominence of heel.

Other Skeletal. Thin posterior ribs with or without missing rib.

Hypoplasia of pelvis with shallow acetabular angle.

Cardiac. Abnormality in 80 per cent with ventricular septal defect, patent ductus arteriosus, auricular septal defect, and dextroposition, in decreasing order of frequency.

Genitalia. Male: cryptorchidism, abnormal scrotum.

Female: bicornuate uterus.

Hematological. Increased frequency of nuclear projections in neutrophils.

Unusual persistence of embryonic and/or fetal type hemoglobin.

Other. Single umbilical artery.

Inguinal or umbilical hernia.

ABNORMALITIES FOUND IN LESS THAN 50 PER CENT OF PATIENTS

Growth. Congenital hypoplasia, mean birth weight, 2480 gm.

Central Nervous System. Hypertonia, hypotonia, agenesis of corpus callosum, hydrocephalus, fusion of basal ganglia, cerebellar hypoplasia, meningomyelocele.

Eyes. Shallow supraorbital ridges, slanting palpebral fissures, absent eyebrows, hypotelorism, hypertelorism, anophthalmos, cyclopia.

Nose, Mouth, and Mandible. Absent philtrum, narrow palate, cleft tongue, micrognathia.

Hands and Feet. Retroflexible thumb, ulnar deviation at wrist, low arch digital dermal ridge pattern, fibular S-shaped hallucal dermal ridge pattern, syndactyly, cleft between first and second toes, hypoplastic toenails, equinovarus, radial aplasia.

Cardiac. Anomalous venous return, overriding aorta, pulmonary stenosis, hypoplastic aorta, atretic mitral and/or aortic valves, bicuspid aortic valve.

Abdominal. Omphalocele, heterotopic pancreatic or splenic tissue, incomplete rotation of colon, Meckel's diverticulum.

Renal. Polycystic (31 per cent), hydronephrosis, horseshoe kidney, duplicated ureters.

Genitalia. Hypospadias, duplication and/or anomalous insertion of fallopian tubes, uterine cysts, hypoplastic ovaries.

Other. Thrombocytopenia, situs inversus of lungs, cysts of thymus, calcified pulmonary arterioles, large gallbladder, radial aplasia, flexion deformity of large joints, diaphragmatic defect.

NATURAL HISTORY. Forty-four per cent of these babies die within the first month and 69 per cent by six months; only 18 per cent survive the first year. Survivors have severe mental defects, often seizures, and fail to thrive. Only one adult, 33 years of age, has been detected. Because of the high infant mortality, surgical or orthopedic corrective procedures should be withheld in early infancy to await the outcome of the first few months. Furthermore, because of the severe brain defect, it is the opinion of the author that no medical means should be utilized to prolong the life of individuals with this syndrome, as should be self-evident from the accompanying illustrations.

ETIOLOGY. Trisomy for all or a large part of a specific D group (13-15) chromosome which is tentatively referred to as number 13. Older maternal age has been a factor in the occurrence of this aneuploidy syndrome, the mean maternal age being 30.9 years. Although no accurate empiric recurrence risk data are presently available, it is presumed that the likelihood for recurrence is of very low magnitude for the full 13 trisomy cases. As with Down's syndrome, chromosomal studies are indicated on 13 trisomy syndrome babies born of young mothers, in order to detect the rare translocation patient having a balanced translocation parent for whom the risk for recurrence would be of major concern.

COMMENT. The defects of mid-face, eye, and forebrain, which occur in variable degree as a feature of this syndrome, appear to be the consequence of a single defect in the early (three weeks) development of the prechordal mesoderm, which is not only necessary for morphogenesis of the mid-face but exerts an inductive role on the subsequent development of the prosencephalon, the forepart of the brain. This type of defect has been referred to as holoprosencephaly or arhinencephaly and varies in severity from cyclopia, to cebocephaly, to less severe forms.

REFERENCES

1. Warburg, M., and Mikkelsen, M.: A case of 13-15 trisomy or Bartholin-Patau's syndrome. Acta Ophth., *41*:321, 1963.
2. Patau, K., Smith, D. W., Therman, E., Inhorn, S. L., and Wagner, H. P.: Multiple congenital anomaly caused by an extra chromosome. Lancet, *1*:790, 1960.
3. Smith, D. W.: Autosomal abnormalities. Am. J. Obstet. & Gynec., *90*:1055, 1964.
4. Warkany, J., Passarge, E., and Smith, L. B.: Congenital malformations in autosomal trisomy syndromes. Am. J. Dis. Children, *112*:502, 1966.

13 TRISOMY SYNDROME

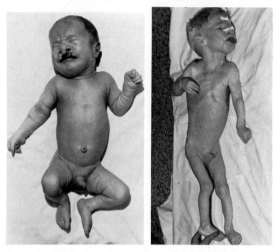

13 Trisomy patient at six weeks (22 inches, 9 pounds) and again at two years (30 inches, 15 pounds).

Some Pathological Features

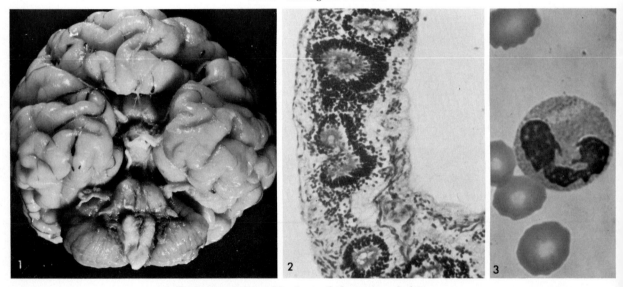

1. Lack of septation of forebrain (holoprosencephaly).
2. Dysplastic retina with rosette formation.
3. Excess nuclear projections in polymorphonuclear leukocyte.

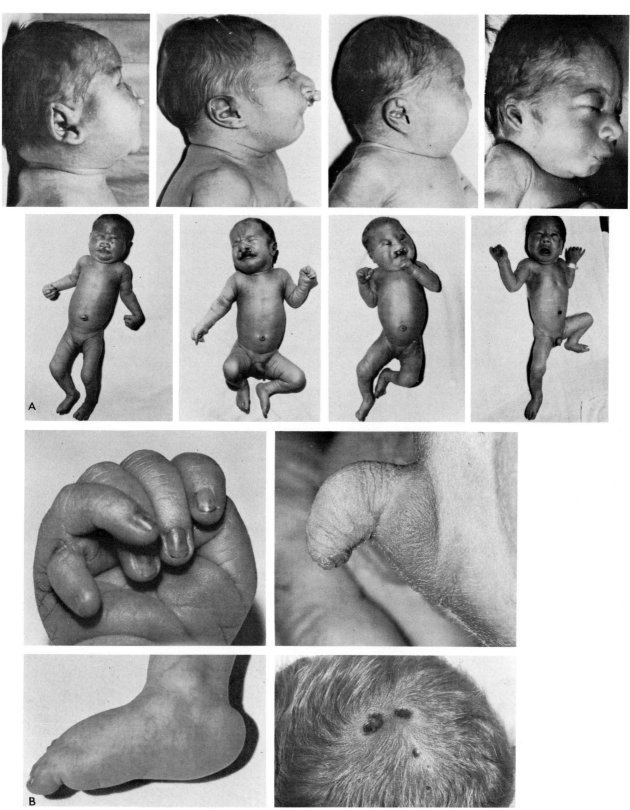

A, Note sloping forehead, variable defect in facial development. (From Smith, D. W., et al.: J. Pediat., *62*:326, 1963.)

B, Narrow hyperconvex fingernails, anomalous scrotum, prominent heel, and posterior scalp lesions. (From Smith, D. W.: Am. J. Obstet. & Gynec., *90*:1055, 1964.)

5. CHROMOSOME NUMBER 4 SHORT ARM DELETION SYNDROME

Ocular Hypertelorism with Broad or Beaked Nose, Microcephaly and/or Cranial Asymmetry, and Low Set, Simple Ear with Preauricular Dimple

After delineation of the cri-du-chat syndrome, occasional patients with deletions of the short arm of a B-group chromosome were found who lacked the typical cry and some other features of that condition. Autoradiographic labeling studies revealed that the deficient chromosome was a number 4 rather than a number 5, and the detection of further cases with consistent clinical findings have allowed the definition of the syndrome.

ABNORMALITIES (12 cases)

Growth. Marked growth deficiency, prenatal onset.

Performance. Feeble fetal activity. Severe mental deficiency; seizures.

Craniofacial. Strabismus, iris deformity, epicanthic folds; cleft lip and/or palate, downturned "fishlike" mouth, short upper lip.

Extremities. Hypoplastic dermal ridges, low dermal ridge count. Simian creases.

Other. Hypospadias, cryptorchidism, sacral dimple or sinus.

OCCASIONAL ABNORMALITIES.

Exophthalmos, defect of the medial half of the eyebrows, cardiac defect, metatarsus equinovarus, absence of pubic rami, delayed bone age, precocious puberty, midline scalp defect.

NATURAL HISTORY.

These children are profoundly mentally defective and tend to have severe grand mal seizures. Those who survive beyond early childhood have shown continued slow growth, with a propensity for respiratory infections. One boy with the syndrome experienced precocious puberty.

ETIOLOGY. Partial deletion of the short arm of chromosome 4. All cases reported to date have been sporadic occurrences, and no parental carriers for the deletion have yet been detected.

COMMENT. Although chromosome analysis may be misleading because of difficulties in discriminating between chromosomes number 4 and 5, this condition can be distinguished from the cri-du-chat syndrome on clinical grounds.

REFERENCES

1. Leao, J. C., et al.: New syndrome associated with partial deletion of short arms of chromosome no. 4. J.A.M.A., *202*:434, 1967.
2. Pfeiffer, R. A.: Neue Dokumentation zur Abgrenzung eines Syndroms der Deletion des kurzen Arms eines Chromosoms Nr. 4. Z. Kinderh., *102*:49, 1968.
3. Wolf, U., and Reinwein, H.: Klinische und cytogenetische Differentialdiagnose de Defizienzen an den kurzen Armen der B-Chromosomen. Z. Kinderh., *98*:235, 1967.

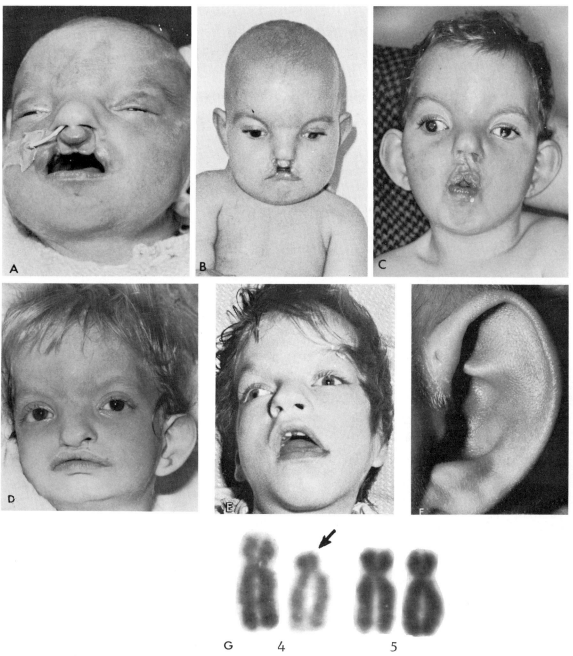

A to C, Two week old, 11 month old, and two and three fourths year old. (From Wolf, U., and Reinwein, H.: Ztschr. für Kinderh., 98:235, 1967.)

D, Five and three fourths year old with height age of ten months, and intelligence quotient of less than 20.

E, Seven year old with height age of three and one half years; performance age of less than six months.

F, Relatively simple form of ear with cutaneous pit.

G, B group of chromosomes from patient shown in E.

6. CRI-DU-CHAT SYNDROME

(Partial Deletion of the Short Arm of Chromosome Number 5)

Cat-Like Cry in Infancy, Microcephaly, Anti-Mongoloid Slant of the Palpebral Fissures

Lejeune et al.[1] first described this condition in 1963 in patients with a similar pattern of malformation who had a partial deletion of the short arm of one of the B group chromosomes. In 1964, German[2] demonstrated by autoradiographic studies that this was chromosome number 5. Further reports have raised to about 30 the number of cases described.

ABNORMALITIES

General. Low birth weight (less than	
2.5 kg.)	72%
Slow growth	100%
Cat-like cry	100%
Performance. Mental deficiency	100%
Hypotonia	78%
Craniofacial. Microcephaly	100%
Round face	68%
Hypertelorism	94%
Epicanthic folds	85%
Downward slanting of the palpebral	
fissures	81%
Strabismus	61%
Low set and/or poorly formed ears	58%
Heart. Congenital heart disease	
(variable in type)	30%
Hands. Simian crease	81%
Distal axial triradius	40%

OCCASIONAL ABNORMALITIES. Cleft lip and cleft palate, preauricular skin tag, facial asymmetry, bifid uvula, short neck, short metacarpals, clinodactyly, inguinal hernia, cryptorchidism, absent kidney and spleen, and hemivertebra.

NATURAL HISTORY. The majority of the reported cases have been young, and thus it is difficult to depict the natural history of this disease at the present time. The mewing cry, ascribed to abnormal laryngeal development, becomes less pronounced with increasing age of the patient, thus making the diagnosis more difficult in older patients.

ETIOLOGY. The underlying chromosomal aberration, partial deletion of the short arm of chromosome number 5, has appeared as a fresh phenomenon in the vast majority of the cases, which have been, therefore, sporadic occurrences within the families. In two cases an inherited translocation has been reported: one by Lejeune et al., in which the patient's mother had a balanced 5/D translocation; and the other by Laurent and Robert,[3] who studied a sibship with three affected brothers whose normal-appearing mother also had a deletion of the short arm of chromosome number 5, her missing piece of number 5 presumably being translocated to an unknown recipient chromosome.

REFERENCES

1. Lejeune, J., Lafourcade, J., Berger, R., Vialatte, J., Boeswillwald, M., Seringe, P., and Turpin, R.: Trois cas de délétion partielle du bras court du chromosome 5. C. Rend. Acad. Sci., *257*:3098, 1963.
2. German, J., Lejeune, J., MacIntyre, M. N., and DeGrouchy, J.: Chromosomal autoradiography in the cri-du-chat syndrome. Cytogenetics, *3*:347, 1964.
3. Laurent, C., and Robert, J. M.: Etude génétique et clinique d'une famille de sept enfants dans laquelle trois sujets son atteints de la "maladie du cri-du-chat." Ann. Genet., *9*:G113, 1966.
4. Berg, J. M., Delhanty, J. D. A., Faunch, J. A., and Ridler, M. A. C.: Partial deletion of short arm of a chromosome of the 4 and 5 group (Denver) in an adult male. J. Ment. Defic. Res., *9*:219, 1965.

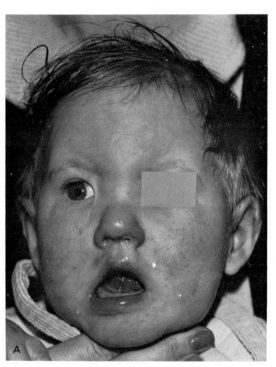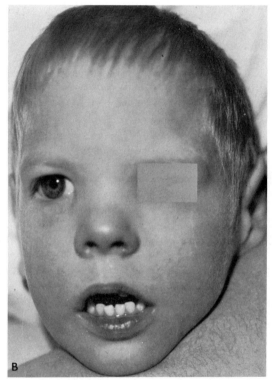

A, Nine month old with height age of 5 months; birth length 18 inches. Note the delay in dentition.

B, Three and five sixths year old, height age of one and one half years. Note the inner epicanthal fold and relatively small cranium with narrow forehead.

(From Smith, D. W.: J. Pediat., *70*:475, 1967.)

7. LONG ARM 18 DELETION SYNDROME

Mid-Facial Hypoplasia, Prominent Antihelix, Whorl Digital Pattern

Discovered by DeGrouchy et al. in 1964, this genetic imbalance syndrome has been documented in more than 24 cases,[6] and a recognizable pattern of malformation has emerged.

ABNORMALITIES[1-6]
Growth. Small stature.
Performance. Mental deficiency with hypotonia, poor coordination, nystagmus, conductive deafness.
Craniofacial. Microcephaly.
  Mid-facial hypoplasia with deep set eyes.
  Carp-shaped mouth, narrow palate.
Ears. Prominent antihelix, antitragus, or both.
  Narrow or atretric external canal.
Limbs. Long hands, tapering fingers and short first metacarpal with proximal thumb.
  High frequency whorl digital pattern, distal axial triradius, simian crease.
  Abnormal toe placement.
  Vertical talus with or without talipes equinovarus.
Genitalia. Female: hypoplastic labia minora.
  Male: cryptorchidism with or without small scrotum and penis.
Other. Eczema (6 of 24).
  Skin dimples over acromion, knuckles.
  Cardiac defect.

ABNORMALITIES OF UNCERTAIN FREQUENCY
Eye. Inner epicanthic folds, slanted palpebral fissures, ocular hypertelorism, microphthalmia, corneal abnormality, cataract, retinal defect, abnormal optic disc.
Ear. Atretic middle ear, low set ears.
Other. Cleft palate, widely spaced nipples, extra rib, horseshoe kidney, lipomata at lateral border of feet.

NATURAL HISTORY. Severe mental deficiency and growth deficiency, coupled with variable visual and hearing problems, may leave these individuals seriously handicapped. However, some patients with this deletion have not been severely affected. For example, a ten year old child studied by Wertelecki et al.[5] was not obviously debilitated.

REFERENCES

1. DeGrouchy, J., Royer, P., Salmon, C., and Lamy, M.: Délétion partielle du bras long du chromosome 18. Path. Biol., *12*:579, 1964.
2. Lejeune, J., Berger, R., Lafourcade, J., and Réthoré, M-O.: La délétion partielle du bras long du chromosome 18. Individualisation d'un nouvel état morbide. Ann. Génét., *9*:32, 1966.
3. Destiné, M. L., Punnett, H. H., Thovichit, S., DeGeorge, A. M., and Weiss, L.: La délétion partielle du bras long du chromosome 18 (syndrome 18Q-). Rapport de deux cas. Ann. Génét., *10*:65, 1967.
4. Insley, J.: Syndrome associated with a deficiency of part of the long arm of chromosome No. 18. Arch. Dis. Childhood, *42*:140, 1967.
5. Wertelecki, W., Schindler, A. M., and Gerald, P. S.: Partial deletion of chromosome 18. Lancet, *2*:641, 1966.
6. Wertelecki, W.: Personal communication.

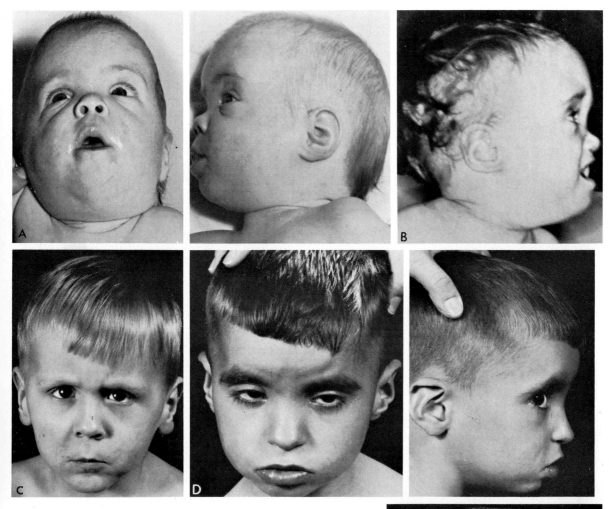

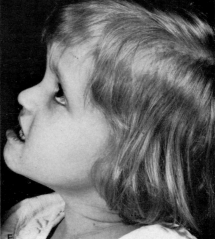

A, Young infant. Note shape of mouth, midfacial hypoplasia, and prominent antihelix. (Courtesy of E. Engel, Vanderbilt University.)

B, Infant. Note prominent antihelix and absence of external auditory canal openings.

C, Note mild slant to palpebral fissures, strabismus, and facial asymmetry.

D, Note mouth and micrognathia.

E, Note prominent forehead in relation to hypoplasia of midface.

(*B* to *E* courtesy of W. Wertelecki, National Cancer Institute—NIH, P. S. Gerald, Boston Children's Hospital.)

51

A. Chromosomal Abnormality Syndromes

8. LONG ARM "21" DELETION SYNDROME

(Antimongolism)

Downslanting Palpebral Fissure, Large Malformed External Ears, Micrognathia

One other case has been reported since Lejeune et al.[1] described this condition in 1964,[2] and a third case has been studied by German.[3]

ABNORMALITIES. Features found in at least two of the three patients:
Growth. Birth weight below 2.5 kg.
Performance. Apparent mental deficiency and hypertonia.
Facies. Blepharochalasis (redundant eyelids), anti-mongoloid slanting of the palpebral fissures, prominent nasal bridge, large external ear with wide external auditory canal, and micrognathia.
Hands. Dysplastic nails, distal axial triradii.
Other. Hypospadias, pyloric stenosis, thrombocytopenia, retarded osseous maturation.

OCCASIONAL ABNORMALITIES. Found in only one of the three patients: seizures; cataracts; absent helix, preauricular tags; cryptorchidism; agenesis of the left kidney; inguinal hernia; hemivertebrae; syndactyly; increased iliac index; eosinophilia; increased leukocyte alkaline phosphatase.

NATURAL HISTORY. Lejeune's[1] and Reisman's[2] patients were both young infants, and we have no information regarding their further clinical course.

ETIOLOGY. The partial deletion, presumably of the long arm of the 21 chromosome, has been of different extent in each of the cases, which may account for some of the variability in phenotypic expression.

COMMENT. This syndrome appears to be a distinct entity, although it will require further definition before a clear pattern of malformation can be set forth.

REFERENCES

1. Lejeune, J., Berger, R., Réthoré, M., Archambault, L., Jerome, H., Thieffry, S., Aicardi, J., Broyer, M., Lafourcade, J., Cruveiller, J., and Turpin, R.: Monosomie partielle pour un petit acrocentrique. C. Rend. Acad. Sci., *259*:4187, 1964.
2. Reisman, L. E.: Anti-mongolism. Studies in an infant with a partial monosomy of the 21 chromosome. Lancet, *1*:394, 1966.
3. German, J.: Personal communication.

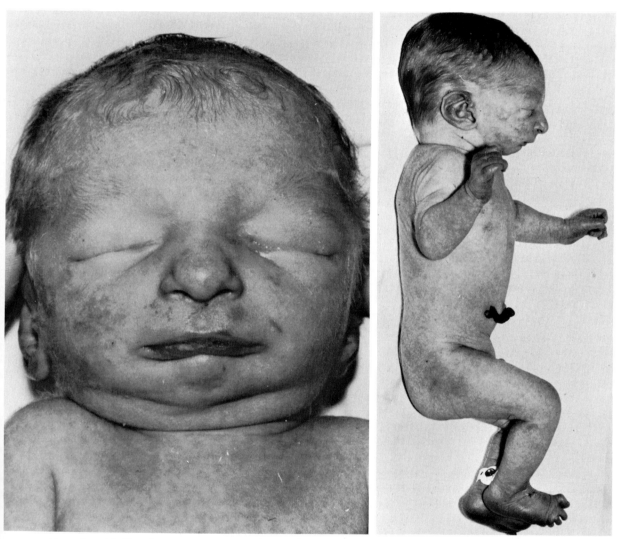

Four day old. Note large ears, micrognathia, and malar hypoplasia with downslanting palpebral fissures. (From Reisman, L. E.: Lancet, *1*:394, 1966.)

9. COLOBOMA OF IRIS AND ANAL ATRESIA SYNDROME — DUE TO SMALL ACROCENTRIC CHROMOSOME

(Cat-Eye Syndrome)

Coloboma of Iris, Downslanting Palpebral Fissures, Anal Atresia

This pattern of malformation and its chromosomal etiology were discovered by Schmid in Zurich and Fraccaro in Pavia, and the condition was briefly reported by Schachenmann et al.[1] in 1965.

ABNORMALITIES. Based on four cases, all females.
Performance. Mild to moderate developmental and/or mental deficiency (four).
Facies. Colobomata of iris (lower vertical) (four).
  Mild hypertelorism and slight downward slant to palpebral fissures (four).
  Preauricular fistula (two).
Intestine. Anal atresia with rectovestibular fistula (three).

OCCASIONAL ABNORMALITIES. Microphthalmos, dislocation of hip, unilateral renal aplasia (one case each).

ETIOLOGY. All four patients had an abnormally small acrocentric extra chromosome, about half the size of a G group autosome. At least part of the abnormal chromosome seems derived from a 13-15 or a 21-22 chromosome because its short arms bear satellites. Two of the patients were a mother and her daughter, demonstrating that reproduction can occur in this disorder allowing for a dominant mode of inheritance.

REFERENCES

1. Schachenmann, G., Schmid, W., Fraccaro, M., Mannini, A., Tiepolo, L., Perona, G. P., and Sartori, E.: Chromosomes in coloboma and anal atresia. Lancet, 2:290, 1965.
2. Schmid, W.: Pericentric inversions (report of two malformation cases suggestive of parental inversion heterozygosity). J. de Génét. Humaine, 16:89, 1967.

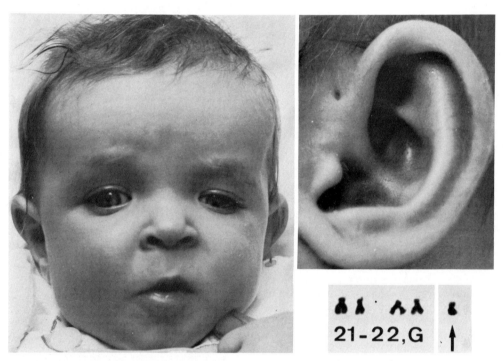

Infant showing downslanting palpebral fissures, colobomata of iris, and preauricular pits. Arrow denotes extra chromosome. (From Schmid, W.: J. de Génét. Humaine, *16*:89, 1967.)

10. PENTA-X SYNDROME

*Upward Slant to Palpebral Fissures, Patent Ductus Arteriosus, Coma,
Small Hands with Clinodactyly of Fifth Fingers*

The first description of an individual with XXXXX was by Kesaree and Wooley[1] in 1963. Subsequently only one other case has been reported.[2]

ABNORMALITIES. Findings common to both patients:

Severe mental deficiency.

Growth deficiency, especially postnatally.

Mild upward slant (mongoloid) to palpebral fissures.

Small hands with mild clinodactyly of fifth fingers.

Patent ductus arteriosus.

ANOMALIES FOUND IN ONE OF THE TWO CASES. Colobomata of iris, hypertelorism, inner canthal folds, low set ears, short neck, simian creases, equinovarus, overlapping toes.

NATURAL HISTORY. One patient was prematurely born. Both failed to thrive; one had frequent vomiting and the other had frequent respiratory infections.

COMMENT AND ETIOLOGY. Of interest is the occurrence in these XXXXX individuals of many of the nonspecific anomalies found in Down's syndrome, a diagnosis which was initially considered in both patients. However, the total pattern of malformation in each case differs from the usual pattern of Down's syndrome. The finding of as many as four sex chromatin bodies in interphase nuclei in conjunction with three extra C group chromosomes in metaphase preparations establishes the presence of 5 X chromosomes.

The maternal ages at birth of the two patients were 42 years and 22 years respectively.

REFERENCES

1. Kesaree, N., and Wooley, P. V.: A phenotypic female with 49 chromosomes, presumably XXXXX. A case report. J. Pediat., *63*:1099, 1963.

2. Brody, J., Fitzgerald, M. G., and Spiers, A. S.: A female child with five X chromosomes. J. Pediat., *70*:105, 1967.

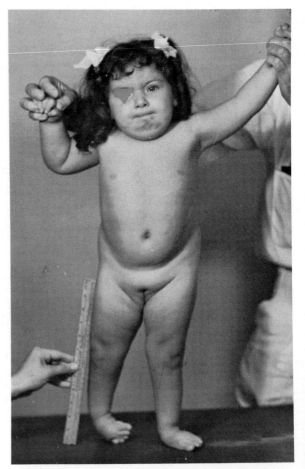

Two and one third year old with height age of 18 months and a performance level of about one year. A patent ductus arteriosus had been repaired. The hands were small with incurved fifth fingers, and the ears were slightly low in placement. (From Brody, J., et al.: J. Pediat., *70*:105, 1967.)

11. XO SYNDROME

(Turner's Syndrome)

*Short Female, Broad Chest with Wide Spacing of Nipples,
Congenital Lymphedema or Its Residua*

An association between small stature and defective ovarian development had been noted as early as 1922 by Rossle,[1] who classified the disorder under "sexagen dwarfism." A more expanded syndrome of small stature, sexual infantilism, webbed neck, and cubitus valgus in seven females was described by Turner[2] in 1938. The discovery of the chromosomal basis for the syndrome led to a more concise and expanded appreciation of the clinical phenotype of the XO syndrome, generally called Turner's syndrome.

Chromosomal studies of spontaneous abortuses have clearly shown that the majority of XO individuals die in the first few prenatal months. The precise reason for this early mortality has not been elucidated. At birth the incidence of sex chromatin negative females, presumably XO individuals, is 0.4 of 1000 females, or about 1 : 5000 newborns. Obviously this does not include many of the XO/XX mosaics or individuals with only a partial deletion of one X, who might be sex chromatin positive.

ABNORMALITIES. The following list of abnormalities, with the approximate precentage for each anomaly, includes those of the full monosomic XO syndrome. Patients with only a part of the cells XO (XX/XO mosaics, XY/XO mosaics with varying degrees of male type genitalia), or in whom only a part of one X is missing (X-isochromosome X or X-deleted X), generally have a lesser degree of malformation and seldom have such features as congenital lymphedema, web neck, or coarctation of the aorta. The most consistent features for the entire group are small stature and gonadal dysgenesis. Because the latter feature is not evident during childhood, a chromosomal study is indicated in any girl with short stature of unknown cause whose clinical phenotype is not incompatible with the XO syndrome.

Growth. Small stature, often evident by birth (100 per cent).

Gonad. Ovarian dysgenesis with hypoplasia to absence of germinal elements (90+ per cent).

Lymph Vessels. Transient congenital lymphedema with residual puffiness over the dorsum of the fingers and toes (80+ per cent).

Thorax. Broad chest with widely spaced nipples which may be hypoplastic, inverted, or both (80+ per cent); often mild pectus excavatum.

Auricles. Anomalous auricles, most commonly prominent (80+ per cent).

Facies. Narrow maxilla (palate) (80+ per cent). Relatively small mandible (70+ per cent). Inner canthal folds (40+ per cent).

Neck. Low posterior hairline, appearance of short neck (80+ per cent). Webbed posterior neck (50 per cent).

Extremities. Cubitus valgus or other anomaly of elbow (70+ per cent). Knee anomalies such as medial tibial exostosis (60+ per cent). Short fourth metacarpal, metatarsal, or both (50+ per cent).

Other Skeletal. Bone dysplasia with coarse trabecular pattern, most evident at metaphyseal ends of long bones (50+ per cent).

Nails. Narrow, hyperconvex and/or deep set nails (70+ per cent).

Skin. Excessive pigmented nevi (50+ per cent). Distal palmar axial triradii (20+ per cent). Loose skin, especially about the neck in infancy (? per cent).

Renal. Most commonly horseshoe kidney, double or cleft renal pelvis, and minor alterations (60+ per cent).

Cardiac. Cardiac defect (20+ per cent), of which 70 per cent are coarctation of aorta.

CNS. Perceptive hearing impairment (50+ per cent).

OCCASIONAL ABNORMALITIES

Skeletal. Abnormal angulation of radius to carpal bones, short mid-phalanx of fifth finger, short third to fifth metacarpals and/or metatarsals, scoliosis, kyphosis, spina bifida, vertebral fusion, cervical rib, abnormal sella turcica.

Eyes. Ptosis (16 per cent), strabismus, blue sclerae, cataract.

CNS. Mental retardation, about 10 per cent. Mean intelligence quotient about 95.

Other. Hemangiomata, rarely of the intestine. Idiopathic hypertension.

NATURAL HISTORY. The congenital lymphedema usually recedes in early infancy, leaving only puffiness over the dorsum of the fingers and toes, although rarely there may be recrudescence of the lymphedema with estrogen replacement therapy. At birth the skin tends to be loose,

(Text continued)

especially in the posterior neck where excess skin may persist as the pterygium colli. Small size is often evident at birth, the mean birth weight being 2900 gm. Linear growth proceeds at about half to three fourths the usual rate, there is usually no adolescent growth spurt, and final height of 50 to 60 inches with a mean of 55 inches is achieved at a usual age despite the roentgen evidence of "retarded osseous maturation." The relative stature of XO individuals is still influenced by the genetic background, the tallest sets of parents having the tallest XO children.

An occasional patient with the XO syndrome may show evidence of estrogen production at adolescence, although this is generally transient; one XO individual was fertile. Generally cyclic estrogen replacement therapy is indicated, beginning at the appropriate psychological time for each individual. At some time between eight years and adolescence they should be told that the ovaries are incompletely developed and they should plan on adopting children and taking "the same kind of medicine the ovary makes" at adolescence.

The actual incidence of early mortality due to congenital heart defect is unknown because there is no large series of cases diagnosed from birth. The types of renal anomalies that occur generally pose no problem to health, which is generally good. Enhancement of physical appearance by plastic surgery for prominent inner canthal folds, protruding auricles, and especially for web neck should be given serious consideration prior to school age. The major psychological problem is usually the adaptation to shortness of stature, for which there is no effective treatment at present.

At the present time we do not have adequate information on longevity and cause of death beyond the age of childhood for individuals with the XO syndrome.

ETIOLOGY. Faulty chromosomal distribution leading to XO individual with 45 chromosomes. The paternal sex chromosome is more likely the one to be missing, as indicated by studies for X-linked gene expressions in the XO individuals and their parents. There has been no significant older maternal age factor for this aneuploidy syndrome. It is generally a sporadic event in a family, although there are as yet no adequate data on risk for recurrence.

REFERENCES

1. Rossle, R. I.: Wachstum und Altern. München, 1922.
2. Turner, H. H.: A syndrome of infantilism, congenital webbed neck, and cubitus valgus. Endocrinology, 23:566, 1938.
3. Lindsten, J.: The nature and origin of X chromosome aberrations in Turner's syndrome. Stockholm, Almquist and Wiksell, 1963.

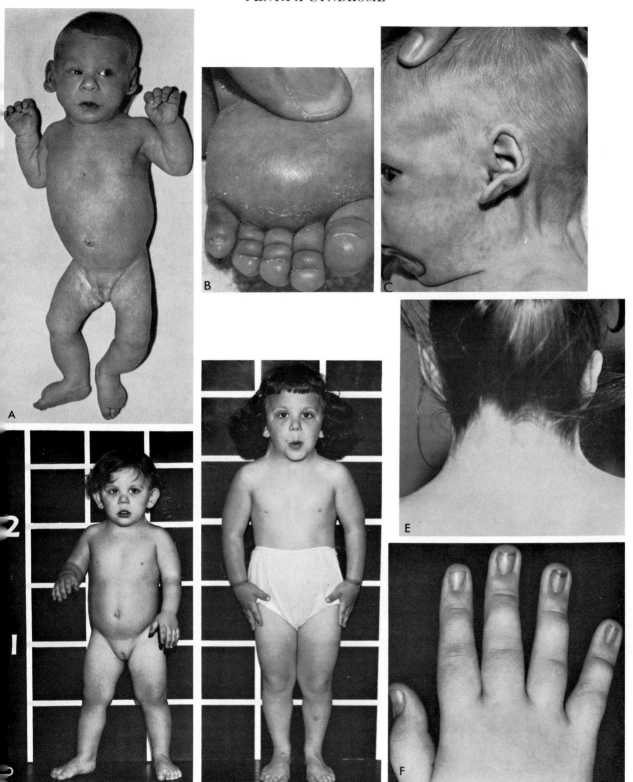

A to C, One month old. Note lymphedema, prominent ears, and loose folds of skin in posterior neck with low hair line.

D, Same girl at two years and at four years, with height ages of 17 months and three years respectively.

E, Low posterior hair line and residual lateral neck web.

F. Narrow, hyperconvex, deep-set fingernails; residual puffiness.

(A to C, E, and F from Lemli, L., and Smith, D. W.: J. Pediat., 63:577, 1963.)

12. TURNER-LIKE SYNDROME

(Male Turner's Syndrome Without Chromosome Abnormality, Noonan's Syndrome)

Webbing of the Neck, Pectus Excavatum, Cryptorchidism, Pulmonic Stenosis

Kobilinsky[1] reported in 1883 a 20 year old male with webbing of the neck, incomplete folding of the ears, and low posterior hairline, but no mention was made of other physical findings. The first complete description appears to be that of Weissenberg[2] in 1928. Several reports during the recent years have raised the number of published cases to about 80.

ABNORMALITIES

Growth. Short stature	86%
Performance. Mental retardation	43%
Facies. Epicanthic folds	30%
Low set and/or abnormal auricles	30%
Neck. Low posterior hairline	40%
Web neck	74%
Thorax. Shield chest	36%
Pectus excavatum	50%
Other Skeletal. Cubitus valgus	51%
Abnormalities of vertebral column*	41%
Heart. Congenital heart disease	
(pulmonic stenosis, septal defects)	48%
Genitalia. Small penis	40%
Cryptorchidism	63%
Small testes, without cryptorchidism	25%

OCCASIONAL ABNORMALITIES. Ptosis of the eyelids, hypertelorism; nerve deafness; high arched palate; hypoplastic nipples; edema of the dorsum of the hands and feet; simian creases; unusual woolly-like consistency of the hair.

NATURAL HISTORY. The natural history of this condition has not been adequately delineated. There is no apparent propensity to any special type of illness. The degree of mental retardation is seldom severe, and the social performance is usually better than anticipated from the intelligence quotient.

The reported findings from testicular biopsies are difficult to interpret in terms of

*Abnormal curvature or abnormal vertebrae (e.g., spina bifida occulta, hemivertebrae).

function because most have been performed in prepubertal or undescended testes.

ETIOLOGY. Unknown. Usually a sporadic occurrence within families. Nora[5] has observed this pattern of malformation in three families with a vertical mode of dominant inheritance, and Migeon[6] has reported a similar syndrome in siblings whose parents were normal. Perhaps closer scrutiny will reveal several clinical entities within the rather loose designation, Turner-like syndrome.

The most likely condition to be confused with this syndrome is the XO/XY mosaicism. The incomplete development of the penis, which many XO/XY individuals have, is helpful in the differential diagnosis.

COMMENT. General differences between this syndrome and the XO Turner's syndrome are clinically evident. Patients with the Turner-like syndrome are more likely to have mental retardation, a serious degree of pectus excavatum, and congenital heart disease is not only a more common feature but is also of different type than in the XO syndrome.

REFERENCES

1. Kobilinsky, O.: Ueber eine flughautahnliche Ausbreitung am Halse. Arch. Anthrop., *14*:343, 1883.
2. Weissenberg, S.: Eine eigentumliche Hautfaltenbildung am Halse. Anthrop. Anz., *5*:141, 1928.
3. Heller, R. H.: The Turner phenotype in the male. J. Pediat., *66*:48, 1965.
4. Chaves-Cabballa, E., and Hayles, A. B.: Ullrich-Turner syndrome in the male: review of the literature and report of a case with lymphocytic (Hashimoto's) thyroiditis. Mayo Clin. Proc., *41*:843, 1966.
5. Nora, J.: Personal communication.
6. Migeon, B. R., and Whitehouse, D.: Familial occurrence of the somatic phenotype of Turner's syndrome. Johns Hopkins Med. J., *120*:78, 1967.

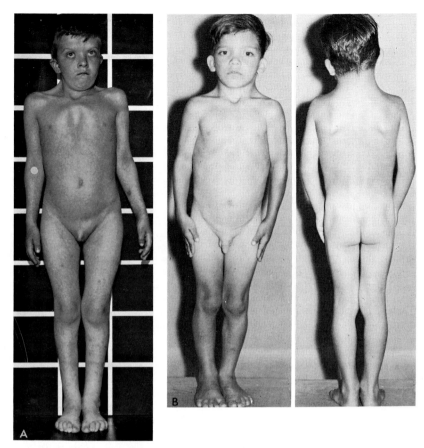

A, Twelve year old with height age of seven years. Mental deficiency but a very affable personality. Cardiac defect. Cryptorchidism. (From Smith, D. W.: J. Pediat., *70:*473, 1967.)

B, Nine year old; height age at ten and one half years was five and two thirds years. Cardiac defect. (From Ferrier, P. E.: Pediatrics, *40:*575, 1967.)

13. CORNELIA DE LANGE SYNDROME

Synophrys of Eyebrows, Thin Downturning Upper Lip, Micromelia

The syndrome was originally described in 1933 by Cornelia de Lange,[1] and although several reports appeared in the following years in the European literature, it was not until 1963 that it came into more general recognition. About 120 cases have been reported.

ABNORMALITIES

Growth. Shortness of stature of	
prenatal onset	100%
Retarded osseous maturation	50%
Performance. Mental retardation and	
sluggish physical activity	100%
Initial hypertonicity	100%
Low pitched weak cry	100%
Cranium. Microbrachycephaly	93%
Eyes. Bushy eyebrows and synophrys	99%
Long, curly eyelashes	100%
Nose. Small nose, anteverted nostrils	100%
Mouth. Characteristic lips and mouth*	100%
High arched palate	50%
Mandible. Micrognathia	97%
Spurs in the anterior angle of the	
mandible, prominent symphysis	66%
Skin. Hirsutism	97%
Cutis marmorata and perioral	
"cyanosis"	64%
Hypoplastic nipples and umbilicus	7/7
Hands and Arms. Micromelia	69%
Phocomelia and oligodactyly	30%
Clinodactyly of fifth fingers	69%
Simian crease	84%
Proximal implantation of thumbs	81%
Flexion contracture of elbows	84%
Feet. Micromelia	99%
Syndactyly of second and third toes	81%
Male Genitalia. Hypoplasia	4/17
Undescended testes	15/26

OCCASIONAL ANOMALIES. Myopia, astigmatism, optic atrophy, coloboma of the optic nerve, proptosis, choanal atresia, low set ears, cleft palate, congenital heart defect, hiatus hernia, duplication of gut, malrotation of colon, brachyesophagus, pyloric stenosis, inguinal hernia, small labia majora, radial hypoplasia, short first metacarpal and absent second to third interdigital triradius.

---

*Thin lips with small midline beak of the upper and corresponding notch in the lower lip; downward curving of the angle of the mouth.

NATURAL HISTORY AND MANAGEMENT. These patients show a marked retardation of growth, evident by the time of birth, and as a rule they fail to thrive. Their intellectual performance is usually severely limited. Episodes of aspiration in infancy, and increased susceptibility to infections appear to constitute the major hazard for survival in these patients. Although no adequate mortality statistics are available, it is apparently unusual for such patients to attain adulthood.

ETIOLOGY AND RECURRENCE RISK. Unknown.

The etiology is uncertain, but the fact that the syndrome is such a homogeneous one, and that the vast majority of the cases are sporadic, makes the hypothesis of its being determined by a single gene mutation very appealing. Because none of these patients have reproduced, this possibility cannot be substantiated.

Chromosomal aberrations of different types have been occasionally found in patients with the Cornelia de Lange syndrome, but they have not been consistent enough to be considered as its mode of determination. However, a small deletion, undetectable with our present laboratory techniques remains a possibility. Another possibility is etiologic heterogeneity, there being more than one mode of cause for this pattern of malformation.

COMMENT. The different functional abnormalities that have been reported in some patients, e.g., endocrine, hematologic, immunologic, represent another indication of the widespread effect of this condition in the patient.

REFERENCES

1. de Lange, C.: Sur un type nouveau de generation (typus Amstelodamensis). Arch. Med. Engant., *36*:713, 1933.
2. Jervis, G. A., and Stimson, C. W.: De Lange syndrome. J. Pediat., *63*:634, 1963.
3. Ptacek, L. J., Opitz, J. M., Smith, D. W., Gerritsen, T., and Waisman, H. A.: The Cornelia de Lange syndrome. J. Pediat., *63*:1000, 1963.
4. Vischer, D.: Typus degenerativus Amstelodamensis (Cornelia de Lange syndrome). Helv. Paediat. Acta, *20*:415, 1965.

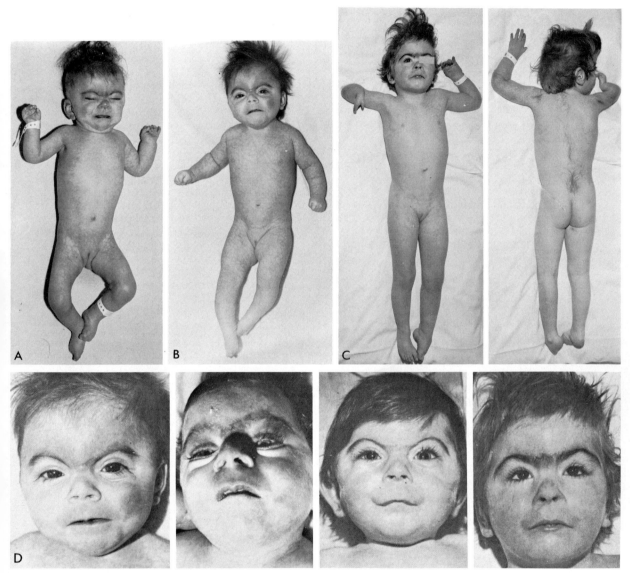

A, Neonate with small hands and feet.
B, Three month old with newborn length.
C, Five and one half year old with height age of two years and severe defect of right distal limb.
D, Similar facies of four affected individuals.
(From Ptacek, L. J., et al.: J. Pediat., *63*:1000, 1963.)

14. RUBINSTEIN-TAYBI SYNDROME

Broad Thumbs and Toes, Slanted Palpebral Fissures, Hypoplastic Maxilla

Rubinstein and Taybi set forth this clinical entity in 1963.[1] More than 24 cases have been reported,[2-4] and Rubinstein is aware of 112 cases.

ABNORMALITIES

Growth. Short stature	79%
Retarded osseous maturation	94%
Performance. I.Q. 17 to 86.	
EEG abnormality	60%
Cranium. Small	84%
Facies. Palpebral fissures slant downward	100%
Maxilla hypoplastic with narrow palate	100%
Beaked nose with nasal septum extending below alae	68%
Epicanthic folds	62%
Strabismus	79%
Refractive error	58%
Auricles low set and/or malformed	84%
Hands and Feet. Broad thumbs with radial angulation and broad toes	100%
Other fingers and toes broad	50%
Excess dermal ridge patterning in thenar and first interdigital areas of palm[5]	50%
Pelvis. Low acetabular angle, flare to ilia	?
Genitalia. Cryptorchidism	100%
Skin. Nevus flammeus	54%

OCCASIONAL ABNORMALITIES

Skeletal.   Prominent forehead, large anterior fontanel, large foramen magnum, parietal foramina, micrognathia, sternal anomalies, unfused arch of first cervical vertebra and other vertebral anomalies, scoliosis, syndactyly, polydactyly, clinodactyly of fifth finger.

Other.   Cataract, coloboma, ptosis of eyelid, long eyelashes and hypertrichosis, simian crease, distal axial triradius, cardiac anomaly, renal anomaly, angulated penis, kyphoscoliosis, seizures, absence of corpus callosum.

NATURAL HISTORY.   Respiratory infections and feeding difficulties are frequent problems in infancy. The degree of mental deficiency is variable, the most usual intelligence quotient being in the 40 to 50 range.

ETIOLOGY.   Unknown. All cases have been a sporadic occurrence in the family with the exception of two siblings reported by Johnson.[3]

REFERENCES

1. Rubinstein, J. H., and Taybi, H.: Broad thumbs and toes and facial abnormalities. A possible mental retardation syndrome. Am. J. Dis. Children, *105*:588, 1963.
2. Coffin, G. S.: Brachydactyly, peculiar facies and mental retardation. Am. J. Dis. Children, *108*: 351, 1964.
3. Johnson, C. F.: Broad thumbs and broad great toes with facial abnormalities and mental retardation. J. Pediat., *68*:942, 1966.
4. McArthur, R. G.: Rubinstein-Taybi Syndrome: a presentation of three cases. Canad. Med. Ass. J., *96*:462, 1967.
5. Giroux, J., and Miller, J. R.: Dermatoglyphics of the broad thumb and great toe syndrome. Am. J. Dis. Children, *113*:207, 1967.

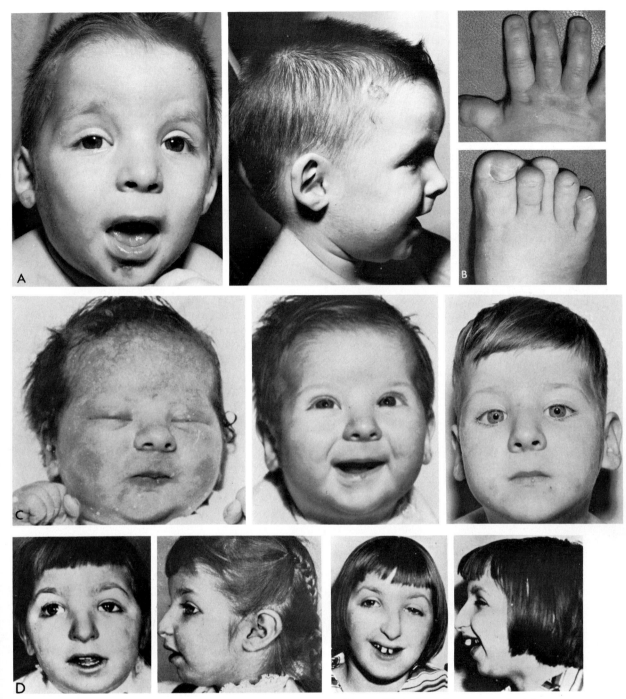

A, Three and one half year old. Height age of two years. IQ, 45. Slight downslant to palpebral fissures.
B, Hand and foot on patient shown in *A*.
C, Change in facies from birth to several years of age. Note broad thumb at birth.
D, Change in facies from three and one half to 14 years.
(*C* and *D* are gratefully acknowledged to J. Rubinstein, Cincinnati.)

15. SILVER'S SYNDROME

Short Stature of Prenatal Onset, Skeletal Asymmetry, Small Incurved Fifth Finger

This pattern of malformation was initially described by Silver[1] in 1959, and he later summarized the findings in 29 patients.[2]

ABNORMALITIES. Based on 29 cases.[2]
Growth and Skeletal. Small

stature, prenatal onset	93%
Immature osseous development	55%
Asymmetry, most commonly of extremities	78%
Short and/or incurved fifth finger	76%

Facies. Turned down corners of

mouth	62%
Triangular facies	52%

Skin. Café-au-lait spots — 45%

OCCASIONAL ABNORMALITIES. Altered pattern of sexual maturation in at least 34 per cent; syndactyly in 38 per cent; mental deficiency, dislocation of hips, dislocation of radius and ulna at the elbow, hypospadias.

NATURAL HISTORY. The patients generally have a consistently slow pace of growth. Because no adults have been reported, it is not possible to state final height attainment. The altered patterns of sexual development observed by Silver have been (1) early advent of gonadotropin, (2) sexual precocity out of accordance with level of osseous maturation, and (3) premature onset of only certain features of adolescence such as estrinization of vaginal mucosa.

ETIOLOGY. Unknown. All cases described to date have been sporadic, with the exception of one family known to Dr. Silver in which the mother of a patient is short of stature, has café-au-lait spots, and had precocious adolescence. The observation raised the question of whether this disorder is due to a single mutant gene with most cases representing fresh mutations.

REFERENCES

1. Silver, H. K.: Congenital asymmetry, short stature, and elevated urinary gonadotropin. A.M.A. J. Dis. Children, *97*:768, 1959.
2. Silver, H. K.: Asymmetry, short stature, and variations in sexual development. A syndrome of congenital malformations. Am. J. Dis. Children, *107*:495, 1964.

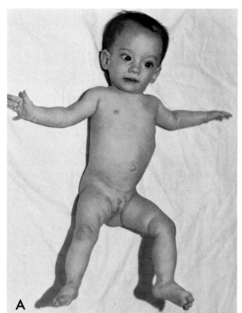
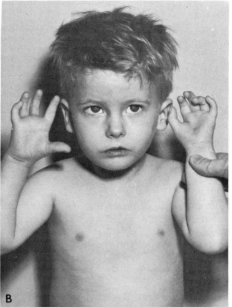
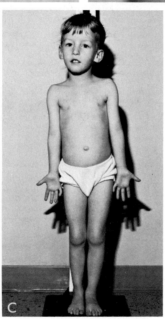

A, Six month old; height age, two months. Asymmetric leg length. (From Smith, D. W.: J. Pediat., *70*:483, 1967.)

B, Three and three fourths year old; height age, one and one half years. Note slight facial asymmetry.

C, Six year old with height age of two years. Note clinodactyly of fifth fingers. (Courtesy of J. Aase, University of Washington.)

16. BLOOM'S SYNDROME

Short Stature, Malar Hypoplasia, Telangiectatic Erythema of the Face

Since Bloom's original description in 1954,[1] about 20 cases of this disorder have been reported.

ABNORMALITIES. Prenatal onset of shortness of stature and facial telangiectatic erythema which involves the butterfly area and is exacerbated by exposure to sunlight. Dolichocephaly with malar hypoplasia with or without a small nose.

OCCASIONAL ABNORMALITIES. Telangiectatic erythema of the dorsa of the hands and forearms. Absence of upper lateral incisors. Prominent ears. Café-au-lait spots, ichthyotic skin, hypertrichosis, pilonidal cyst, sacral dimple. Syndactyly, polydactyly, clinodactyly of fifth finger, short lower extremity, club foot, Propensity to develop lymphoreticular malignancy.

NATURAL HISTORY. These patients show a consistently slow pace of growth. Feeding problems are frequent during infancy. The facial erythema is very seldom present at birth, usually appearing during infancy following exposure to sunlight; it may excoriate, but improves after childhood. These are pleasant children with normal intelligence.

Malignancy has been the major known cause of death. Three patients are known to have died of leukemia, and another is reported to have a solid malignant tumor, out of 23 cases studied.

Of interest is the in vitro tendency to chromosomal breakage and rearrangements found in cultured leukocytes and fibroblasts from all patients studied and, to a lesser extent, in some of their parents.

GENETICS. Autosomal recessive, with the majority of individuals being of Ukrainian Jewish ancestry. The excess of affected males to females is unexplained.

COMMENT. The relation of the in vitro chromosomal breakage and the development of malignancies is not well understood at present. The same type of chromosomal breakage has been observed in Fanconi's pancytopenia syndrome, in which there is also an increased frequency of leukemia among affected individuals and close relatives.

REFERENCES

1. Bloom, D.: Congenital telangiectatic erythema resembling lupus erythematosus in dwarfs. Am. J. Dis. Children, *88*:754, 1954.
2. Bloom, D.: The syndrome of congenital telangiectatic erythema and stunted growth. J. Pediat., *68*:103, 1966.
3. Sawitsky, A., Bloom, D., and German, J.: Chromosomal breakage and acute leukemia in congenital telangiectatic erythema and stunted growth. Ann. Int. Med., *65*:487, 1966.

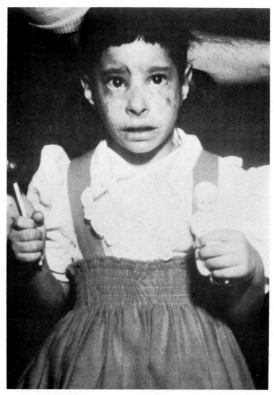

Four and one half year old. Height age, two and one half years. Died of leukemia at 13 and one half years. (Courtesy of D. Bloom, M.D.)

17. SECKEL'S SYNDROME

Severe Short Stature, Microcephaly, Prominent Nose

Reported by Mann and Russell[1] in 1959, this condition was extensively studied by Seckel in 1960.[2]

ABNORMALITIES

Growth. Prenatal onset of marked growth deficiency.

CNS. Mental deficiency.

Cranium. Microcephaly with premature synostosis.

Facies. Hypoplasia with prominent nose.

Auricle. Low set, malformed, or both; especially lack of lobule.

Upper Extremity. Clinodactyly of fifth finger, simian crease, absence of some phalangeal epiphyses, hypoplasia of proximal radius.

Lower Extremities. Dislocation of hip, hypoplasia of proximal fibula, gap between first and second toes.

Thorax. Only 11 ribs.

Genitalia. Cryptorchidism (male).

OCCASIONAL ABNORMALITIES.

Facial asymmetry, strabismus, partial anodontia, enamel hypoplasia, sparse hair, scoliosis, club foot, pes planus, hypoplastic external genitalia.

NATURAL HISTORY.

Gestational timing may be prolonged. Birth length, 13.5 to 17 inches; birth weight, 1 to 4.3 pounds. Final height, about 3 to 3½ feet. Moderate to severe mental deficiency, though early motor progress may be near normal. The cerebrum is small with a simple primitive convolutional pattern resembling that of a chimpanzee. Though they tend to be friendly and pleasant, these patients are often hyperkinetic and easily distracted. Poor joint development and support may be evident by dislocations of the hip, elbow, or both, and by later development of scoliosis, kyphosis, or both. Survival to an age of 75 years has been recorded.

ETIOLOGY. Probable autosomal recessive.

COMMENT.

This pair of mutant genes presumably retards the pace of mitosis, leading to congenital hypoplasia with a continued slow pace of growth.

REFERENCES

1. Mann, T. P., and Russell, A.: Study of a microcephalic midget of extreme type. Proc. Roy. Soc. Med., *52*:1024, 1959.
2. Seckel, H. P. G.: Bird-Headed Dwarfs. Springfield, Ill., Charles C Thomas, 1960, p. 241.
3. Harper, R. G., Orti, E., and Baker, R, K.: Bird-headed dwarfs (Seckel's syndrome). A familial pattern of developmental, dental, skeletal, genital, and central nervous system anomalies. J. Pediat., *70*:799, 1967.
4. McKusick, V. A., Mahloudji, M., Abbott, M. H., Lindenberg, R., and Kepan, D.: Seckel's bird-headed dwarfism. New England J. Med., *277*: 279, 1967.

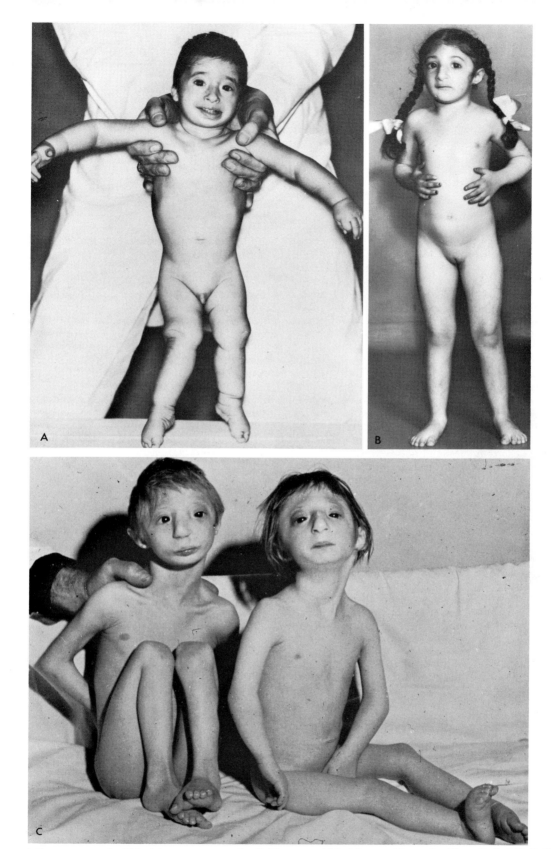

A, Fourteen month old; height age, two months. B, Five year old; height age, 19 months. (From Seckel, H. P. G.: Bird-Headed Dwarfs. Springfield, Ill., Charles C Thomas, 1960.)

C, Mentally deficient brother (six year old) and sister (three year old) with height ages of 11 months and four months respectively. (From Harper, R. G., et al.: J. Pediat., 70:799, 1967.)

18. HALLERMAN-STREIFF SYNDROME

(Oculomandibulodyscephaly with Hypotrichosis)

Microphthalmia, Small Pinched Nose, Hypotrichosis

The first report was by Audry,[1] who described an incomplete case in 1893. Hallerman, in 1948, and Streiff, in 1950, independently described three cases, recognizing this syndrome as a separate entity. In 1958 Francois[2] collected all the previously published cases and emphasized the cardinal features of the condition. About 50 cases have been reported in the literature.

ABNORMALITIES

Growth. Proportionate small stature.

Craniofacial. Brachycephaly with frontal and parietal bossing, thin calvarium, and delayed ossification of the sutures.

Malar hypoplasia; micrognathia, with hypoplasia of the rami and anterior displacement of the temporomandibular joint.

Bilateral microphthalmia; congenital cataracts, total or incomplete, which may resorb spontaneously.

Nose thin, small, and pointed, with hypoplasia of the cartilage, becoming parrot-like with age.

Microstomia, narrow and high arched palate.

Dentition: hypoplasia of the teeth and/or malimplantation, neonatal teeth and partial anodontia.

Atrophy of the skin, most prominent over the nose and sutural areas of the scalp; thin and light hair, with hypotrichosis, especially of the scalp, eyebrows, and eyelashes.

OCCASIONAL ABNORMALITIES.

Scaphocephaly, microcephaly, platybasia, shallow sella turcica, absence of the mandibular condyles, double cutaneous chin. Blue sclerae, nystagmus, strabismus, upward slant to palpebral fissures, optic disc coloboma, and various chorioretinal pigment alterations. Syndactyly, winging of the scapulae, lordosis, scoliosis, spina bifida, funnel chest. Mental retardation. Hypogenitalism, cryptorchidism in the male.

NATURAL HISTORY. Because the majority of the literature pertains to the ocular defect, there are insufficient data upon which to base the natural history in terms of the growth defect or mortality in infants. During early infancy, they may have feeding and respiratory problems, even necessitating tracheostomy. Respiratory infections may contribute to the cause of death. The peculiar physiognomy and shortness of stature may impair their psychological adjustment, though the major handicap is the ocular defect, which usually culminates in blindness despite surgery. The vast majority of the reported patients have been of normal intelligence, but motor and mental deficit have been noted in some.

ETIOLOGY. Until Guyard et al.[4] reported an apparently affected father and daughter, the etiology was undetermined. Now the most likely hypothesis is that of a single mutant gene (dominant), most cases representing fresh mutations.

REFERENCES

1. Audry, C.: Variete d'alopecie congenitale; alopecie suturale. Ann. Dermat. et Syph. (ser. 3), *4*:899, 1893.
2. Francois, J.: A new syndrome: dyscephalis with bird face and dental anomalies, nanism, hypotrichosis, cutaneous atrophy, microphthalmia and congenital cataract. Arch. Ophth., *60*:842, 1958.
3. Hoefnagel, D., and Bernirschke, K.: Dyscephalia mandibulo-oculo-facialis. (Hallerman-Streiff syndrome). Arch. Dis. Children, *40*:57, 1965.
4. Guyard, M., Perdriel, G., and Ceruti, F.: Sur deux cas de syndrome dyscéphalizue a tête d'oiseau. Bull. Soc. Ophth. France, *62*:443, 1962.

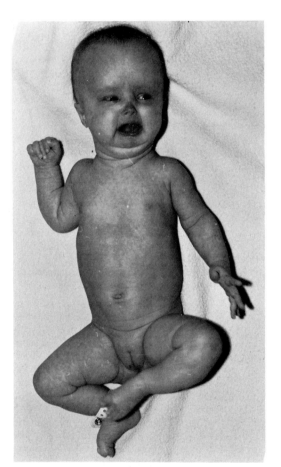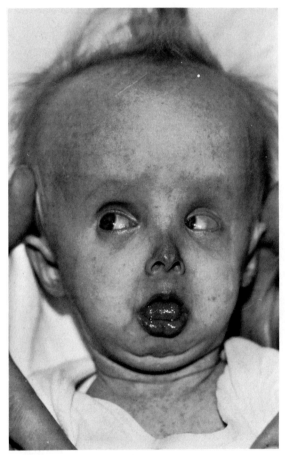

Left, Two and one half month old with height age of one month.
Right, Same patient at ten months showing changes in facies.
(From Smith, D. W.: J. Pediat., *70*:481, 1967.)

19. PROGERIA

(Hutchinson-Gilford Syndrome)

Alopecia, Atrophy of Subcutaneous Fat, Skeletal Hypoplasia and Dysplasia

The following entry was recorded in the *St. James Gazette* in 1754: "March 19, 1754 died in Glamorganshire of mere old age and a gradual decay of nature at seventeen years and two months, Hopkins Hopkins, the little Welshman, lately shown in London. He never weighed more than 17 pounds but for three years past no more than twelve. The parents have still 6 children left, all of whom in no way differ from other children except one girl of twelve years of age, who weighs 18 pounds and bears upon her all the marks of old age, and in all respects resembles her brother at that age." Whether or not this description was of progeria remains unknown.

In 1886 Hutchinson[1] described the "congenital absence of hair and mammary glands with atrophic condition of the skin and its appendages in a boy whose mother had been almost bald from alopecia areata from the age of six." Later Gilford[2] studied this boy and another patient with a remarkably similar phenotype and he termed the condition progeria, meaning premature aging. Since then, only about 40 cases have been recorded.

ABNORMALITIES. These include the development of the following conditions.

Alopecia. Onset birth to 18 months with degeneration of hair follicles.

Thin Skin. Onset early to midinfancy, also smooth tongue and thin intestinal epithelium have been noted.

Hypoplasia of Nails. Onset in infancy, nails may be brittle, curved, yellowish.

Loss of Subcutaneous Fat (Including Ear Lobule). Onset in infancy, last areas of adipose atrophy are cheeks and pubic area.

Periarticular Fibrosis. Onset at one to two years, stiff, or partially flexed prominent joints, or both; leads to "horse-riding" stance.

Skeletal Hypoplasia, Dysplasia, and Degeneration. Deficient growth, which becomes evident from six to 18 months; subsequent growth rate one-half to one-third normal rate or less; skeletal hypoplasia most obvious in facial hypoplasia with micrognathia, slim tubular bones and ribs with small thoracic cage, and thin calvarium with marked delay in ossification of fontanels; skeletal dysplasia evident in coxa valga and tendency toward ovoid vertebral bodies; skeletal degeneration evident in loss of bone in clavicle and distal phalanges.

Dentition. Delayed eruption with first deciduous tooth ten months to two and one-half years and marked delay in permanent dentition; crowding of teeth.

Atherosclerosis. As early as five years, onset of generalized atherosclerosis, especially evident in coronary arteries, aorta, and mesenteric arteries; at later age may have cardiac murmur, left ventricular hypertrophy.

Metabolic Alterations. Mild to moderate elevation of serum cholesterol.

OCCASIONAL ABNORMALITIES. Scleroderma, irregular brownish-yellow skin pigmentation, perceptive hearing deficit, congenital or acquired cataract, absent breast and nipples, relatively large thymus and lymphoid and reticular hyperplasia, elevated serum lipoproteins, aminoaciduria.

NATURAL HISTORY. Though the onset of disease manifestations is usually stated as one to two years, there may be subtle indicators of disease within the first year. The average birth weight for 17 cases was a relatively low 2.7 kg. One patient whose scalp was shaved at six weeks had no regrowth of hair; also delayed eruption of teeth is a common feature. The deficit of growth becomes severe after one year of age and eventual stature seldom exceeds that of a five year old. Because of the loss of fat, skeletal hypoplasia, and relative muscle hypoplasia, the weight is usually less than is expected for the height. The tendency to fatigue easily is a factor that might limit full participation in childhood activities. The life span is shortened by the early advent of relentless arterial atheromatosis and the usual cause of death is coronary occlusion. The life expectancy for 13 cases was seven to 27 years with an average of 14.2 years. Since intelligence and brain development do not appear to be impaired, children with progeria should be allowed as normal a social life as possible.

At the present time there is no effective therapy; however, the cosmetic use of a wig is recommended.

(Text continued)

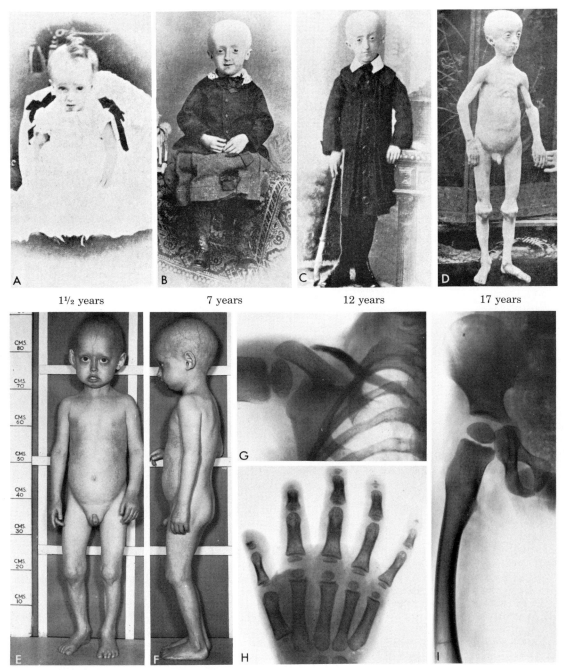

1½ years	7 years	12 years	17 years

A to *D*, Gilford's original patient. (From Gilford, H.: Practitioner, *73*:188, 1904.)

E to *I*, Three year old showing loss of outer clavicle, distal phalanges, and straight femur. (From Macleod, W.: Brit. J. Radiol., *39*:224, 1966.)

ETIOLOGY. The character of this disease and the striking similarity between affected patients is suggestive of a genetic mode of determination. The occurrence of this condition in two siblings of first cousin parentage is indicative of autosomal recessive inheritance;[4] however, the lack of other reports of sibship occurrence, except for Hopkins Hopkins (see historical introduction), or consanguinity leaves the question of transmission unresolved.

COMMENT. This condition might be classified as an abiotrophic disease since tissues that initially were fairly well developed have undergone hypoplastic, atrophic, or degenerative change, resulting in the multiple defects. The total clinical picture is different in many ways from the normal process of senile aging and the term progeria therefore seems inappropriate.

REFERENCES

1. Hutchinson, J.: Congenital absence of hair and mammary glands with atrophic condition of the skin and its appendages in a boy whose mother had been almost wholly bald from alopecia areata from the age of six. Trans. Med. Chir. Soc. Edinburgh, *69*:473, 1886.
2. Gilford, H.: Progeria: a form of senilism. Practitioner, *73*:188, 1904.
3. Rosenthal, I. M., Bronstein, I. P., Dallenbach, F. D., Pruzansky, S., and Rosenwald, A. K.: Progeria. Report of a case with cephalometric roentgenograms and abnormally high concentrations of lipoproteins in the serum. Pediatrics, *18*:565, 1956.
4. Gabr, M., Hashem, M., Fahmi, A., and Saforth, M.: Progeria. A pathologic study. J. Pediat., *57*:70, 1960.
5. Macleod, W.: Progeria. Brit. J. Radiol., *39*:224, 1966.

C. Senile-Like Appearance with Associated Defects

20. WERNER'S SYNDROME

Late Childhood to Early Adult Onset of Cataract, Thin Skin with Thick Fibrous Subcutaneous Tissue, Gray Sparse Hair

The subject of Werner's doctoral thesis in 1904,[1] this disease is usually not diagnosed until young adult life. More than 125 cases have been recorded.

ABNORMALITIES
Growth. Short stature; mean stature of affected males, 61 inches; females, 57.5 inches.
Deterioration. Loss of subcutaneous fat; slim spindly extremities with small hands and feet; pinched facies with beak nose.
Thick fibrous subcutaneous tissue with thin dermis.
Osteoporosis, atherosclerosis with calcification.
Muscle hypoplasia with patchy areas of fibrosis.
Gray sparse hair, premature balding.
Cataract, retinal degeneration.
Premature loss of teeth.
Hypogonadism, reduced fertility.
High pitched voice, fibrous thickening in submucosal tissues.
Liver atrophy.
Adult-type diabetes (44 per cent).

OCCASIONAL ABNORMALITIES. Propensity toward malignancy (10 per cent), especially sarcoma. Mild hyperthyroidism. Adrenal atrophy. Valvular sclerosis. Hyperkeratosis of palms and soles.

NATURAL HISTORY. Often noted to be slim with a slow rate of growth in latter childhood, these individuals have no adolescent growth spurt and reach their final height at ten to 18 years, usually around 13 years. Gray hair develops at around 20 years, and cataract about 25 years; and old age appearance is evident by 30 to 40 years, with the mean age of survival being 47 years. Calcification occurs not only in the atheromatous vessels but in the thick subcutaneous tissues as well.

ETIOLOGY. Autosomal recessive. Epstein et al.[2] noted a decreased rate of cell division plus a limited total number of mitotic divisions per cell in cultured fibroblasts from a patient with Werner's syndrome, thereby suggesting a basic defect in cell life capacity resulting in severe disease which resembles, but is not the same as, aging.

REFERENCES

1. Werner, O.: Über Katarakt in Verbindung mit Sklerodermie. (Doctoral dissertation, Kiel University.) Kiel, Schmidt and Klaunig, 1904.
2. Epstein, C. J., Martin, G. M., Schultz, A. L., and Motulsky, A. G.: Werner's syndrome. Medicine, *45*:177, 1966.

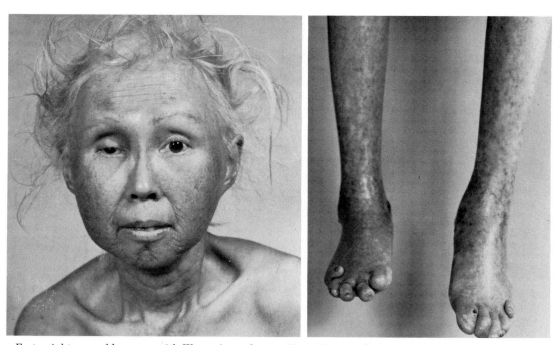

Forty-eight year old woman with Werner's syndrome. (From Epstein, C. J., et al.: Medicine, *45*:177, 1966.)

21. COCKAYNE'S SYNDROME

Senile-Like Changes Beginning in Infancy, Retinal Degeneration and Impaired Hearing, Photosensitivity of Thin Skin

Cockayne[1] reported this disorder in siblings in 1946. Subsequently more than 16 other cases have been documented.

ABNORMALITIES[1-5]

Growth.   Growth deficiency with loss of adipose by mid to late infancy.

Performance.   Mental deficiency with unsteady gait; sometimes tremor.

Moderate deafness.

Craniofacial.   Salt and pepper retinal pigmentation, optic atrophy.

Relatively small cranium with thick calvarium, loss of facial adipose with slender nose, moderately sunken eyes, and thin skin which is photosensitive. Carious teeth.

Extremities.   Cool hands and feet, sometimes cyanotic.

Mild to moderate joint limitation.

Trunk.   Relatively short, with biconvex flattening of vertebrae and tendency toward dorsal kyphosis.

Other.   Hepatomegaly. Ohno and Hirooka[5] discovered albuminuria with hyalinization of glomeruli, atrophy of tubules, and interstitial fibrosis in renal biopsies from three affected individuals.

OCCASIONAL ABNORMALITIES.   Intracranial calcification, small sella turcica, cataract, nystagmus, decreased sweating and tearing, some "marble" epiphyses in digits, asymmetrical fingers, short second toes, infolding of iliac crest, cryptorchidism. Graying of sparse hair.

NATURAL HISTORY.   Growth and development proceed at a more normal rate in early infancy, and it is not until two to four years of age that the pattern of defect is clearly evident. The personality and behavior tend to be similar to the normal for mental age, which is defective. Photosensitivity of skin may lead to problems on exposure to sunlight.

INHERITANCE.   Autosomal recessive.

REFERENCES

1. Cockayne, E. A.: Dwarfism with retinal atrophy and deafness. Arch. Dis. Childhood, *21*:52, 1946.
2. Neill, C. A., and Dingwall, M. M.: A syndrome resembling progeria: a review of two cases. Arch. Dis. Childhood, *25*:213, 1950.
3. MacDonald, W. B., Fitch, K. D., and Lewis, I. C.: Cockayne's syndrome. An heredo-familial disorder of growth and development. Pediatrics, *25*:997, 1960.
4. Spark, H.: Cachectic dwarfism resembling the Cockayne-Neill type. J. Pediat., *66*:41, 1965.
5. Ohno, T., and Hirooka, M.: Renal lesions in Cockayne's syndrome. Tohoku J. Exp. Med., *89*:151, 1966.

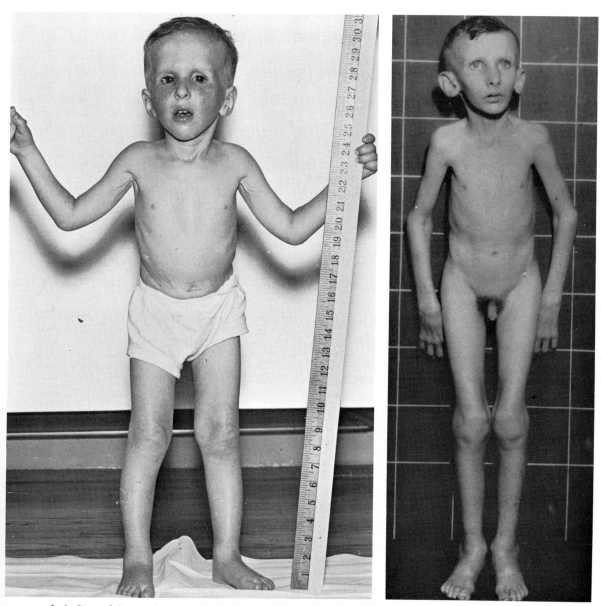

Left, Six and five sixths year old. Height age, 16 months. (From Windmiller, J.: Am. J. Dis. Children, *105*:204, 1963.)

Right, Fourteen and one half year old. Height age, three and one half years. Bone age, 16 years. (Courtesy of R. M. Blizzard. From Wilkins, L.: Diagnosis and Treatment of Endocrine Disorders in Childhood and Adolescence. 3rd ed. Springfield, Ill., Charles C Thomas, 1965.)

22. FAMILIAL DWARFISM AND STIFF JOINTS

(Moore-Federman Syndrome)
Short Stature of Childhood Onset, Stiff Joints, Hyperopia

Moore and Federman[1] described this pattern of altered connective tissue development in six individuals in three generations of one family in 1965. They recognized the similarity of their patients to those with Leri's syndrome of "familial pleonosteosis";[2] however, it is not presently possible to be certain whether they represent the same entity.

ABNORMALITIES. Based on six cases.[1]
Growth. Short stature, onset in childhood.
Joints. Limited motility at elbow, knee, wrist, and fingers, especially at thickened distal phalangeal joints.
Skin. Taut and somewhat thickened over joints.
Eye. Hyperopia (five).
Other. Asthma (four), hoarse voice (three), hepatomegaly (three).

NATURAL HISTORY. Apparently normal at birth; slow growth and joint stiffness noted by three to five years, with gradual progression and eventual inability to clench the hand completely. The span tends to be less than height; adult height varied from 54 to 57 inches. Other than slightly widened phalangeal metaphyses and diminished height of vertebrae, no alteration in bony form was noted. Glaucoma, cataract, and retinal detachment developed in one adult and may represent a serious threat to vision in later life. Asthma, especially in association with respiratory infections, was a frequent feature in later childhood (after five years).

ETIOLOGY. Autosomal dominant.

COMMENT. Studies for abnormal mucopolysaccharide or amino acid excretion have been negative in this disorder.

REFERENCES

1. Moore, W. T., and Federman, D. D.: Familial dwarfism and "stiff joints." Report of a kindred. Arch. Int. Med., *115*:398, 1965.
2. Leri, A.: Une maladie congénitale et héréditaire de l'ossification: la pléonostéose familiale. Presse Méd., *30*:13, 1922.

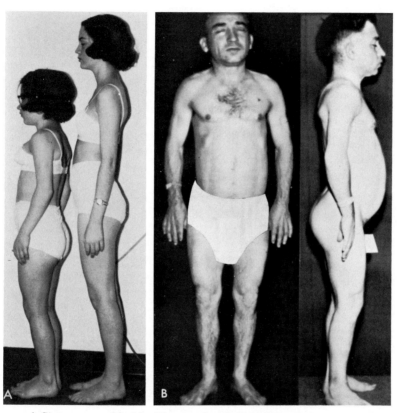

A, Sixteen year old girl with normal girl of similar age.

B, Father of affected girl in A, showing short stature and stiff joints. (From Moore, W. T., and Federman, D. D.: Arch. Int. Med., *115*:398, 1965.)

D. Joint Dysplasia with Associated Defects

23. LERI'S PLEONOSTEOSIS

Broad Thumb, Joint Limitation, Upward Slant to Palpebral Fissures

Leri[1] described this disease in 1922. Though many instances have been reported in the French literature, it has received little recognition in the English literature.

ABNORMALITIES[2, 3]

Joints and Fibrous Tissues. Postnatal onset of thickened joint contractures, especially hands.

Thick palms and soles.

Skeletal. Broad thumbs and great toes with short "spade-like" hand.

Posterior neural arches increased in height.

Large paranasal sinuses.

Facies. Mild upward slant to palpebral fissures.

NATURAL HISTORY. The joint limitations apparently begin in childhood and can progress into adult life.

ETIOLOGY. Autosomal dominant with full penetrance and varying expressivity.

REFERENCES

1. Leri, A.: Une maladie congénitale et héréditaire de l'ossification: la pléonostéose familiale. Presse Méd., *30*:13, 1922.
2. Rukavina, J. G., Falls, H. F., Holt, J. F., and Block, W. D.: Leri's pleonosteosis. A study of a family with a review of the literature. J. Bone Joint Surg., *41-A*:397, 1959.
3. McKusick, V.: Hereditable Disorders of Connective Tissue. 3rd ed. St. Louis, C. V. Mosby Co., 1966, p. 419.

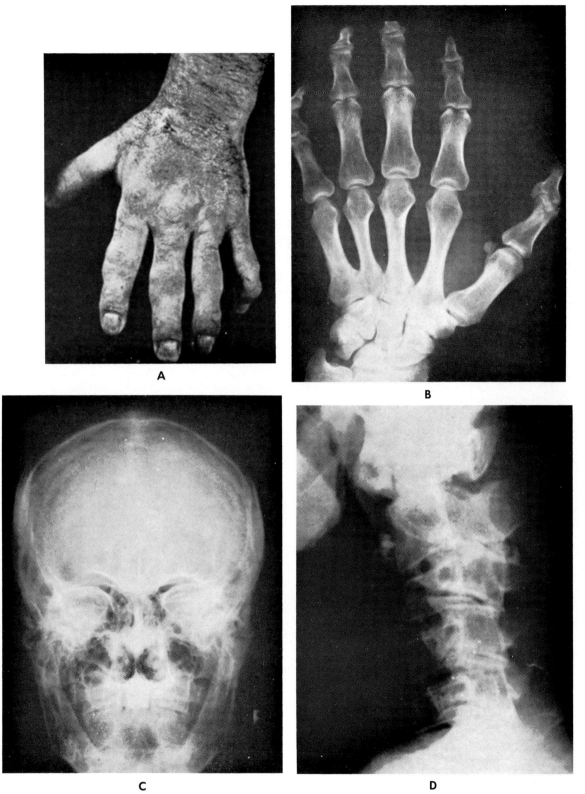

Forty year old male with Leri's pleonosteosis.
A, Multiple nodules on deformed fingers.
B, Short and relatively broad deformed metacarpals and phalanges.
C, Large paranasal sinuses.
D, Increased height of posterior neural arches of cervical vertebrae.
(From Rukavina, J. G., et al.: J. Bone Joint Surg., *41-A*:397, 1959.)

D. Joint Dysplasia with Associated Defects

24. STICKLER'S SYNDROME

(Progressive Arthro-Ophthalmopathy)
Joint Pain and Stiffness, Myopia, Deafness

Stickler et al.[1] reported the initial observations in 1965 on affected individuals in five generations of one family, and later published additional findings.[2]

ABNORMALITIES
Eye. Progressive myopia (8 to 18 diopters), frequently leading to retinal detachment during first decade. Secondary glaucoma and blindness may develop.

Ear. Sensorineural deafness.

Joints. Bony enlargement with irregular articular surface.

Pain and stiffness; may be swollen and red, may have crepitation.

Severe arthropathy by third to fourth decade.

Spine. Mildly flattened vertebral bodies with irregular epiphyseal surfaces and narrow intervertebral area.

Kyphosis and, less commonly, scoliosis.

OCCASIONAL ABNORMALITY. Subluxation of hip.

ETIOLOGY. Autosomal dominant, complete penetrance.

REFERENCES

1. Stickler, G. B., Belau, P. G., Farrell, F. J., Jones, J. D., Pugh, D. G., Steinberg, A. G., and Ward, L. E.: Hereditary progressive arthro-ophthalmopathy. Mayo Clin. Proc., *40*:433, 1965.
2. Stickler, G. B., and Pugh, D. G.: Hereditary progressive arthro-ophthalmopathy. II. Additional observations on vertebral abnormalities, a hearing defect, and a report of a similar case. Mayo Clin. Proc., *42*:495, 1967.

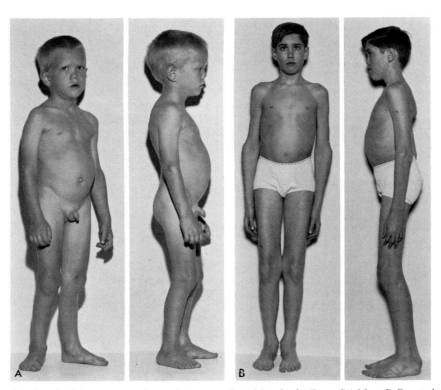

A and *B*, Child and adolescent, members of a large affected kindred. (From Stickler, G. B., et al., Mayo Clin. Proc., *40*:433, 1965.)

25. LAURENCE-MOON-BIEDL SYNDROME

Retinal Pigmentation, Obesity, Polydactyly

The variable manifestations of this syndrome were initially described by Laurence and Moon in 1865,[1] and the clinical phenotype was further delineated and popularized by Bardet and Biedl in the 1920's. Subsequently more than 300 cases have been reported.

PRINCIPAL ABNORMALITIES

Obesity	83%
Mental deficiency	80%
Polydactyly, syndactyly, or both	75%
Retinitis pigmentosa	68%
Genital hypoplasia, hypogonadism, or both	60%

OTHER DEFECTS. Renal defect (including a chronic glomerulonephritis type of lesion) and nerve deafness are features observed in this syndrome; however, their incidence is unknown. Occasional defects include nystagmus, strabismus, diabetes insipidus, clinodactyly of the fifth finger, cardiac defect, hypospadias, and anal atresia. Moderate shortness of stature may also be a feature.

NATURAL HISTORY. The natural history of this condition is poorly outlined in the literature. The mental deficiency is usually mild to moderate, and the retinal degeneration generally results in problems of night vision during childhood, even by three years of age. There may also be neurological evidence of spinocerebellar degeneration or cranial nerve palsy. Apparently the obesity does not become a problem until early childhood. Hypogonadism has been described as primary germinal hypoplasia and also as hypogonadotropic in type. It is important to appreciate that many of the patients undergo a spontaneous adolescent change.

ETIOLOGY. The finding of a high incidence (27 per cent) of parental consanguinity and the multiple sib involvement are indicative of autosomal recessive mode of inheritance. An occasional parent or collateral relative may show a partial expression, suggesting that the heterozygote may sometimes show abnormality.

COMMENT. The extent of abnormality may vary considerably between affected siblings, and it may be impossible to make the diagnosis of Laurence-Moon-Biedl syndrome in an isolated case demonstrating only a part of the syndrome, especially only mental retardation, obesity, and genital hypoplasia.

REFERENCES

1. Laurence, J. Z., and Moon, R. C.: Four cases of "retinitis pigmentosa," occurring in the same family, and accompanied by general imperfections of development. Ophth. Rev., *2*:32, 1865.
2. Bell, J.: The Laurence-Moon syndrome. Part 3 of Vol. 5, The Treasury of Human Inheritance, edited by L. S. Penrose, London, Cambridge University Press, 1958.
3. Blumel, J., and Kniker, W. T.: Laurence-Moon-Bardet-Biedl syndrome. Texas Reports Biol. Med., *17*:391, 1959.

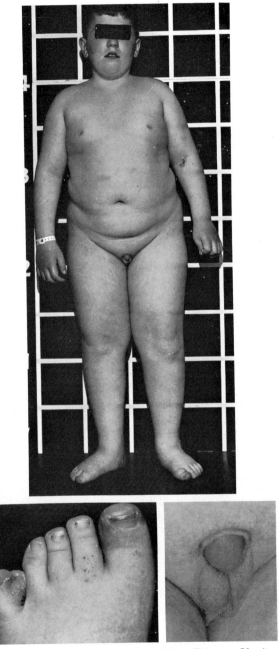

Ten year old male with retinal pigmentation and renal insufficiency. Obesity from birth. I.Q., 52.

26. PRADER-WILLI SYNDROME

Hypotonia, Obesity, Small Hands and Feet

Prader, Labhart, and Willi[1] reported this pattern of abnormality in nine children in 1956, and subsequently over 30 cases have been recorded.[2, 3]

ABNORMALITIES
Small Stature.   May be small at birth, occasionally normal stature until later childhood.
Obesity.   Onset from infancy to six years.
Mental Deficiency.   Intelligence quotient 20 to 80, most commonly 40 to 60.
Hypotonia.   Severe in early infancy.
Strabismus.
Small Hands and Feet.   One patient wore size 3 shoes at 23 years.
Small Penis and Cryptorchidism.   Frequent hypogonadism.
Dental Caries.   Frequent; may have enamel hypoplasia.
Diabetic Glucose Tolerance Response.   Frequent; may only be evident with hydrocortisone provocation.

OCCASIONAL ABNORMALITIES.   Microcephaly, clinodactyly, syndactyly, hypoplasia of auricular cartilage.

NATURAL HISTORY.   The mother may have noted feeble fetal activity. The hypotonia is most severe in early infancy when there may be respiratory and feeding problems, not uncommonly necessitating tube feeding. The degree of mental deficiency may appear to be greater in infancy than at a later age because of the severity of the hypotonia hindering developmental performance. Regarding behavior, these patients have been noted to be cheerful and good natured. Birth weight tends to be low, and failure to thrive is frequent in early infancy with obesity presenting as a later feature, especially over the lower abdomen, buttocks, and thighs.

The reason for a diabetic glucose tolerance response is unknown. The condition may progress to diabetes mellitus after the first ten years of life. Such patients differ from the usual childhood diabetes mellitus in that the diabetic state is not labile, there is no ketosis, and insulin is generally not required.

ETIOLOGY.   Unknown. All cases have been sporadic. If the Prader-Willi syndrome is always due to the same etiology, one possibility is a single mutant gene which represents a fresh mutation in each instance. Because affected individuals generally do not reproduce, this hypothesis will be difficult to substantiate. The present excess of reported males to females may be due to the ascertainment bias of the hypogenitalism in the male.

REFERENCES

1. Prader, A., Labhart, A., and Willi, H.: Ein Syndrom von Adipositas, Kleinwuchs, Kryptorchismus und Oligophrenie nach myatonieartigem Zustand im Neugeborenenalter. Schweiz. Med. Wschr., 86:1260, 1956.
2. Evans, P. R.: Hypogenital dystrophy with diabetic tendency. Guy's Hosp. Rep., 113:207, 1964.
3. Hooft, C., Delire, C., and Casneuf, J.: Le syndrome de Prader-Labhardt-Willi-Fanconi. Étude clinique, endocrinologique et cytogenetique. Acta Paediat. Belg., 20:27, 1966.
4. Laurance, B. M.: Hypotonia, mental retardation and cryptorchidism associated with dwarfism and diabetes in children. Arch. Dis. Childhood, 42: 126, 1967.

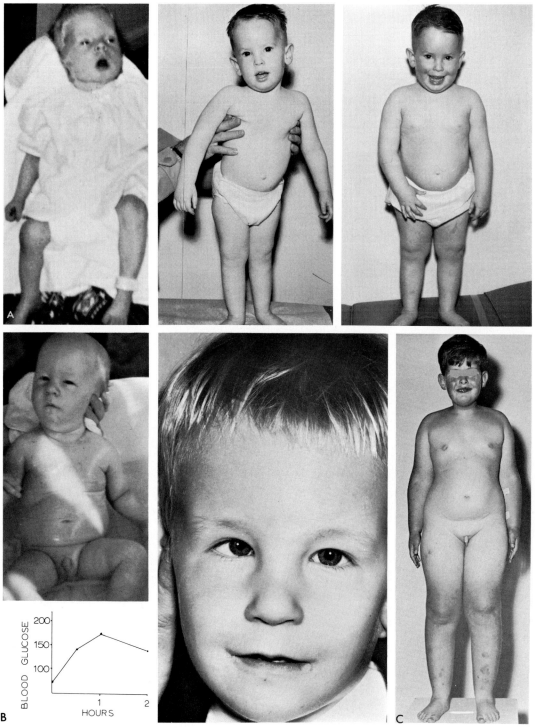

A, Same patient as neonate, at one and five sixths years, and at two and five sixths years (height age, two and one third years; developmental quotient, 60).

B, Same patient at five months and at four and one sixth years, at which time height age was three and one sixth years, developmental quotient was 50, and response to an oral glucose load was abnormal.

C, Nine and one half year old with height age of seven and one half years and mental age of five years.

(Courtesy of Prof. A. Prader, University Kinderspital, Zurich.)

27. LARSEN'S SYNDROME

Multiple Joint Dislocation, Flat Facies, Short Fingernails

Larsen, Schottstaedt, and Bost[1] described six sporadic cases of this condition in 1950, and the author has been unable to discover any subsequent reports.

ABNORMALITIES. Based on six cases.
Facies. Flat, with depressed nasal bridge and prominent forehead.
Joints. Dislocations of elbows, hips, and knees.
Hands. Spatulate thumbs, short nails, shortened metacarpals.
Feet. Equinovalgus or varus.

OCCASIONAL ABNORMALITIES. Cleft palate, abnormal segmentation of vertebrae.

NATURAL HISTORY. Inadequate information. Mentally normal.

ETIOLOGY. Unknown. All six cases sporadic.

REFERENCE

1. Larsen, L. J., Schottstaedt, E. R., and Bost, F. C.: Multiple congenital dislocations associated with characteristic facial abnormality. J. Pediat., *37*:574, 1950.

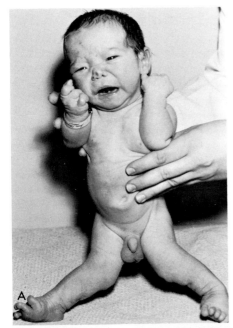

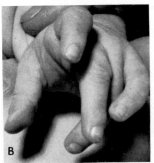

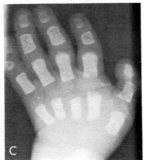

A to D, Two week old with dislocations of elbow, hip, and knee; altered hand positioning and short metacarpals; and flat facies.

E and F, Features from patients described by Larson et al.: J. Pediat., 37:574, 1950.

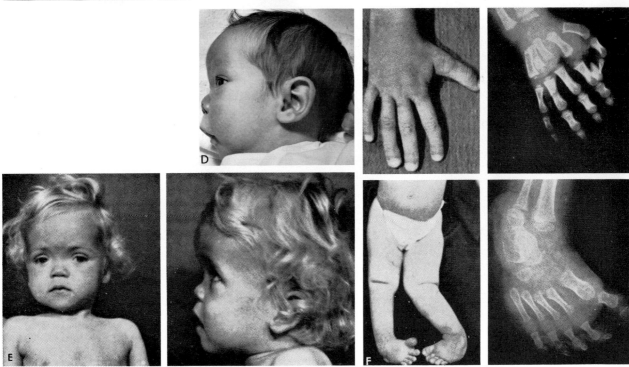

28. CEREBRO-HEPATO-RENAL SYNDROME

Hypotonia, High Forehead with Flat Facies, Hepatomegaly

Bowen et al.[1] and Smith et al.[2] independently reported siblings with this pattern of malformation in 1964 and 1965, and Passarge and McAdams[3] further delineated the syndrome in five siblings, bringing the number of reported cases to nine.

ABNORMALITIES

General. Growth deficiency; mean birth weight, 3300 gm. Hypotonia.

Craniofacial. High forehead with shallow supraorbital ridges and flat facies. Inner epicanthic folds. Mild upslanting of palpebral fissures.

Liver. Hepatomegaly with dysgenesis, including cirrhotic change.

Kidney. Albuminuria. Small cysts, chiefly of glomeruli.

Cardiac. Patent ductus arteriosus, with or without septal defect.

Brain. Macrogyria and polymicrogyria noted; also incomplete myelinization and sudanophilic leukodystrophy, mainly in astrocytes.

OCCASIONAL ABNORMALITIES.
Open metopic suture, early closure of sagittal suture, abnormal auricles, cataract, glaucoma, partial simian crease, camptodactyly of third and fourth fingers, cubitus valgus, equinovarus, inability to fully extend knee, deep sacral dimple, hypospadias, cryptorchidism, hypertrophied pylorus.

NATURAL HISTORY.
Most of these babies were born in the breech presentation. They failed to thrive. Four developed persisting icterus and four had bloody stools, possibly related to hypoprothrombinemia. All died from one day to six months after birth. It has not been possible to accurately determine whether mental deficiency is a feature, but judging from both early performance and autopsy findings serious mental deficiency would be likely.

ETIOLOGY.
Presumed autosomal recessive on the basis of occurrence in siblings of both sexes born to normal parents. No definite consanguinity in the three families.

COMMENT.
Several of these babies were mistakenly identified initially as having Down's syndrome. Chromosomal studies have been normal.

Opitz[4] has discovered evidence of excess iron storage in several babies with this syndrome.

REFERENCES

1. Bowen, P., Lee, C. S. N., Zellweger, H., and Lindenberg, R.: A familial syndrome of multiple congenital defects. Bull. Hopkins Hosp., *114*:402, 1964.
2. Smith, D. W., Opitz, J. M., and Inhorn, S. L.: A syndrome of multiple developmental defects including polycystic kidneys and intrahepatic biliary dysgenesis in two siblings. J. Pediat., *67*:617, 1965.
3. Passarge, E., and McAdams, A. J.: Cerebro-hepatorenal syndrome. J. Pediat., *71*:691, 1967.
4. Opitz, J.: Personal communication.

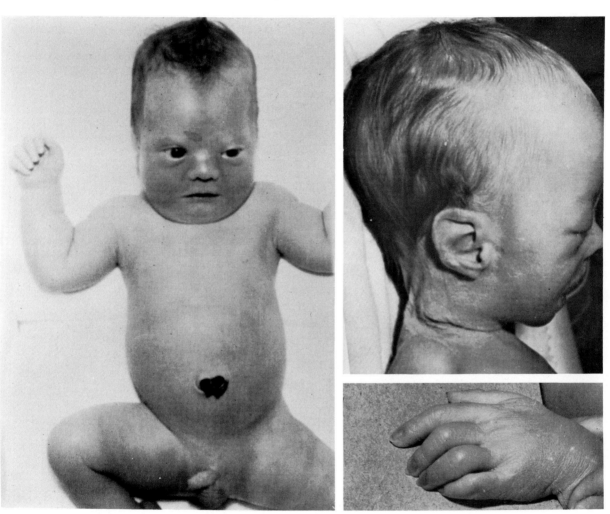

Affected siblings at one day of age (left) and post-mortem at ten weeks of age (right). Note camptodactyly of third, fourth and fifth fingers. (From Smith, D. W., et al.: J. Pediat., 67:617, 1965.)

29. OCULO-CEREBRO-RENAL SYNDROME OF LOWE

Hypotonia, Cataract, Renal Tubular Dysfunction

Lowe et al.[1] recognized this disease in 1952; subsequently more than 50 cases have been reported.

ABNORMALITIES

General. Hypotonia and joint hypermotility, with diminished to absent deep tendon reflexes and muscle hypoplasia with fatty infiltration.

Hyperactivity. Mental deficiency, moderate to severe with diffuse EEG abnormality. Postnatal growth deficiency.

Eye. Cortical cataract with or without glaucoma.

Renal and Bone. Renal tubular dysfunction with limited ammonium production and hyperchloremic acidosis, phosphaturia tending toward hypophosphatemia, and generalized aminoaciduria. Albuminuria. Moderate to severe osteoporosis and sometimes rickets. There is also organic aciduria of unknown cause.

Gonad. Cryptorchidism.

OCCASIONAL ABNORMALITIES. Seizures.
Pectus excavatum. Craniosynostosis. Dental cysts. Fracture.

NATURAL HISTORY. Failure to thrive. Both growth rate and bone mineralization may improve by administration of sodium-potassium citrate in adequate quantity to correct the acidosis. The prognosis for survival with such treatment is not known. However, the prognosis for brain function is poor.

ETIOLOGY. X-linked, with many of the heterozygote females showing fine lenticular opacities by slit lamp examination and occasionally a frank cataract.

REFERENCES

1. Lowe, C. U., Terrey, M., and MacLachland, E. A.: Organic-aciduria, decreased renal ammonia production, hydrophthalmos, and mental retardation. Am. J. Dis. Children, *83*:164, 1952.
2. Illig, R., Dumermuth, G., and Prader, A.: Das oculo-cerebro-renale Syndrom (Lowe). Helvet. Paediat. Acta, *18*:173, 1963.
3. Richards, W., Donnell, G. N., Wilson, W. A., Stowens, D., and Perry, T.: The oculo-cerebro-renal syndrome of Lowe. Am. J. Dis. Children, *109*:185, 1965.

30. RIEGER'S SYNDROME

Iris Dysplasia, Hypodontia, Myotonic Dystrophy

Rieger[1] described this association of anomalies in 1935. All the reported subsequent cases have been from Europe.

ABNORMALITIES[2,3]

Eye. Dysplasia of iris including hypoplasia, mesenchymal tissue filling in the angle of the anterior chamber, and aberrant synechiae of iris.

Teeth. Hypodontia, partial anodontia, or both.

Neurological. Myotonic dystrophy.

OCCASIONAL ABNORMALITIES.
Eye: glaucoma, microcornea, corneal opacity, ectopia lentis, aniridia, optic atrophy. Mental deficiency.

ETIOLOGY.
Autosomal dominant with rather wide variance in expression. Because of this variability it is difficult to know whether all cases described as Rieger's syndrome are the same eti-

ological entity. However, families such as one with affected individuals in five generations indicate that there is at least one specific disease entity.

COMMENT.
Iris dysplasia of the type noted by Rieger has been reported as a dominantly inherited anomaly without any other defect.[3]

REFERENCES

1. Rieger, H.: Beiträge zur Kenntnis seltener Missbildungen der Iris. Arch. Ophth., *133*:602, 1935.
2. Busch, G., Weiskopf, J., and Busch, K.-T.: Dysgenesis mesodermalis et ectodermalis Rieger oder Rieger'sche Krankheit. Klin. Monatsbl. Augenh., *136*:513, 1960.
3. Pearce, W. G., and Kerr, C. B.: Inherited variation in Rieger's malformation. Brit. J. Ophth., *49*:530, 1965.

31. STEINERT'S SYNDROME

(Myotonic Dystrophy)

Myotonia with Muscle Atrophy, Cataract, Hypogonadism

The text by Caughey and Myrianthopoulos[1] presents the manifold abnormalities that may occur as features of this single mutant gene. Many hundreds of cases have been documented.

ABNORMALITIES[1-4]

Muscle Degeneration. Myotonia (difficulty in relaxing a contracted muscle), often best appreciated in the hand or jaw. Degeneration of swollen muscle cells giving way to thin and atrophic muscle fibers.

Cataract. Cataract, often only evident as "myotonic dust" by slit lamp inspection.

Gonadal Insufficiency. Testicular atrophy (80 per cent) in males. Amenorrhea, dysmenorrhea, ovarian cyst in females.

Scalp. Premature frontal recession, especially in males.

Cardiac. Conduction defects with arrhythmias.

OCCASIONAL ABNORMALITIES. Hypotonia in infancy, mental deficiency, microcephaly, club foot, clinodactyly, hernia, kyphoscoliosis, hyperostotic cranial bones, atrophic thin skin, macular abnormality, blepharitis, keratitis sicca, goiter, thyroid adenomata, diabetes mellitus.

NATURAL HISTORY. The age of onset is stated as eight to 47 years, with an average of 27 years.[1] Initial signs of the disease are variable. Myotonia may be so mild as to be detected only when specifically tested for. Muscle wasting and weakness, occasionally asymmetrical, most often involve the facial and temporal muscles, yielding the expressionless "myopathic facies." Other involved muscles are the anterior cervical and those of the arms, thighs, and anterior lower leg, with progression from proximal to distal. Ptosis of the eyelids is frequent and pseudohypertrophy is an occasional feature. One of the most sensitive early indications of muscle dysfunction is the roentgen evidence of partial retention of radiopaque material in the pharynx after swallowing. Mental deterioration may also be a feature. There is increasing debility with death, usually by the fifth or sixth decade, as a consequence of pneumonia, cardiac failure, or intercurrent illness.

Pruzanski[3] and Calderon[4] both emphasize disease manifestations in pre-adolescent life. Some patients have been hypotonic and "floppy" with apparent mental defect during infancy.

ETIOLOGY. Autosomal dominant with wide variability in degree and extent of expression. One important question is whether the maternal environment of an affected pregnant woman may have an adverse effect on fetal development, especially of the central nervous system.

REFERENCES

1. Caughey, J. E., and Myrianthopoulos, N. C.: Dystrophia Myotonica and Related Disorders. Springfield, Ill., Charles C Thomas, 1963.
2. Pruzanski, W.: Myotonic dystrophy—a multisystem disease; report of 67 cases and a review of the literature. Psychiat. Neurol., *149*:302, 1965.
3. Pruzanski, W.: Variants of myotonic dystrophy in pre-adolescent life (the syndrome of myotonic dysembryoplasia). Brain, *89*:563, 1966.
4. Calderon, R.: Myotonic dystrophy: a neglected cause of mental retardation. J. Pediat., *68*:423, 1966.

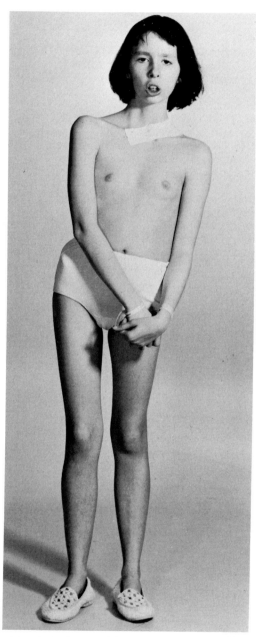

Fourteen year old with relatively immobile facies, scoliosis, and I.Q. performance of 58.

32. FREEMAN-SHELDON SYNDROME

Mask-Like "Whistling" Facies, Hypoplastic Alae Nasi, Club Feet

This disorder was described in two patients by Freeman and Sheldon[1] in 1938; the author was able to find only two other reported cases.[2, 3]

ABNORMALITIES. Based on four cases.[1–3]

Facies. Full forehead and mask-like facies with small mouth giving a "whistling" appearance.

Deep set eyes, broad nasal bridge, epicanthus, small nose, hypoplastic alae nasi, long philtrum.

H-shaped cutaneous dimpling on chin.

High palate, small tongue, limited palatal movement with nasal speech.

Extremities. Ulnar deviation of hands, thick skin over flexor surface of proximal phalanges.

Equinovarus with contracted toes.

OCCASIONAL ABNORMALITIES. Blepharophimosis, ptosis, strabismus, subcutaneous ridge across lower forehead, small stature, low birth weight, scoliosis.

NATURAL HISTORY. Vomiting and swallowing difficulty may lead to failure to thrive in infancy. Eventual intelligence is said to be in the normal range.

ETIOLOGY. Sporadic, with the exception of one of Freeman's original patients who has subsequently had a child with identical deformities,[4] indicating a dominant mode of inheritance.

REFERENCES

1. Freeman, E. A., and Sheldon, J. H.: Cranio-carpo-tarsal dystrophy. An undescribed congenital malformation. Arch. Dis. Childhood, *13*:277, 1938.
2. Otto, F. M. G.: Die "Cranio-carpo-tarsal Dystrophie" (Freeman-Sheldon). Ein kasuistischer Beitrag. Z. Kinderh., *73*:240, 1953.
3. Burian, F.: The "whistling face" characteristic in a compound cranio-facio-corporal syndrome. Brit. J. Plast. Surg., *16*:140, 1963.
4. Freeman, E. A.: Personal communication.

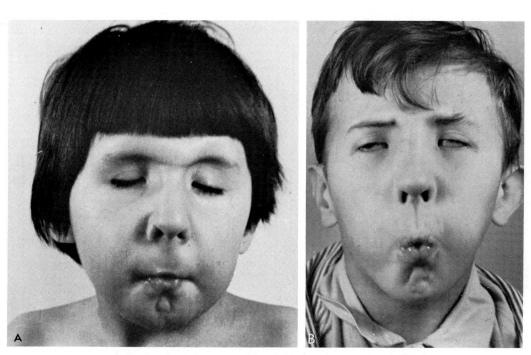

A, Five and one half year old girl. Note crease pattern in chin.
B, Older boy. Note the retraction of the alae nasi.
(From Burian, F.: Brit. J. Plast. Surg., *16*:140, 1963.)

33. SCHWARTZ'S SYNDROME

Myotonia, Blepharophimosis, Joint Limitation

Schwartz and Jampel[1] described a brother and sister with this condition in 1962, and later Aberfeld et al.[2] reported further observations on the same patients.

ABNORMALITIES. Based on two cases.
Growth. Small stature, one with prenatal onset.
Muscle. Myotonia with sad, fixed facies.
  Hypoplasia with atrophy and small muscle fibers.
Joint. Limitation in hips, wrist, fingers, toes, and spine.
  Equinovarus (one patient).
Osseous. Vertical shortness of vertebrae with short neck.
  Fragmentation and flattening of femoral epiphyses.
  Pectus carinatum.
Larynx. Small with high pitched voice.
Eye. Blepharophimosis, myopia.
  Long eyelashes in irregular rows.
Other. Low hairline, low set ears, small testicles.

NATURAL HISTORY. Onset of progressive myotonia, muscle wasting, and orthopedic problems during infancy with slow linear growth.

ETIOLOGY. Autosomal recessive considered the most likely mode of etiology.

COMMENT. This disease appears to be a specific disorder of connective tissue in which deterioration occurs during infancy and childhood.

REFERENCES

1. Schwartz, O., and Jampel, R. S.: Congenital blepharophimosis associated with a unique generalized myopathy. Arch. Ophth. *68*:52, 1962.
2. Aberfeld, D. C., Hinterbuchner, L. P., and Schneider, M.: Myotonia, dwarfism, diffuse bone disease and unusual ocular and facial abnormalities (a new syndrome). Brain, *88*:313, 1965.

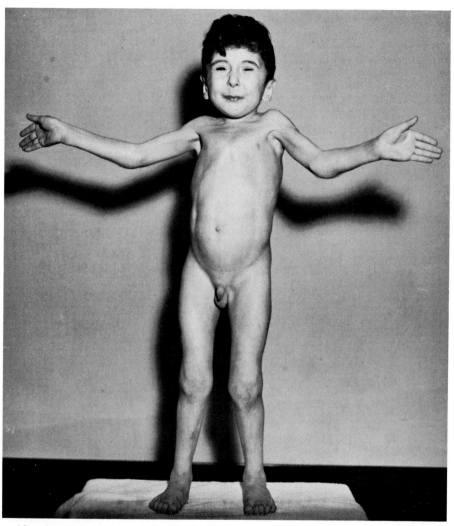

Six year old male with height age of three and one half years. A female sibling had the same disorder and the parents appeared normal. (From Schwartz, O., and Jampel, R. S.: Arch. Ophth., *68*:52, 1962.)

34. MARINESCO-SJÖGREN SYNDROME

Cerebellar Ataxia, Hypotonia, Cataracts

This condition was described by Marinesco et al.[1] in 1931 and further delineated by Sjögren[2] in 1947. Only about 50 cases have been reported.

ABNORMALITIES[1-4]

Growth.   Mild to moderate growth deficiency.

Performance.   Moderate to severe mental deficiency with cerebellar ataxia, weakness with or without hypotonia, and tendency toward nystagmus and dysarthria.

Eye.   Cataracts, usually evident from early life.

OCCASIONAL ABNORMALITIES.   Strabismus, development of kyphoscoliosis.

ETIOLOGY.   Autosomal recessive with high incidence of parental consanguinity.

COMMENT.   Todorov's pathological studies indicated a degenerative process, most severe in the cortical areas of the cerebellum.[4]

REFERENCES

1. Marinesco, G., Draganesco, S., and Vasiliu, D.: Nouvelle maladie familiale caracterisé par une cataracte congénitale et un arrêt du développement somato-neuro-psychique. Encephale, *26*:97, 1931.
2. Sjögren, T.: Hereditary congenital spinocerebellar ataxia combined with congenital cataract and oligophrenia. Acta Psychiat. Scand. Suppl., *46*: 286, 1947.
3. Andersen, B.: Marinesco-Sjögren syndrome: spinocerebellar ataxia, congenital cataract, somatic and mental retardation. Develop. Med. Child. Neurol., 7:249, 1965.
4. Todorov, A.: Le syndrome de Marinesco-Sjögren. Premiere etude anatomo-clinique. J. de Génét. Humaine, *14*:197, 1965.

35. BIEMOND'S SYNDROME

Short Third and Fourth Metacarpals, Ataxia

A syndrome of brachydactyly, with short fourth metacarpal and third metatarsal bones, associated with ataxia and nystagmus was reported by Biemond in 1934 as occurring in four generations of a family. Presumed autosomal dominant with lack of expression in at least two heterozygotes.

REFERENCE

1. Biemond, A.: Brachydactylie, nystagmus en cere-
   bellaire ataxie als familiair syndroom. Nederl.
   T. Geneesk., 78:1423, 1934.

36. ATAXIA-TELANGIECTASIA

(Louis-Bar Syndrome)

Ataxia, Telangiectasia, Lymphopenia and Immune Deficit

Though this disease was initially described by Louis-Bar in 1941, it has only recently received broader recognition, with well over 100 cases having been reported since 1958.

ABNORMALITIES
Growth.   Deficiency, variable in age of onset.
CNS.   Progressive ataxia and other evidence of degeneration of CNS function.
Skin and Conjunctiva.   Telangiectasia in bulbar conjunctiva and later over bridge of nose, auricles, elsewhere.
Respiratory.   Catarrh, frequent respiratory infections; bronchiectasis may develop.
Immune System.   Deficiency in cellular immunity .with thymic hypoplasia, hypoplasia of tonsil and adenoid lymphoid tissue, lymphopenia, and often low to absent gamma 1-A globulin in the serum.

OCCASIONAL FEATURES
Skin and Hair.   Areas of altered skin or hair pigmentation, including café-au-lait spots. Sclerodermatous changes.
Lymphoreticular System.   Malignancy, including leukemia, sarcoma, and Hodgkin's disease.
Gonad.   Sexual immaturity. Ovarian dysgerminoma or hypoplasia.

NATURAL HISTORY.   Growth deficiency, though it may be prenatal in onset, more commonly becomes evident in latter infancy or in childhood. Progressive ataxia usually develops during infancy and is usually accompanied by features of choreoathetosis, and by dysrhythmic speech, drooling, aberrant ocular movements such as fixation nystagmus, a stooped posture plus dull sad facies, and occasionally seizures. Instability, suggesting vestibular deficit, often becomes so severe that ambulation is no longer possible in later childhood. These children are usually affable and pleasant despite their progressive handicap. Mental deficiency, though difficult to assess, is considered a feature in about 50 per cent of cases, especially in later stages of this fatal disease. The immune deficiency probably contributes to the frequent respiratory infections and bronchiectasis; however, the persistent catarrh and the progressive generalized bronchiectasis are relatively unresponsive to antibiotic management, and there may be a basic problem in the mucous membranes besides the cellular immune deficit. Death is usually a consequence of lung infection, neurological deficit, or both. Affected patients seldom survive later childhood, and the oldest survivor was 30 years.

ETIOLOGY.   Autosomal recessive.

COMMENT.   The general hypoplasia of the whole individual and immune deficit with abiotrophic features of deterioration in the central nervous system, skin, and respiratory tract indicate the severe pleiotrophic effect of this pair of mutant genes. No common cellular metabolic defect has yet been detected; however, it is of interest to note certain common features between Fanconi's syndrome, Bloom's syndrome, and ataxia-telangiectasia. In each of these disorders there is generalized growth deficiency, skin disorder, and a propensity to develop lymphoreticular malignancy, plus a high frequency of chromosomal breakage in cultured leukocytes.[6]

REFERENCES

1. Louis-Bar, D.: Sur un syndrome progressif comprenant des télangiectasies capillaires cutanées et conjonctivales, à disposition naevoïde et des troubles cérébelleux. Confin. Neurol., *4*:32, 1941.
2. Boder, E., and Sedgwick, R. P.: Ataxia-telangiectasia. A familial syndrome of progressive cerebellar ataxia, oculocutaneous telangiectasia and frequent pulmonary infection. Pediatrics, *21*:526, 1958.
3. Tadjoedin, M. K., and Fraser, F. C.: Heredity of ataxia-telangiectasia (Louis-Bar Syndrome). Am. J. Dis. Children, *110*:64, 1965.
4. Eisen, A. H., Karpati, G., Laszlo, T., Andermann, F., Robb, J. P., and Bacal, H. L.: Immunologic deficiency in ataxia-telangiectasia. New England J. Med., *272*:18, 1965.
5. Karpati, G., Eisen, A. H., Andermann, F., Bacal, H. L., and Robb, J. P.: Ataxia-telangiectasia. Further observations and report of eight cases. Am. J. Dis. Children, *110*:51, 1965.
6. Hecht, F., Koler, R. D., Rigas, D. A., Dahnke, G. S., Case, M. P., and Tisdale, V.: Leukaemia and lymphocytes in ataxia-telangiectasia. Lancet, *2*: 1193, 1966.

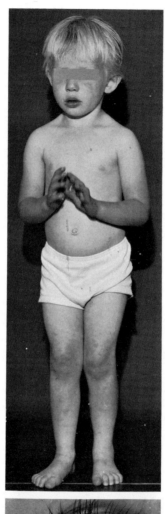

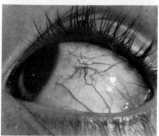

Nine and one half year old. Height age, eight years. (From Smith, D. W.: J. Pediat., *70*:487, 1967.)

37. SJÖGREN-LARSSON SYNDROME

Ichthyosis, Mental Deficiency, Spasticity

Sjögren and Larsson[1] reported this entity in 28 Swedish individuals in 1957, and others with the same condition have been recognized subsequently.[2, 3]

ABNORMALITIES

Central Nervous System. Mental retardation; I.Q., 30 to 60 or less.

Spasticity, most pronounced in lower extremities.

Skin. Ichthyosis (see natural history).

Growth. Short stature.

OCCASIONAL ABNORMALITIES.
Pigmentary retinal degeneration (30 per cent), seizures, diminished sweating except face and dorsum of hands, hypoplasia of teeth, enamel hypoplasia, hypertelorism, kyphosis.

NATURAL HISTORY.
Erythema of skin in early infancy with scaling and hyperkeratosis in most areas except face. Lichenification with exaggerated skin markings most evident in axillae and folds of neck. The mental defect usually includes speech problems of dysarthria, monosyllables, or no speech. The electroencephalogram may show slow paroxysmal activity.

ETIOLOGY.
Autosomal recessive. Sjögren and Larsson tentatively traced all the Swedish cases back to one heterozygote 600 years ago.

REFERENCES

1. Sjögren, T., and Larsson, T.: Oligophrenia in combination with congenital ichthyosis and spastic disorders. Acta Psychiat., 32:Suppl. 113:1, 1957.
2. Zaleski, W. A.: Congenital ichthyosis, mental retardation and spasticity (Sjögren-Larsson syndrome). Canad. Med. Ass. J., 86:951, 1962.
3. Selmanowitz, V. J., and Porter, M. J.: The Sjögren-Larsson syndrome. Am. J. Med., 42:412, 1967.

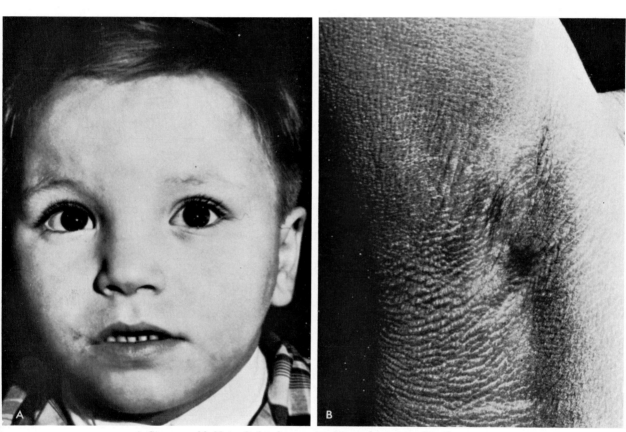

A, Six year old. Note slight changes in skin and spacing of teeth.
B, Fourteen year old, showing thickened, ridged skin in axillary area.
(From Selmanowitz, V. J., and Porter, M. J.: Am. J. Med., *42*:412, 1967.)

38. MENKES' SYNDROME

Progressive Cerebral Deterioration with Seizures, Twisted and Fractured Hair

Menkes et al.[1] described five related male infants with this disease in 1962. Subsequently, at least three other families with affected males have been reported.[2–4]

ABNORMALITIES

Growth. Deficiency, sometimes small at birth.

Central Nervous System. Severe degenerative process in cerebral cortex with gliosis and atrophy. Profound and progressive neurological deficit from one to two months with hypertonia, irritability, seizures, and feeding difficulties.

Hair. Sparse stubby white hair that, by magnified inspection, shows twisting and partial breaking.

Skin. Occasionally thick and relatively dry.

NATURAL HISTORY. Progressive deterioration beginning in early infancy with death in infancy or as late as three years. O'Brien and Sampson[4] have found decreased brain polyunsaturated glycerophosphatids, but the nature of the underlying metabolic defect is unknown.

ETIOLOGY. X-linked recessive.

REFERENCES

1. Menkes, J. H., Alter, M., Steigler, G. K., Weakley, D. R., and Sung, J. H.: A sex-linked recessive disorder with retardation of growth, peculiar hair, and focal cerebral and cerebellar degeneration. Pediatrics, 29:764, 1962.
2. Breg, P. F.: Sex-linked neurodegenerative diseases associated with monilethrix. Pediatrics, 36:417, 1965.
3. Aguilar, M. J., Chadwick, D. L., Okuyama, K., and Kamoshita, S.: Kinky hair disease. I. Clinical and pathological features. J. Neuropath. Exp. Neurol., 25:507, 1966.
4. O'Brien, J. S., and Sampson, E. L.: Kinky hair disease. II. Biochemical studies. J. Neuropath. Exp. Neurol., 25:523, 1966.

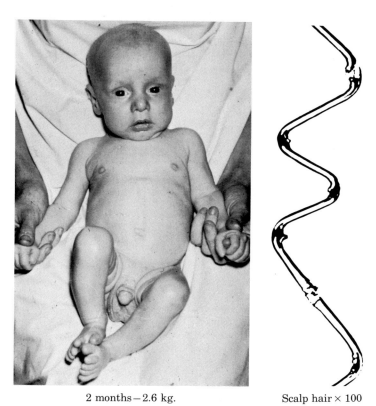

2 months — 2.6 kg.   Scalp hair × 100

(From Menkes, J. H., et al.: Pediatrics, *29*:764, 1962.)

39. TREACHER COLLINS SYNDROME

(Mandibulofacial Dysostosis, Franceschetti-Klein Syndrome)

Malar Hypoplasia with Downslanting Palpebral Fissures, Defect of Lower Lid, Malformation of External Ear

Although Thomson[1] reported the first case in 1846, the syndrome has been associated with Treacher Collins, who described two cases in 1900. Franceschetti, Zwahlen, and Klein made extensive reports on this condition and called it mandibulofacial dysostosis (1940's). More than 250 cases have been reported.

ABNORMALITIES

Antimongoloid slanting palpebral fissures	89%
Malar hypoplasia	81%
Mandibular hypoplasia	78%
Lower lid coloboma	69%
Partial to total absence of lower eyelashes	53%
Malformation of auricles	77%
External ear canal defect	36%
Conductive deafness	40%
Projection of scalp hair onto lateral cheek	26%

OCCASIONAL ABNORMALITIES. Coloboma of the upper lid. Microphthalmia. Macrostomia, microstomia, choanal atresia. Cleft palate. Blind fistulas and skin tags between auricle and angle of the mouth. Absence of the parotid gland. Congenital heart defect, cervical vertebral anomalies, malformation of the extremities, cryptorchidism. Mental deficiency has been reported in only 5 per cent of the cases.

NATURAL HISTORY. As the great majority of these patients are of normal intelligence, the early recognition of deafness and its correction with hearing aids or surgery, when possible, are of great importance for development.

The growth of the facial bones during infancy and childhood results in some cosmetic improvement which may be enhanced by plastic surgery.

ETIOLOGY. Autosomal dominant with 60 per cent of the cases representing presumed fresh mutations. Analysis of affected families shows a regular autosomal dominant inheritance with almost 100 per cent of penetrance. An excess of affected offspring from affected females and of normal offspring from affected males has been found. There is wide variability in expression but moderate similarity within a given sibship.

COMMENT. The wide variance in expression which allows for different clinical forms of the condition has led to erroneous interpretations of some cases, which have been described as separate entities. Franceschetti and Klein have emphasized this phenotypic variability.

REFERENCES

1. Thomson, A.: Notice of several cases of malformation of the external ear, together with experiments on the state of hearing in such persons. Month. J. Med. Sci., 7:420, 1846.
2. Treacher Collins, E.: Case with symmetrical congenital notches in the outer part of each lower lid and defective development of the malar bones. Trans. Ophth. Soc. U.K., 20:190, 1900.
3. Franceschetti, A., and Klein, D.: The mandibulofacial dysostosis, a new hereditary syndrome. Copenhagen, E. Munksgaard, 1949.
4. Rovin, S., Dachi, S. F., Borenstein, D. B., and Cotter, W. B.: Mandibulofacial dysostosis, a familial study of five generations. J. Pediat., 65:215, 1964.

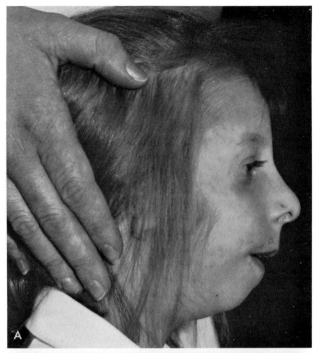

A, Six year old. Note the hair extending onto the lateral cheek.

B, Pre-adolescent girl. Note the defect of lower eyelid and the malar hypoplasia.

C, Same as *B*, post-adolescent. Note the improvement in mandible and plastic surgery to auricle.

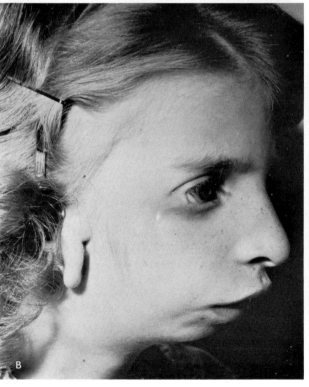

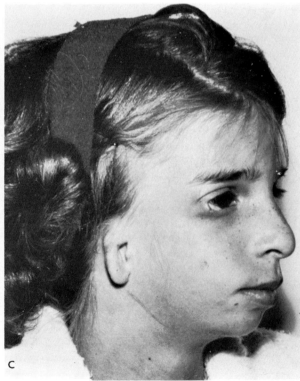

40. GOLDENHAR'S SYNDROME

(Oculo-Auriculo-Vertebral Syndrome)

Malformed External Ear, Epibulbar Lipodermoid and/or Dermoid, Malar Hypoplasia

Originally noted by Von Arlt[1] in 1845, this condition was set forth as a distinct entity by Goldenhar[2] in 1952. More than 40 cases have been reported.

ABNORMALITIES

Eye. Epibulbar conjunctival lipodermoid and/or dermoid.

Cleft of upper eyelid (60 per cent).

Ear. Incomplete external auricle, often with conductive deafness.

Pre-auricular cutaneous and cartilaginous appendages.

Face. Hypoplasia of zygomatic arches with lack of malar prominence and variable downward slant to palpebral fissures.

Mandibular hypoplasia (60 per cent).

Macrostomia (40 per cent).

Vertebral. Occipitalization of atlas.

Cervical and occasionally thoracic or lumbar defects, usually subclinical.

Other. Dental malocclusion.

OCCASIONAL ABNORMALITIES.

Mental deficiency (10 to 15 per cent), frontal bossing, ocular hypertelorism, microphthalmos, cleft of lower eyelid, hypoplasia or aplasia or colobomata of iris, cataract, hypoplasia, cleft and/or cutaneous appendages of external nares, fibrous band from corner of mouth to tragus area of auricle, bifid tongue, cleft lip with or without palate, narrow palate, aplasia of parts of mandible, low hairline, rib anomalies, umbilical and/or inguinal hernia.

NATURAL HISTORY. Conductive deafness is a major concern if both external auditory canals are incompletely developed, in which case hearing aids should be utilized from early infancy. Plastic surgery is usually indicated for the auricles, and occasionally an external canal can be created. Reconstructive surgery may be indicated in the zygomatic area, mandible, or both, after there has been an adequate opportunity to assess the degree of spontaneous improvement during early childhood. Dental care for crowding of teeth is usually necessary. All these measures are thoroughly indicated because these individuals usually have normal potential for intelligence and are healthy.

ETIOLOGY. Unknown. ? Autosomal recessive, but most reported cases have been a sporadic occurrence in the family.

REFERENCES

1. Von Arlt, F.: Klinische Darstellung der Krankheiten des Auges. Vol. 3, Wien, 1845, p. 376; cited by Van Duyse.
2. Goldenhar, M.: Associations malformatives de l'oeil et de l'oreille. J. de Génét. Humaine, 1:243, 1952.
3. Gorlin, R. J., and Pindborg, J. J.: Oculo-auriculo-vertebral dysplasia. In Syndromes of the Head and Neck. New York, McGraw-Hill Co., 1964, p. 419.
4. Dumars, K., and Charles, M. A.: Oculo-auriculo-vertebral dysplasia—Goldenhar's syndrome. Rocky Mountain Med. J., 65:44, 1968.

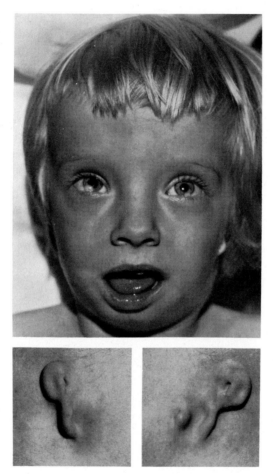

Two and one half year old. A laryngeal cyst was excised at four months of age. She has a 40 to 50 decibel hearing deficit by air conduction but normal reception by bone conduction. Note the epibulbar lipodermoids.

41. FAMILIAL BLEPHAROPHIMOSIS

Inner Canthal Fold, Lateral Displacement of Inner Canthi, Ptosis

This entity, predominantly a dysplasia of the eyelids, was apparently first described by Vignes[1] in 1889 and recently brought to medical attention again by Sacrez et al.[2] and Johnson.[3]

ABNORMALITIES

Eyes. Inverted inner canthal fold between upper and lower lid, short palpebral fissures with lateral displacement of inner canthi, low nasal bridge and ptosis of eyelids.

OTHER ABNORMALITIES.

Possible general hypotonia, strabismus, nystagmus.

NATURAL HISTORY.

Plastic surgery is indicated both for cosmetic reasons and for improvement of ocular function.

ETIOLOGY.

Autosomal dominant, apparently with complete penetrance.

COMMENT.

The facial appearance may initially suggest a condition with associated mental retardation; however, the affected individuals are not generally mentally deficient. Sacrez et al.[2] reported I.Q.'s from 75 to 100, with a mean value of 86.

REFERENCES

1. Vignes: Epicanthus héréditaire. Rev. Gén. Ophth. (Paris), *8*:438, 1889.
2. Sacrez, R., Francfort, J., Juif, J. G., and de Grouchy, J.: Le blépharophimosis compliqué familial. Étude des membres de la famille Ble. Ann. Pediat., *10*:493, 1963.
3. Johnson, C. C.: Surgical repair of the syndrome of epicanthus inversus, blepharophimosis and ptosis. Arch. Ophth., *71*:510, 1964.

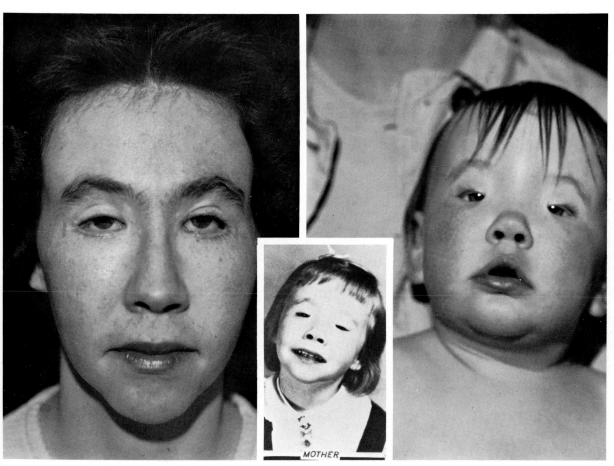

Mother and infant daughter, with insert of the mother as a child, prior to surgical repair.

42. LOWER LIP FISTULAS WITH OR WITHOUT CLEFT LIP, CLEFT PALATE, OR BOTH

Over 150 cases of mid or lower lip fistulas have been reported, and the association with clefts of lip and palate has been noted.[1, 2] The lower lip fistula tract leads to embedded mucous glands, sometimes with acini. They may be found as an isolated anomaly or, in some families, are inherited in a dominant fashion with variable expression for cleft lip, cleft palate, or both. Among such families Van der Woude[2] found that 57 per cent of those with lip fistula had cleft lip, cleft palate, or both. It is important to appreciate that commissural pits at the corners of the mouth are fairly common (0.2 per cent) and bear no such relationship with cleft lip and palate.

Surgical removal of the fistulas is recommended, because they may have a watery mucous discharge that can be embarrassing to the individual.

REFERENCES

1. Gorlin, R. J., and Pindborg, J. J.: Syndromes of the Head and Neck. New York, McGraw-Hill Book Co., 1963, p. 113.
2. Van der Woude, A.: Fistula labii inferioris congenita and its association with cleft lip and palate. Am. J. Human Genet., 6:244, 1954.

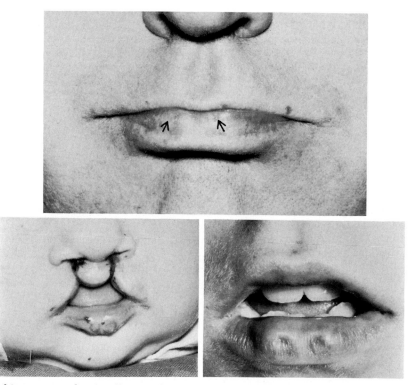

Father and his two sons showing lip pits (denoted by arrows for the father), with cleft lip expression in the infant son.

43. POPLITEAL WEB SYNDROME

Popliteal Web, Cleft Palate, Lower Lip Pits

This disorder was first reported by Trelat[1] in 1869; about 30 cases have been recorded.

ABNORMALITIES

Oral.   Cleft palate with or without cleft lip.
   Salivary lower lip pits.
Extremities.   Popliteal web, in extreme form from heel to ischium.
   Toenail dysplasia.

OCCASIONAL ABNORMALITIES.   Oral frenula, cutaneous webs between eyelids, inter-crural pterygium, syndactyly of fingers or toes, hypoplasia or aplasia of digits, fusion of distal interphalangeal joints, valgus deformity of feet, pyramidal form to skin over hallux, hypoplasia of tibia, bifid or absent patella, posterior dislocation of fibulae, low acetabular angle, spina bifida occulta, other vertebral anomalies, scoliosis, cryptorchidism, bifid scrotum, hypoplastic labia majora, ambiguous external genitalia, inguinal hernia, abnormal scalp hair, mental retardation (two cases).

NATURAL HISTORY.   There is usually a dense fibrous cord in the posterior portion of the popliteal pterygium, and extreme care must be exercised in the surgical repair because this cord may contain the tibial nerve. There may be associated defects of muscle in the lower extremities, with limitation of function despite repair of the pterygium. Other webbing across the eyelids or in the mouth may require excision. The palate tends to be short, such that, even with repair of the cleft, function is impaired. Intelligence is usually normal, these individuals are otherwise healthy, and cosmetic and orthopedic corrective procedures are merited.

ETIOLOGY.   Of 23 pedigrees there have been seven with more than one sibling affected, and in four instances a parent showed partial expression, usually cleft palate with or without cleft lip and lip pits. The question remains open as to whether this disease is autosomal recessive with partial expression in an occasional heterozygote, or whether it is a single gene autosomal dominant with wide variance in expression.

REFERENCES

1. Trelat, U.: Sur un vice conformation très-rare de la levre-inferiure. J. Med. Chir. Prat., *40*:442, 1869.
2. Wolff, J.: Ueber einen Fall von angeborener Flughautbildung. Arch. Klin. Chir., *38*:66, 1889.
3. Hecht, F., and Jarvinen, J. M.: Heritable dysmorphic syndrome with normal intelligence. J. Pediat., *70*:927, 1967.

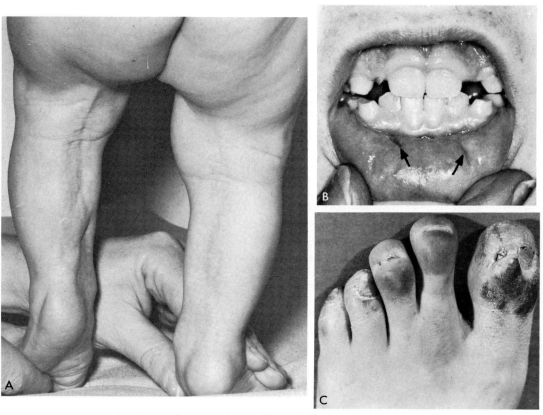

A, Infant with popliteal web. Note rod-like taut core.
B, Boy with lower lip pits (arrows).
C, Toenail dysplasia, a variable feature.
(From Hecht, F., and Jarvinen, J. M.: J. Pediat., *70:*927, 1967.)

44. ORAL-FACIAL-DIGITAL (OFD) SYNDROME

Oral Frenula and Clefts, Hypoplasia of Alae Nasi, Digital Asymmetry

Papillon-Leage and Psaume[1] set this condition forth as a clinical entity in 1954.

ABNORMALITIES

Oral. Webbing between buccal mucous membrane and alveolar ridge.

Partial clefts in mid-upper lip, tongue, alveolar ridges (at area of lateral incisors which may be missing), between premaxilla and lateral hard palate, with or without irregular complete cleft of soft palate.

Facial. Hypoplasia of alar cartilages, short philtrum, lateral placement of inner canthi.

Digital. Asymmetrical shortening of digits with clinodactyly with or without syndactyly.

Scalp. Dry rough hair and dry scalp.

CNS. Variable; mental deficiency with average intelligence quotient of 70.

Cranium. Increased naso-sella-basion angle at base of cranium.

OCCASIONAL ABNORMALITIES

Oral. Enamel hypoplasia, supernumerary teeth, hamartoma of tongue, fistula in lower lip.

Facial. Frontal bossing, malar hypoplasia.

Digital. Polydactyly.

Skeletal. Nonprogressive metaphyseal rarefaction.

CNS. Trembling, hydrocephalus.

Hair. Alopecia.

Ear. Milia on skin of auricle during infancy.

NATURAL HISTORY. Management is directed toward plastic surgical correction of oral clefts and dental care, including dentures when indicated. Psychometric evaluation is merited, because about half the reported patients have mental deficiency.

ETIOLOGY. Dominant mutant gene with a lethal effect in the XY male. The ratio of female to male offspring of affected women has been 2 : 1, and no affected woman has been known to have a son with the OFD syndrome. Therefore the risk for the OFD mother having an affected offspring is one in three. Present data do not allow for a distinction between an X-linked gene, lethal in the hemizygote, and an autosomal mutant which is an early lethal in the male.

REFERENCES

1. Papillon-Léage, Mme., and Psaume, J.: Une malformation héréditaire de la muqueuse buccale: brides et freins anormaux. Rev. Stomatol., *55*: 209, 1954.
2. Gorlin, R. J., and Psaume, J.: Orodigitofacial dysostosis — a new syndrome. J. Pediat., *61*:520, 1962.
3. Gorlin, R. J., and Pindborg, J. J.: Syndromes of the Head and Neck. New York, McGraw-Hill Book Co., 1964, p. 438.
4. Doege, T. C., Thuline, H. C., Priest, J. H., Norby, D. E., and Bryant, J. S.: Studies of a family with the oral-facial-digital syndrome. New England J. Med., *271*:1073, 1964.

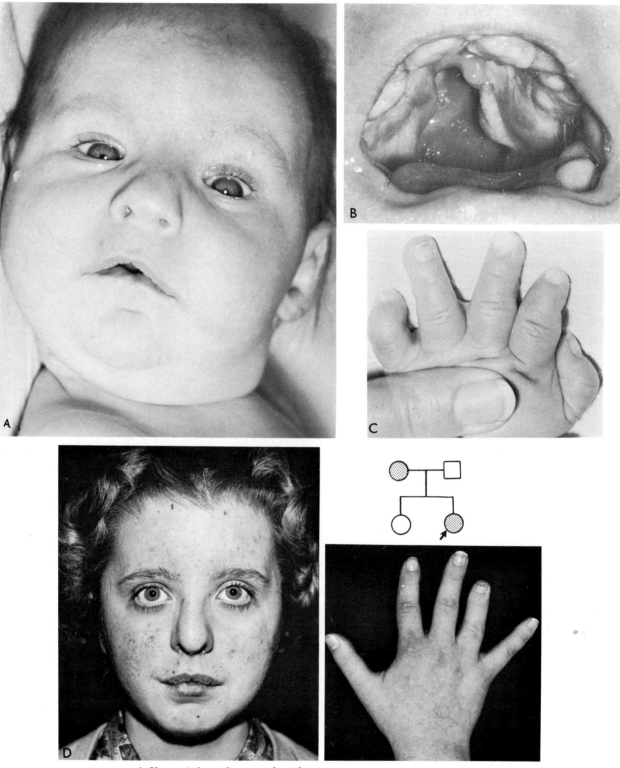

A, Young infant of a normal mother.
B, Irregular clefts in alveolar ridge, palate, and tongue.
C, Short third finger; partial syndactyly of third and fourth fingers.
D, Seventeen year old daughter of affected mother.

45. MOHR SYNDROME

Cleft Tongue, Conductive Deafness, Partial Reduplication of Hallux

Mohr[1] described this pattern in several male siblings in 1941, and recently Rimoin and Edgerton[2] reported an affected brother and sister.

ABNORMALITIES

General. Mild shortness of stature.

Conductive deafness due apparently to defect of incus.

Facies and Mouth. Low nasal bridge with lateral displacement of inner canthi.

Broad nasal tip, sometimes slightly bifid.

Midline partial cleft of lip.

Hypertrophy of usual frenula.

Midline cleft of tongue, nodules on tongue.

Flare to alveolar ridge.

Hypoplasia of zygomatic arch, maxilla, and body of mandible.

Extremities. Partial reduplication of hallux, first metatarsal, cuneiform, and cuboid.

Relatively short hands with clinodactyly of fifth finger.

Metaphyseal flaring and irregularity.

OCCASIONAL ABNORMALITIES. Wormian

cranial bones, missing central incisors, cleft palate, pectus excavatum, scoliosis.

NATURAL HISTORY. These patients apparently have normal intelligence, and plastic surgery is indicated for the clefts, frenula, and partial reduplication of the hallux. A surgical attempt to reconstruct the auditory ossicles was unsuccessful in one case.

ETIOLOGY. Presumed autosomal recessive.

COMMENT. This condition may easily be confused with the oral-facial-digital syndrome.

REFERENCES

1. Mohr, O. L.: A hereditary sublethal syndrome in man. Skr. Norske Vidensk. Akad., I. Mat. Naturv. Klasse, *14*:3, 1941.
2. Rimoin, D. L., and Edgerton, M. T.: Genetic and clinical heterogeneity in the oral-facial-digital syndromes. J. Pediat., *71*:94, 1967.

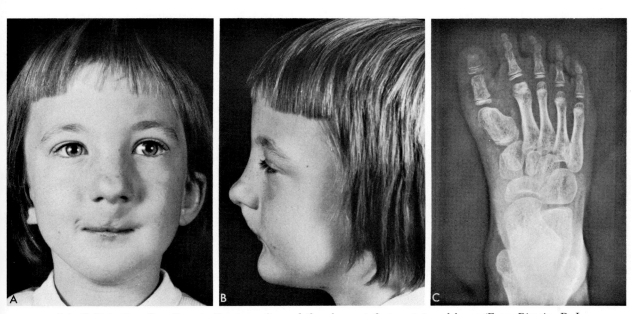

A to *C,* Note the alterations in the upper lip and the aberrant first metatarsal bone. (From Rimoin, D. L., and Edgerton, M. T.: J. Pediat., *71*:94, 1967.)

46. MIETENS' SYNDROME

Corneal Opacity, Narrow Nose, Flexion Contracture at Elbow

In 1966, Mietens and Weber[1] recorded this pattern of malformation in four of six siblings born of normal unrelated parents.

ABNORMALITIES

General.   Dull mentality, with intelligence quotients of 70 to 81.

Small stature (prenatal onset in at least one instance).

Facies.   Corneal opacity, horizontal and rotatory nystagmus and strabismus.

Narrow nose with hypoplasia of alae nasi.

Extremities.   Short forearms and dislocation of proximal radius with flexion contracture at elbow.

OCCASIONAL ABNORMALITIES.   Pes valgus, inability to fully extend knee, dislocation of hip, pectus excavatum, arterial aneurysm.

NATURAL HISTORY.   Because of the impaired vision plus the limitation of function of the arms, it is difficult to know whether the 70 to 80 intelligence quotients are a valid indicator of mental defect or not. Vascular anomalies may be a serious feature in this syndrome. The older girl (illustration) died from rupture of an aneurysm of the right anterior cerebral artery.[2]

ETIOLOGY.   Undetermined. ? Autosomal recessive.

REFERENCES

1. Mietens, C., and Weber, H.: A syndrome characterized by corneal opacity, nystagmus, flexion contracture of the elbows, growth failure, and mental retardation. J. Pediat., *69*:624, 1966.
2. Mietens, C.: Personal communication.

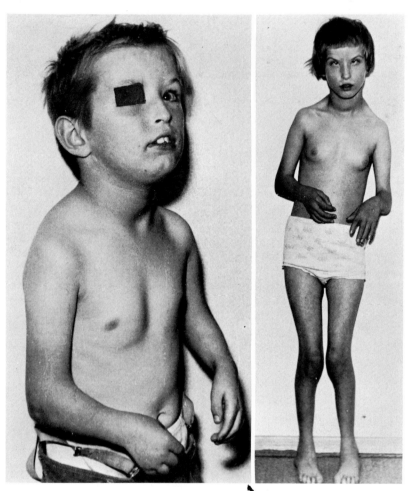

Affected siblings. Note the hypoplasia of the alae nasi and the position of the dislocated elbows. (From Mietens, C., and Weber, H.: J. Pediat., *69*:624, 1966.)

47. OCULODENTODIGITAL SYNDROME

Microphthalmos, Enamel Hypoplasia, Camptodactyly of Fifth Fingers

Originally described in 1920 by Lohmann,[1] this pattern was more fully characterized by Gorlin, Meskin, and St. Geme[2] in 1963. Only 12 cases have been reported.

ABNORMALITIES. Based on 12 cases.

Eye. Microphthalmos, microcornea, fine porous iris.

Nose. Thin, hypoplastic alae nasi with small nares.

Teeth. Enamel hypoplasia.

Hands and Feet. Syndactyly of fourth and fifth fingers, third and fourth toes. Camptodactyly of fifth fingers. Mid-phalangeal hypoplasia or aplasia of one or more fingers, toes.

Hair. Fine, dry, and/or sparse and slow growing.

Other Skeletal. Broad tubular bones and mandible with wide alveolar ridge.

OCCASIONAL ABNORMALITIES. Small palpebral fissures, epicanthic folds, glaucoma, partial anodontia, microdontia, premature loss of teeth, cleft lip and palate, conductive hearing impairment, cubitus valgus, hip dislocation, osteopetrosis, poor posture.

NATURAL HISTORY. Inadequate information. Mentally normal.

ETIOLOGY. Present evidence indicates autosomal dominant with variable expressivity.

REFERENCES

1. Lohmann, W.: Beitrag zur Kenntnis des reinen Mikrophthalmus. Arch. Augenh., *86*:136, 1920.
2. Gorlin, R. J., Meskin, L. H., and St. Geme, J. W.: Oculodentodigital dysplasia. J. Pediat., *63*:69, 1963.
3. Gillespie, F. D.: A hereditary syndrome: "dysplasia oculodentodigitalis." Arch. Ophth., *71*:187, 1964.
4. Eidelman, E., Chosack, A., and Wagner, M. L.: Oro-digitofacial dysostosis and oculodentodigital dysplasia. Two distinct syndromes with some similarities. Oral Surg., *23*:311, 1967.

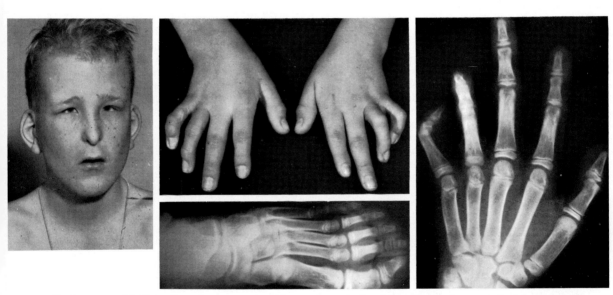

Twelve year old. Note the microcornea, small eyes, hypoplasia of the alae nasi, camptodactyly, repaired syndactyly of the fourth and fifth fingers, and bony abnormalities. (From Gorlin, R. J., et al.: J. Pediat., *63*:69, 1963.)

48. OTO-PALATO-DIGITAL SYNDROME

(Taybi's Syndrome)

Deafness, Cleft Palate, Broad Distal Digits

Three siblings were described by Taybi[1] in 1962, and a fourth case was reported by Dudding, Gorlin, and Langer.[2]

ABNORMALITIES. Based on four cases.

Performance. Mild mental deficiency; I.Q., 75 to 90.

Growth. Small stature, all below tenth percentile for age.

Hearing. Moderate conductive deafness.

Cranium. Frontal and occipital prominence with thick frontal bone and thick base of skull having a steep naso-basal angulation. Absence of frontal and sphenoid sinuses.

Facies. Facial bone hypoplasia and hypertelorism with small nose and mouth.

Mouth. Partial anodontia, impacted teeth, or both. Cleft soft palate, small tonsils.

Mid-Skeletal. Small trunk, pectus excavatum, failure of neural arch fusion, small iliac crests.

Extremities. Limited elbow extension, inward bowing tibiae. Short broad distal phalanges of thumbs and toes, to a lesser extent for other digits. Fusion of hamate and capitate. Accessory ossification center at the base of the second metatarsal.

OCCASIONAL ABNORMALITIES. Delayed closure of anterior fontanel, hip dislocation, limited knee flexion, syndactyly of toes, hallucal nail dystrophy.

NATURAL HISTORY. Speech development is retarded on the basis of hearing impairment, mental deficiency, or both.

ETIOLOGY. Familial, the three cases of Taybi[1] being male siblings. Autosomal dominant or X-linked inheritance is suggested by a family observed by Aase[3] to have three affected male siblings and a partial expression in their mother. However, Gorlin[4] has observed sibship occurrence, including an affected female of normal parentage, and considers autosomal recessive inheritance most likely. It will require more information to resolve this question.

REFERENCES

1. Taybi, H.: Generalized skeletal dysplasia with multiple anomalies. Am. J. Roentgenol., *88*:450, 1962.
2. Dudding, B. A., Gorlin, R. J., and Langer, L. O.: The oto-palato-digital syndrome. A new symptom-complex consisting of deafness, dwarfism, cleft palate, characteristic facies, and a generalized bone dysplasia. Am. J. Dis. Children, *113*:214, 1967.
3. Aase, J.: Personal communication.
4. Gorlin, R.: Personal communication.

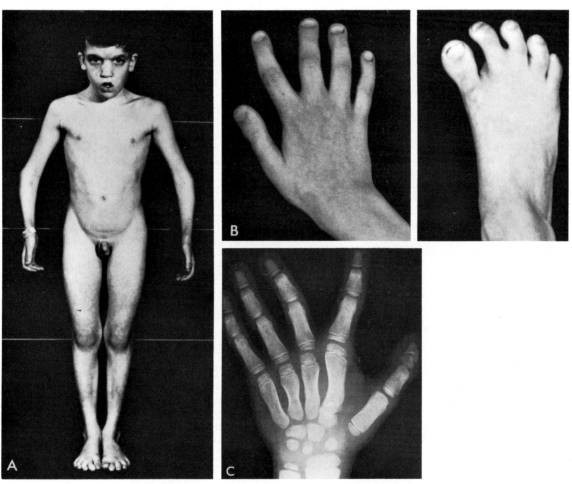

A to *C*, Note irregular length and form of distal phalanges, especially thumb. (From Dudding, B. A., Gorlin, R. J., and Langer, L. O.: Am. J. Dis. Children, *113*:214, 1967.)

49. FANCONI'S SYNDROME OF PANCYTOPENIA AND MULTIPLE ANOMALIES

Hypoplasia of Radial Side of Distal Upper Extremity, Hyperpigmentation, Pancytopenia

Since Fanconi's[1] original description of three affected siblings in 1927, over 160 case have been reported.

ABNORMALITIES. Percentage of patients noted to have each defect.[2]

Small stature	56%
Small cranium	43%
Hypoplasia to aplasia of thumb	78%

Pancytopenia: because marrow failure has generally been an essential prerequisite to the diagnosis, it is difficult to know its true incidence; however, it is presumably a usual feature.

Splenic hypoplasia is a frequent autopsy finding.

Brownish pigmentation of skin is a frequent feature.

Small penis, small testes, and/or cryptorchidism are found in 44 per cent of males.

OCCASIONAL ABNORMALITIES. Mental deficiency (20+ per cent), ptosis of eyelid, strabismus, nystagmus, microphthalmos, auricular anomaly, deafness, osteoporosis, aplasia of radius (15 per cent), duplication of thumb, broad base of proximal phalanges, hypoplasia to aplasia of first metacarpal, diminished carpal centers, syndactyly, dislocation of hip, congenital heart defect, hypospadias, and leukemia (acute monocytic).

NATURAL HISTORY. The majority of patients are relatively small at birth. Respiratory infections may be a frequent problem. The uneven brownish pigmentation of the skin tends to increase with age, being most evident in the anogenital area, groin, axilla, and trunk. Development of bleeding, pallor and/or recurring infection usually appears between five and ten years of age, although pancytopenia may occur in infancy or as late as the third decade. There are nests of hematopoiesis in the generally hypoplastic marrow. Some erythrocytes are macrocytic, there is a high percentage of fetal hemoglobin, and the red cell life span is shortened. The leukopenia is predominantly granulocytopenia. Previously the survival following discovery of pancytopenia was seldom more than two years, although recently combined therapy with testosterone and hydrocortisone analogue has extended the survival period.

ETIOLOGY. The frequent occurrence of affected siblings plus the finding of consanguinity in 20 per cent of the familial cases is indicative of autosomal recessive determination. The findings of greater than 25 per cent affected siblings and the 2 : 1 incidence of affected males to females are presently unexplained. However, the ascertainment bias tends toward detection of families with multiple affected offspring, especially for this condition in which there may be rather wide variance in expression between affected siblings. What is needed is an assessment of the frequency and sex of affected individuals born after the oldest propositus. An occasional parent may have malformation (one case), slight pancytopenia (one case), or neutropenia; leukemia was found in an otherwise normal relative in four of 48 affected families,[3] all possible heterozygote manifestations.

COMMENT. A curious and consistent finding has been undue fragility of the chromosomes of in vitro cultured lymphocytes from patients with this syndrome,[4] a finding which may be related to the propensity to develop leukemia. Chromosomal breaks, gaps, and rearrangements were not a frequent feature of in vivo cells such as those obtained from the marrow.[4]

REFERENCES

1. Fanconi, G.: Die familiäre Panmyelopathie. Schweiz. Med. Wschr., *94*:1309, 1964.
2. Nilsson, L. R.: Chronic pancytopenia with multiple congenital abnormalities (Fanconi's anaemia). Acta Paediat., *49*:518, 1960.
3. Garriga, S., and Crosby, W. H.: The incidence of leukemia in families of patients with hypoplasia of the marrow. Blood, *14*:1008, 1959.
4. Schmid, W. K., Scharer, K., Baumann, T., and Fanconi, G.: Chromosomenbruchigkeit bei der familiären Panmyelopathie (Typus Fanconi). Schweiz. Med. Wschr., *95*:1461, 1965.

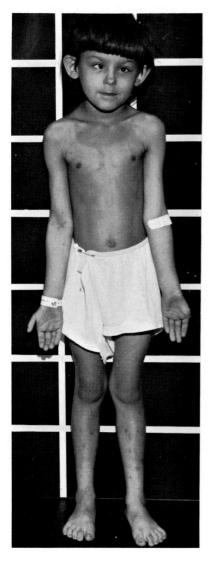

+ Pigmentation (brown) of skin

+ Short stature

+ Small cranium

+ Mental retardation

+ Strabismus

+ Abnormal ears

+ Abnormal thumbs

+ Renal anomaly

+ Hypoplasia of marrow, with time

Seven year old with a height age of three and one half years who has the anomalies listed above. The pedigree notes two affected siblings and one otherwise normal brother who died of leukemia during infancy. (From Smith, D. W.: J. Pediat., 70:479, 1967.)

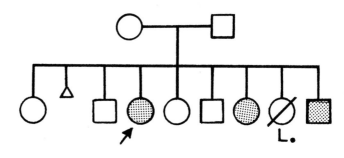

50. RADIAL APLASIA–THROMBOCYTOPENIA

Gross, Groh, and Weippl[1] described this entity in siblings in 1956; subsequently over 20 cases have been reported. Shaw and Oliver[2] and others have clearly distinguished this disorder from Fanconi's pancytopenia with associated malformations.

ABNORMALITIES
Hematological. Most severe in early infancy.
  Thrombocytopenia with absence or hypoplasia of megakaryocytes (absent in 66 per cent, decreased in 12 per cent, inactive in 12 per cent).
  "Leukemoid" granulocytosis in 62 per cent of cases, especially during bleeding episodes. Eosinophilia in 53 per cent.
  Anemia, often out of proportion to apparent blood loss.
Absence or Hypoplasia of Radius. Usually bilateral; often with associated ulnar hypoplasia and defects of the hand, legs, and/or feet.

OCCASIONAL ABNORMALITIES. About 25 per cent have a congenital heart defect. Small stature, genu varum, renal anomaly, and spina bifida have been noted in at least two cases, and individual cases have been reported with brachycephaly, strabismus, micrognathia, syndactyly, short humerus, hypoplastic shoulder girdle, dislocation of the hip, talipes foot deformity and Meckel's diverticulum. One patient developed leukemia, indicating that this unstable hematological disorder may predispose toward development of leukemia.

NATURAL HISTORY. About 40 per cent of the patients have expired, usually as a result of hemorrhage during early infancy. With advancing age the severity of the hematological disorder usually becomes less profound, and therefore vigorous early management is indicated. Hydrocortisone analogue therapy, though it may lessen the likelihood of hemorrhage, has not had a consistently beneficial effect on the thrombocytopenia.

ETIOLOGY. There have been three reports of affected siblings, the sex incidence is about equal, and autosomal recessive mode of determination is considered likely, though parental consanguinity has not been reported. Of interest is the fact that an uncle of one patient died of leukemia.

REFERENCES

1. Gross, H., Groh, C., and Weippl, G.: Congenitale hypoplastische Thrombopenie mit Radialaplasie. Neue Osterr. Z. Kinderh., *1*:574, 1956.
2. Shaw, S., and Oliver, R. A. M.: Congenital hypoplastic thrombocytopenia with skeletal deformities in siblings. Blood, *14*:374, 1956.
3. Gmyrek, D., Otto, F. M. G., and Sylim-Rapoport, I.: Über das familiäre Auftreten von Fanconi-Anämie und Thrombocytopenie mit Missbildungen (Bemerkungen zur Therapie der Fanconi-Anämie). Mschr. Kinderh., *113*:542, 1965.
4. Hunter, R.: Congenital megakaryocytic hypoplasia with radial aplasia. Personal communication.

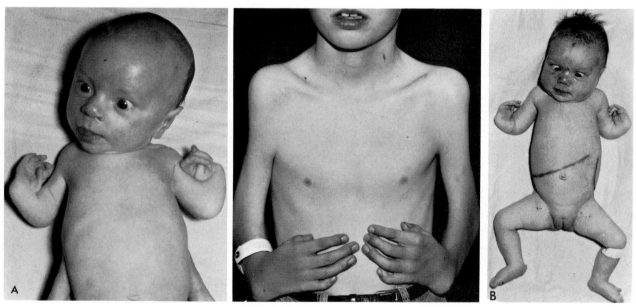

A, Same patient as infant and young boy.
B, Young infant with serious bleeding and hepatosplenomegaly. Patient also had a cardiac defect.
(Courtesy of J. M. Opitz, University of Wisconsin, and R. Hunter, University of Washington.)

51. HOLT-ORAM SYNDROME

(Cardiac-Limb Syndrome)

Upper Limb Defect, Cardiac Anomaly, Narrow Shoulders

This syndrome of skeletal and cardiovascular abnormality was first described by Holt and Oram in 1960.[1]

ABNORMALITIES

Skeletal. Hypoplasia and proximal placement of the thumb is the most common defect, but hypoplasia of the radius and even phocomelia may occur.

Hypoplasia of the clavicles with narrow shoulders.

Cardiovascular. Auricular septal defect, sometimes with arrhythmia, and ventricular septal defect have been the most common defects, and about one third of the patients have had other types of congenital heart defects.

OCCASIONAL ABNORMALITIES. Absent
pectoralis major muscle. Small scapulae. Triphalangeal thumb. Skin tag over lower sternum.

ETIOLOGY. Autosomal dominant with variable expression, tending to be more severe in the female.

REFERENCES

1. Holt, M., and Oram, S.: Familial heart disease with skeletal malformations. Brit. Heart J., 22:236, 1960.
2. Lewis, K. B., Bruce, R. A, Baum, D., and Motulsky, A. G.: The upper limb–cardiovascular syndrome. An autosomal dominant genetic effect on embryogenesis. J.A.M.A., 193:1080, 1965.
3. Gall, J. C., Stern, A. M., Cohen, M. M., Adams, M. S., and Davidson, R. T.: Holt-Oram syndrome: clinical and genetic study of a large family. Am. J. Human Genet., 18:187, 1966.

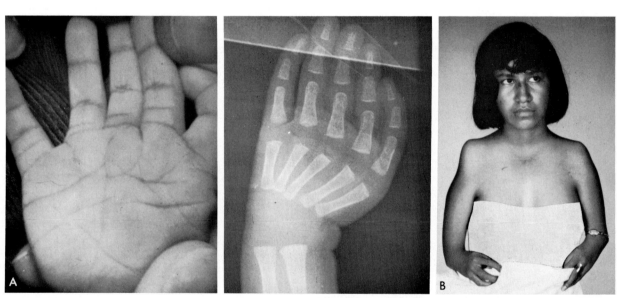

A, Finger-like thumb (to right) in an infant with the Holt-Oram syndrome. (From M. Feingold, Tufts Medical School.)

B, Fifteen year old with auricular septal defect. Note severe forearm hypoplasia, absence of thumbs, and altered shoulder girdle.

52. SMITH-LEMLI-OPITZ SYNDROME

Anteverted Nostrils and/or Ptosis of Eyelid, Syndactyly of Second and Third Toes, Hypospadias and Cryptorchidism in Male

Four patients with this disorder were described by Smith et al.[1] in 1964, and subsequently at least nine further cases have been documented.[2-5]

ABNORMALITIES. Based on 13 cases.

Growth. Moderately small at birth with subsequent failure to thrive.

Performance. Moderate to severe mental deficiency with variable altered muscle tone.

Craniofacial. Microcephaly with relative scaphocephaly, auricles slanted or low set, ptosis of eyelids, inner epicanthic folds, strabismus, broad nasal tip with anteverted nostrils, broad maxillary alveolar ridges, micrognathia.

Extremities. Simian crease, high frequency of digital whorl dermal ridge patterning, syndactyly of second and third toes.

Genitalia. Male: cryptorchidism, hypospadias, mild to severe.

Other Abnormalities. Observed in one or two cases but not evaluated in most cases. EEG abnormality, dysplasia epiphysealis punctata, acrocyanosis of hands and feet, hypoplasia of thymus, cleft palate, polydactyly, vertical talus.

OCCASIONAL ABNORMALITIES. Broad nasal bridge, clenched hand with index finger overlying third, asymmetrical short finger, distal palmar axial triradius, metatarsus adductus, dislocated hip, deep sacral dimple, pit anterior to anus, wide-spread nipples, cardiac defect, inguinal hernia, pyloric stenosis, dilated renal calyces.

NATURAL HISTORY. Feeding difficulty and vomiting have been frequent problems in early infancy, and seven of the 13 patients have died at from two to 14 months of age, with the survivors ranging in age from 18 months to 11 years. Death appeared related to pneumonia in five of the seven patients, one of whom had a hemorrhagic necrotizing pneumonia with varicella, suggesting an increased susceptibility to serious infection. Irritable behavior with shrill screaming may pose a problem during infancy.

ETIOLOGY. ? Autosomal recessive, based on sibship occurrence and normal parents. No consanguinity noted. The prevalence of affected males versus females (11 of 13) may simply be related to the ascertainment bias of the genital anomaly.

REFERENCES

1. Smith, D. W., Lemli, L., and Opitz, J. M.: A newly recognized syndrome of multiple congenital anomalies. J. Pediat., *64*:210, 1964.
2. Gibson, R.: A case of the Smith-Lemli-Opitz syndrome of multiple congenital anomalies in association with dysplasia epiphysealis punctata. Canad. Med. Ass. J., *92*:574, 1965.
3. Pinsky, L., and DiGeorge, A. M.: A familial syndrome of facial and skeletal anomalies associated with genital abnormality in the male and normal genitals in the female. J. Pediat., *66*:1049, 1965.
4. Blair, H. R., and Martin, J. K.: A syndrome characterized by mental retardation, short stature, craniofacial dysplasia, and genital anomalies occurring in siblings. J. Pediat., *69*:457, 1966.
5. Dallaire, L., and Fraser, F. C.: The syndrome of retardation with urogenital and skeletal anomalies in siblings. J. Pediat., *69*:459, 1966.

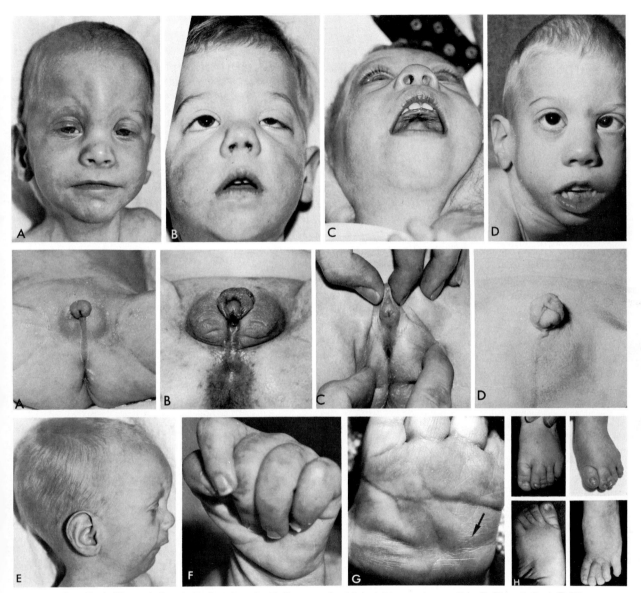

    A to D: A, Young infant raised as female. *B,* Ten month old; height age six months. *C,* Older infant. *D,* Five year old; height age, 18 months. Note ptosis, nasal configuration, and wide secondary alveolar ridge.

    E, Lateral view of patient *A.* Note prominent mid-forehead (glabella), micrognathia.

    F, Clenched hand (patient *A*), a variable feature.

    G, Simian crease and distal palmar axial triradius (arrow).

    H, Unusual appearance of syndactyly of the second and third toes in three of four patients.

    (*B, C, D, G,* and *H* from Smith, D. W., et al.: J. Pediat., *64*:210, 1964.)

137

53. FRASER SYNDROME

Cryptophthalmos,* Defect of Auricle, Genital Anomaly

The association of multiple other malformations in patients with the rare anomaly of cryptophthalmos had been appreciated[1] prior to 1962, when a rather distinctive syndrome found in two sets of siblings was set forth by Fraser.[2] Subsequently two similar cases have been reported,[3, 4] but the syndrome needs further definition and the following represents a preliminary depiction of this condition.

PATTERN OF ABNORMALITY. The most consistent features have been the following:
Eyes. Cryptophthalmos.
Ears. Auricular defect.
Genitalia. Male: hypospadias, cryptorchidism.
  Female: bicornuate uterus, vaginal atresia.

INCONSISTENT FEATURES. Flat nasal bridge, hypertelorism, lacrimal duct defect, palatal defect, partial mid-facial cleft, atresia of external ear canal, defect of middle ear, laryngeal stenosis or atresia, widely spaced nipples, syndactyly, renal anomaly, umbilical anomaly, anal atresia.

---

*Cryptophthalmos (hidden eye) fundamentally means absence of the palpebral fissure but usually includes varying absence of eyelashes and eyebrows and defects of the eye, especially the anterior part.

NATURAL HISTORY. Two of the four patients reported by Fraser[2] were stillborn. As yet no clear statement as to survival or mental retardation can be set forth. Because the defect of eyelid development is frequently accompanied by ocular anomaly, the likelihood of achieving adequate visual perception is small.

ETIOLOGY. Preliminary evidence favors autosomal recessive mode of etiology, as indicated by occurrence in siblings, parental consanguinity in one case, and absence of evident chromosomal abnormality in at least two cases.[2, 4]

REFERENCES

1. Brodsky, I., and Waddy, G.: Cryptophthalmos or ablepharia: a survey of the condition with a review of the literature and the presentation of a case. Med. J. Aust., *1*:894, 1940.
2. Fraser, C. R.: Our genetical 'load.' A review of some aspects of genetical variation. Ann. Human Genet., *25*:387, 1962.
3. Gupta, S. P., and Saxena, R. C.: Cryptophthalmos. Brit. J. Ophth., *46*:629, 1962.
4. François, J.: Syndrome malformatif avec cryptophthalmie. (Note préliminaire.) Ophthalmologica, *150*:215, 1965.

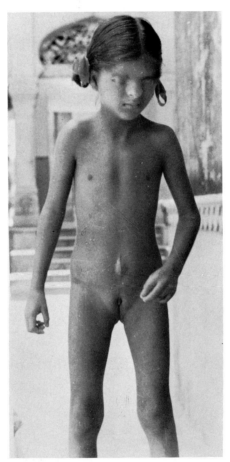

A genetic male with cryptophthalmos, malformed ears with atresia of external auditory canals, aberrant umbilicus, and incomplete development of external genitalia. (Courtesy of S. P. Gupta, University of Lucknow.)

54. HYPERTELORISM-HYPOSPADIAS SYNDROME

(Opitz Syndrome)

Hypertelorism, Hypospadias

Opitz, Summitt, and Smith[1,2] recently reported this dominantly inherited condition in three families in which affected males usually have apparent ocular hypertelorism and hypospadias, whereas affected females have only hypertelorism, there being no opportunity for expression of the penile malformation in the female.

ABNORMALITIES. Apparent ocular hypertelorism in both sexes; varying degrees of hypospadias in the male.

Less Consistent Features in Affected Individuals. Mild to moderate mental deficiency, inguinal hernia, cryptorchidism, anomaly of external ear, cardiac defect.

ETIOLOGY. ? Autosomal dominant with sex limitation for penile malformation. One probable instance of male-to-male transmission tentatively excludes X-linked inheritance.

REFERENCES

1. Opitz, J. M., Smith, D. W., and Summitt, R. L.: Hypertelorism and hypospadias. (Abstract.) J. Pediat., 67:968, 1965.
2. Opitz, J. M., Summitt, R. L., and Smith, D. W.: The BBB Syndrome. Familial Telecanthus with Associated Anomalies. First Conference on Clinical Delineation of Birth Defects. D. Bergsma, Editor. Vol. 5, 86-94, 1969, The National Foundation.

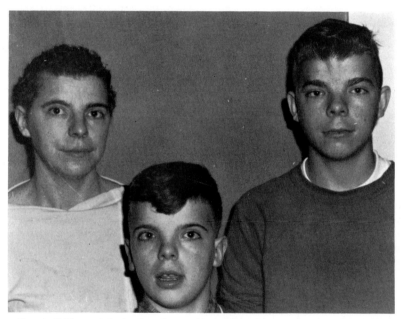

An affected mother (mild hypertelorism) and two of her affected boys who show hypertelorism and also have hypospadias. (From the B. O. family pedigree of Opitz et al.)[2]

55. WAARDENBURG'S SYNDROME

Lateral Displacement of Medial Canthi, Partial Albinism, Deafness

Waardenburg[1] set forth this pattern of malformation in 1951. He found this syndrome in 1.4 per cent of congenitally deaf children and from these data estimated the incidence to be about 1 : 42,000 in Holland.

ABNORMALITIES

Lateral displacement of median canthi	99%
Broad and high nasal bridge	78%
Medial hyperplasia, eyebrows	45%
Partial albinism	37%
Deafness	20%

OCCASIONAL ABNORMALITIES. Flattened alae nasi, rounded tip of nose, full lips with accentuated "cupid's bow" to upper lip, cleft lip and palate, limb defect.

NATURAL HISTORY. The partial albinism is most commonly expressed as a white forelock and/or isochromic pale blue eyes with hypoplastic iral stroma; however, it may be present as heterochromia of the iris, areas of viteligo on the skin, patches of white hair other than the forelock, and/or mottled peripheral pigmentation of the retina. The white forelock may be present at birth only to become pigmented early in life; the hair may become prematurely gray or white.

Congenital deafness is the most serious feature and if present is usually bilateral and severe. The defect appears to be in the organ of Corti with atrophic changes in the spiral ganglion and nerve.

ETIOLOGY. Autosomal dominant. Five of the 16 propositi of Waardenburg were considered to represent fresh mutations, a calculated mutation rate of 0.4×10^{-5} per gamete.

COMMENT. The association of dominantly inherited albinism and deafness was noted in cats as early as 1769 and subsequently in the horse and several types of dog.

REFERENCES

1. Waardenburg, P. J.: A new syndrome combining developmental anomalies of the eyelids, eyebrows and nose root with pigmentary defects of the iris and head hair and with congenital deafness. Am. J. Human Genet., *3*:195, 1951.
2. DiGeorge, A. M., Olmsted, R. W., and Harley, R. D.: Waardenburg's syndrome. J. Pediat., *57*:649, 1960.

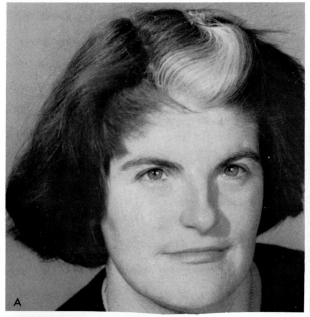
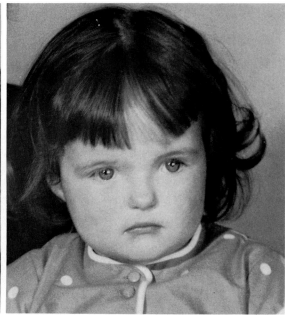
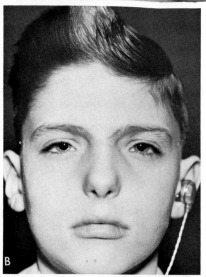
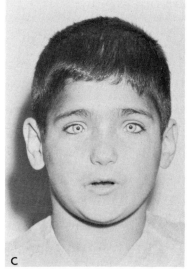
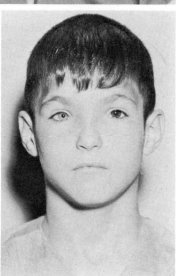
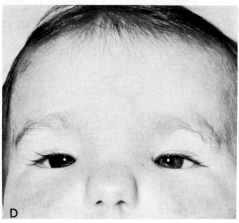

A, Mother and daughter. Note the isochromic light iris. (From Partington, M. W.: Arch. Dis. Childhood, *34:*154, 1959.)

B, Ten year old with congenital deafness. Note prominent nasal root, small alae nasi. (From DiGeorge, A. M.: J. Pediat., *57:*649, 1960.)

C, Brothers, only one of whom has deafness. Note the lack of a white forelock.

D, Four month old infant who had a white forelock at birth which is now pigmented. Note heterochromia of irises, lateral placement of inner canthi, and small alae nasi.

56. RUBELLA SYNDROME

Deafness, Cataract, Patent Ductus Arteriosus

Gregg[1] first called attention in 1941 to the permanent residua of fetal rubella acquired from the mother during the first trimester of gestation. Culture of the viral agent during the severe 1964 epidemic resulted in an appreciation of the "expanded rubella syndrome" as the consequence of widespread chronic disease.

ABNORMALITIES. Fetal death may occur. The following are tissues affected and consequent abnormalities noted in the 1964 epidemic.

The asterisks (*) indicate permanent residua.

Tissue	Abnormality
General hypoplasia	Growth deficiency
Central nervous system	*Mental deficiency, microcephaly
Cochlea	*Deafness
Lens	*Cataract
Other parts of eye	*Glaucoma, corneal opacity, chorioretinitis
Blood vessels	*Patent ductus arteriosus, peripheral pulmonic stenosis
Myocardium	*Septal defects, myocardial disease

Early Infancy

Tissue	Abnormalities
Marrow elements	Thrombocytopenia, anemia
Reticuloendothelial	Hepatosplenomegaly
Liver	Obstructive jaundice
Bone	Osteolytic metaphyseal lesions
Lung	Interstitial pneumonia

OCCASIONAL ABNORMALITIES. Renal disease, hemolytic anemia, large anterior fontanel, late eruption of teeth, hypospadias, cryptorchidism, meningocele, dermatoglyphic alterations.

NATURAL HISTORY. The frequency of fetal infection from mothers having rubella during the first trimester is about 50 per cent. Cultures for rubella virus in excretions were positive in 63 per cent of neonates with evidence of the Rubella syndrome; 31 per cent of cultures were still positive at five to seven months, 7 per cent at ten to 13 months, and none past the age of three years. However, rubella virus was recovered from a cataract removed from a two and one half year old. Thus the disease is chronic and although the neonate has prenatal antibodies to the rubella agent, the intracellular rubella virus may persist for a long period of time.

The extent to which mental deficiency and growth deficiency will persist as permanent residua of the 1964 epidemic remains to be determined. Certainly these features appear to be more frequent residua in this epidemic than in those of the past, in which deafness was the most common residua of fetal rubella (31 per cent).

Prevention of maternal rubella via widespread administration of attenuated rubella vaccine is throughly merited. Beyond this, the occurrence of validated maternal rubella during the first trimester of pregnancy merits serious consideration toward early termination of that pregnancy.

ETIOLOGY. Rubella virus.

REFERENCES

1. Gregg, N. McA.: Congenital cataract following German measles in the mother. Trans. Ophth. Soc. Aust., 3:35, 1941.
2. Heggie, A. D.: Rubella: current concepts in epidemiology and teratology. Pediat. Clin. North America, 13:251, 1966.
3. Cooper, L. Z., and Krugman, S.: Diagnosis and management: congenital rubella. Pediatrics, 37:335, 1966.

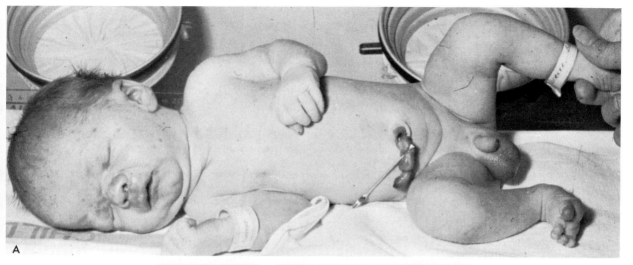

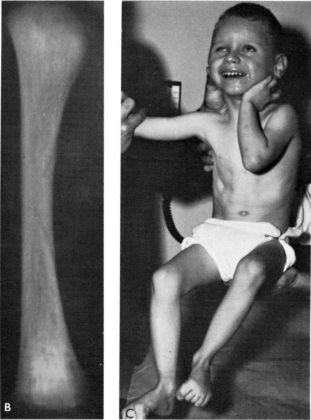

A, Newborn, clinically sick with lethargy, petechiae, and hepatosplenomegaly. (From Smith, D. W.: J. Pediat., *70*:517, 1967.)

B, Osseous lesions in the femur of five day old baby. Note coarse trabecular pattern and subperiosteal rarefaction.

C, Three and three fourths year old with height age of two and three fourths years and mental deficiency. The patient has cataracts, chorioretinitis, hearing impairment, and cryptorchidism—all the apparent residua of congenital rubella.

145

57. Leprechaunism

(Donohue's Syndrome)

Prenatal Adipose Deficiency, Full Lips, Enlarged Phallus

This somewhat puzzling entity was initially described as dysendocrinism by Donohue[1] in 1948. Later Donohue and Uchida[2] reported two siblings under the term leprechaunism. Subsequently only seven other cases have documented, and it is difficult to be sure that they all represent the same entity.

ABNORMALITIES
Growth. Prenatal growth deficiency with retarded osseous maturation and marked lack of adipose tissue; mean birth weight, about 2.6 kg.

Facies. Small with prominent eyes, wide nostrils, thick lips, large ears.

Endocrine. Large phallus, breast hyperplasia in female, Leydig cell hyperplasia (male), follicular development with cystic ovary, increased pituitary gonadotropes, hyperplasia of islets of Langerhans.

Other. Body and facial hirsuitism.

Apparent motor and mental retardation.

Iron deposition in liver.

NATURAL HISTORY. Usually severe failure to thrive and frequent infections with death in early infancy. One patient survived to two and one fourth years of age. Hypoglycemia occurs following prolonged fast. The basic defect in metabolism is undetermined.

ETIOLOGY. Autosomal recessive inheritance is implied by consanguinity and sibship occurrence.

REFERENCES

1. Donohue, W. L.: Dysendocrinism. J. Pediat., *32*:739, 1948.
2. Donohue, W. L., and Uchida, I.: Leprechaunism. A euphuism for a rare familial disorder. J. Pediat., *45*:505, 1954.
3. Salmon, M. A., and Webb, J. N.: Dystrophic changes associated with leprechaunism in a male infant. Arch. Dis. Childhood, *38*:530, 1963.
4. Rogers, D. R.: Leprechaunism (Donohue's syndrome). A possible case, with emphasis on changes in the adenohypophysis. Am. J. Clin. Path., *45*:614, 1966.

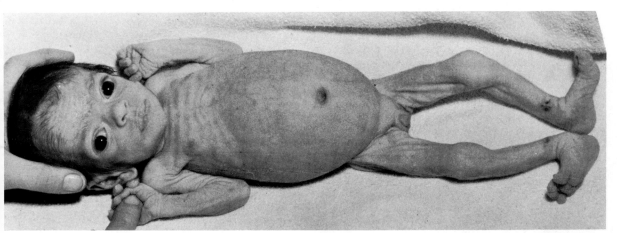

Six week old; birth weight, 3 pounds, 14 ounces. (From Donohue, W. L., and Uchida, I.: J. Pediat., *45*:505, 1954.)

58. BERARDINELLI'S LIPODYSTROPHY SYNDROME

Lipoatrophy, Phallic Hypertrophy, Hepatomegaly and Hyperlipemia

Berardinelli[1] reported this unusual lipodystrophic syndrome in 1954. Although more than 20 cases have subsequently been recorded, the metabolic defect responsible for this inborn error of metabolism has not been determined.

ABNORMALITIES

Performance. Mental deficiency as a variable feature.

Growth. Accelerated growth and maturation, enlargement of hands and feet, phallic enlargement, hypertrophy of muscle with excess glycogen, lack of adipose from early life.

Skin. Coarse with hyperpigmentation, especially in axillae.

Hair. Hirsutism with curly scalp hair.

Vessels. Large superficial veins.

Liver. Hepatomegaly with excess neutral fat, glycogen, and eventual cirrhosis.

Plasma. Hyperlipidemia (neutral fats). Insulin-resistant nonketotic hyperglycemia may develop.

OCCASIONAL ABNORMALITIES.
Cardiomegaly, corneal opacities, hyperproteinemia, hyperinsulinemia.

NATURAL HISTORY.
The accelerated growth and hyperlipidemia are most prominent in early childhood and hyperglycemia may develop in later childhood. The oldest reported patient, 16 years of age, was diabetic. Cirrhosis of the liver with esophageal varices may become a fatal complication.

COMMENT.
Although the accelerated growth and maturation plus the muscle hypertrophy and enlargement of the phallus are suggestive of androgen effect, neither androgens nor gonadotropins are elevated and the hirsutism does not include pubic and axillary hair.

ETIOLOGY.
Autosomal recessive as indicated by sibship occurrence and parental consanguinity.

REFERENCES

1. Berardinelli, W.: An undiagnosed endocrinometabolic syndrome: report of two cases. J. Clin. Endocrin. Metab., *14*:193, 1954.
2. Seip, M., and Trygstad, O.: Generalized lipodystrophy. Arch. Dis. Childhood, *38*:447, 1963.
3. Senior, B., and Gellis, S. S.: The syndromes of total lipodystrophy and of partial lipodystrophy. Pediatrics, *33*:593, 1964.

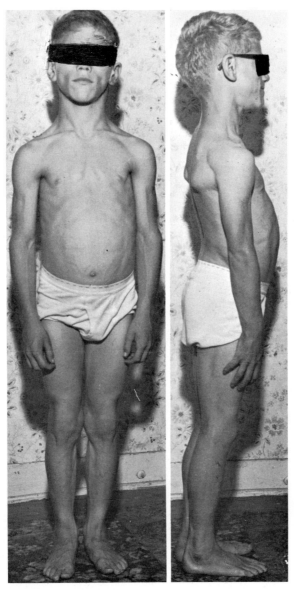

Boy of preadolescent age. Note the hypertrophied muscle and relative lack of subcutaneous fat. (Courtesy of Central Wisconsin Colony and Training School.)

59. INFANTILE HYPERCALCEMIA, PECULIAR FACIES, SUPRAVALVULAR AORTIC STENOSIS

By 1958, certain infants with hypercalcemia were noted to have a peculiar facies and mental retardation,[1] subsequently supravalvular aortic stenosis, and peripheral pulmonic stenosis were also found in such patients.[2, 3]

ABNORMALITIES. Varying features from the following:

Growth. Short stature, sometimes low birth weight.

Performance. Mental deficiency, moderate to severe.

Facies. Broad maxilla and mouth with full prominent upper lip, anteverted small nose. Tendency toward full forehead, hypertelorism, inner epicanthic folds, small mandible, prominent ears.

Vascular. Supravalvular aortic stenosis or hypoplasia and/or peripheral pulmonary artery stenoses.

Skeletal. Osteosclerosis, most evident at base of skull and metaphyses.

Dentition. Hypoplasia.

Metabolic. Hypercalcemia in infancy with symptoms and signs such as hypotonia, constipation, anorexia, vomiting, polyuria, polydysplasia, renal insufficiency and vicarious calcification.

OCCASIONAL ABNORMALITIES. Raucous voice, strabismus, craniosynostosis, partial anodontia, elevated serum cholesterol.

NATURAL HISTORY. The hypercalcemia, when detected, is generally only present in infancy and may be suspected on the basis of failure to thrive with hypotonia, anorexia, constipation, or evidence of renal impairment and slow developmental progress. Therapeutic or spontaneous resolution of the hypercalcemia will be accompanied by improvement in these symptoms, although there may be permanent residua of mental defect, renal insufficiency, or both. Whether the peculiar facies and large vessel abnormalities are the consequence of prolonged hypercalcemia in early life remains to be determined. The production of aortic endothelial abnormalities in young animals rendered hypercalcemic has heightened the suspicion that the vascular defects are secondary to hypercalcemia.

ETIOLOGY. Unknown. All cases have been sporadic. As mentioned previously, the major question is whether all signs and symptoms are the consequence of hypercalcemia in early life or whether the same adverse factor which leads to peculiar facies and the vessel anomalies also enhances the likelihood for hypercalcemia in infancy.

REFERENCES

1. Joseph, M. C., and Parrott, D.; Severe infantile hypercalcaemia with special reference to the facies. Arch. Dis. Childhood, *33*:385, 1958.
2. Beuren, A. J., Schulze, C., Eberle, P., Harmjanz, D., and Opitz, J.: The syndrome of supravalvular aortic stenosis, peripheral pulmonary stenosis, mental retardation and similar facial appearance. Am. J. Cardiol., *13*:471, 1964.
3. Fraser, D., Langford Kidd, B. S., Kooh, S. W., and Paunier, L.: A new look at infantile hypercalcemia. Pediat. Clin. North America, *13*:503, 1966.
4. Coleman, E. N.: Infantile hypercalcemia and cardiovascular lesions. Evidence, hypothesis and speculation. Arch. Dis. Childhood, *40*:535, 1965.

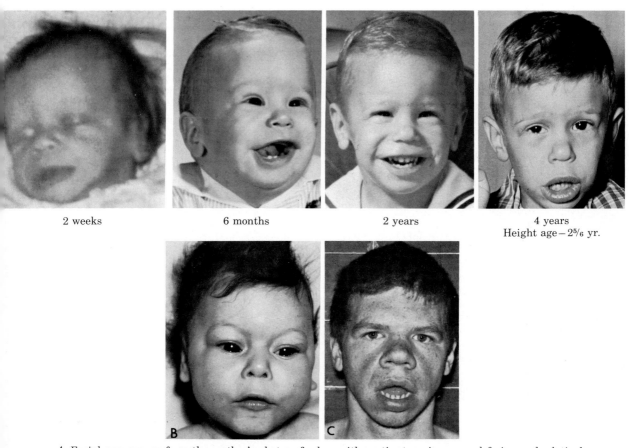

2 weeks   6 months   2 years   4 years
Height age—2⁵⁄₆ yr.

A, Facial appearance from the mother's photos of a boy with aortic stenosis, unusual facies, and relatively slow developmental progress. The serum calcium is presently normal; unknown during infancy.

B, Four and one half month old with severe hypercalcemia whose height age was four months at seven months of age when the baby died. Necropsy showed nonspecific fibrous thickening in the intima of the aortic valve. (From Joseph, M. C., and Parrott, D.: Arch. Dis. Childhood, *33:*385, 1958.)

C, Seventeen year old mentally deficient boy of short stature who has evidence of supravalvular aortic stenosis. (Courtesy of A. Reichert, Rainier State Training School, Buckley, Washington.)

60. WIEDEMANN-BECKWITH SYNDROME

Macroglossia, Omphalocele, Macrosomia, Cytomegaly of Fetal Adrenal

Wiedemann[1] and Beckwith et al.[2] reported this distinct clinical entity in 1964, and numerous cases have subsequently been recognized.

ABNORMALITIES

Performance. Unknown incidence of mild to moderate mental deficiency; may be normal.

Growth. Macrosomia with large muscle mass and thick subcutaneous tissue.

Craniofacial. Macroglossia.

Prominent eyes with *relative* infraorbital hypoplasia.

Capillary nevus flammeus, central forehead and eyelids.

Metopic ridge, central forehead.

Prominent occiput.

Malocclusion with tendency to mandibular prognathism.

Unusual linear fissures in lobule of external ear.

Hyperplasia and Dysplasia. Large kidneys with renal medullary dysplasia.

Pancreatic hyperplasia, including excess of islets.

Fetal adrenocortical cytomegaly—*a consistent feature.*

Interstitial cell hyperplasia, gonads.

Pituitary amphophil hyperplasia.

Other. Neonatal polycythemia.

Hypoglycemia in early infancy (about one third to one half of cases).

Omphalocele or other umbilical anomaly.

Posterior diaphragmatic eventration.

Cryptorchidism.

OCCASIONAL ABNORMALITIES.

Hepatomegaly, mild microcephaly, skeletal asymmetry, adrenal carcinoma, Wilms' tumor, clitoromegaly, large ovaries, hyperplastic uterus and bladder, bicornuate uterus.

NATURAL HISTORY.

Hydramnios and a relatively high incidence of prematurity provide further indication of the rather profound prenatal alterations. Severe problems of neonatal adaptation may occur, with apnea, cyanosis, and seizures as symptoms. Repair of an omphalocele is obviously indicated, but preoperative studies should be carried out to determine if the neonate has this syndrome, which accounted for at least 11.7 per cent of the cases of omphalocele reviewed by Irving.[5] The large tongue may partially occlude respiration and lead to feeding difficulties. Placing the baby on its side or face down may help respiration, and a large soft nipple may facilitate feeding. Detection and treatment of hypoglycemia in any newborn with features of this syndrome are critical. The hypoglycemia is responsive to hydrocortisone analogue therapy, which is usually required for only one to four months. Polycythemia might also merit therapeutic intervention during the early neonatal period. Cautious follow-up for the detection of abdominal tumor is indicated, and pneumonia has been a frequent enough complication during infancy to warrant concern toward its early detection and treatment. All these measures are indicated because affected individuals who survive infancy generally are healthy and all six (of 11) surviving children in Irving's[5] study were considered mentally normal at four to eight and one half years of age; however, Beckwith has noted mild to moderate mental deficiency in survivors.

Early postnatal growth may be slow, but thereafter macrosomia is the rule with growth around the ninetieth percentile and advanced skeletal maturation. Growth may allow adequate oral room for the large tongue. Partial glossectomy was performed in two of Irving's[5] six surviving cases with good results. The prognosis beyond childhood is presently unknown.

ETIOLOGY.

Autosomal recessive inheritance is suspected by the occurrence in siblings,[2-5] although more data is necessary.

COMMENT.

The search for the primary factor in the pathogenesis of this bizarre syndrome is of basic interest as well as of potential importance toward the treatment of these patients. Extensive endocrine and metabolic studies are indicated in individuals with this syndrome, especially looking for abnormal adrenocortical steroids in early infancy. The placenta should be studied and part of it frozen on any such patient, because no placental studies have yet been carried out in this disorder.

REFERENCES

1. Wiedemann, H. R.: Complexe malformatif familial avec hernie ombilicale et macroglossie—un "syn-

(Text continued)

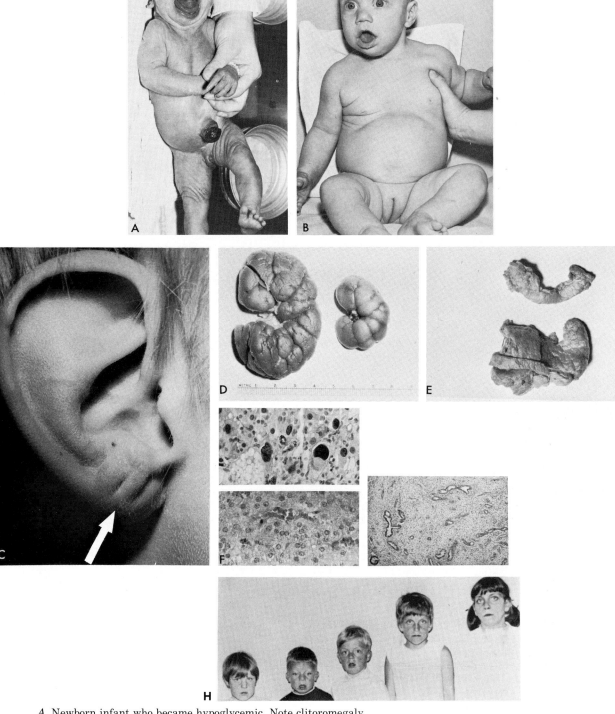

A, Newborn infant who became hypoglycemic. Note clitoromegaly.

B, Six month old large infant. Note scar of repaired omphalocele.

C, Unusual linear creases in the lobulus of the ear.

D and E, Kidney (D, left) and pancreas (E, lower) of patient compared to normal.

F and G, Fetal adrenal cytomegaly (above) compared to normal and renal medullary dysplasia (G). (From Beckwith, J. B.)[6]

H, Similar facial appearance of five surviving children from four to eight years of age, who tend to be large for age with advanced skeletal maturation.

(C and H from Irving, I. M.: J. Pediat. Surg., 2:499, 1967.)

drome nouveau"? J. de Génét. Humaine, *13*:223, 1964.
2. Beckwith, J. B., Wang, C., Donnell, G. N., and Gwinn, J. L.: Hyperplastic fetal visceromegaly, with macroglossia, omphalocele, cytomegaly of the adrenal fetal cortex, postnatal somatic gigantism, and other abnormalities; a newly recognized syndrome. Abstract read by title, at Annual Meeting of American Pediatric Society, Seattle, Washington, June 16–18, 1964.
3. Wiedemann, H. R., et al.: Uber das Syndrom Exomphalos - Macroglossie - Gigantismus, über generalisierte Muskelhypertrophie, progressive

Lipodystrophie, und Miescher-Syndrom im Sinne diencephalischer Syndrome. Z. Kinderh., *102*:1, 1968.
4. Combs, J. T., et al.: New syndrome of neonatal hypoglycemia. New England J. Med., *275*:236, 1966.
5. Irving, I.: Exomphalos with macroglossia: A study of 11 cases. J. Pediat. Surg., *2*:499, 1967.
6. Beckwith, J. B.: Macroglossia, Omphalocele, Adrenal Cytomegaly, Gigantism, and Hyperplastic Visceromegaly. The First Conference on the Clinical Delineation of Birth Defects. Part II, Malformation Syndromes. D. S. Bergsma, Editor. Vol. 5, 188, 1969, The National Foundation.

L. Presumed Metabolic Aberrations Affecting Morphogenesis

61. CEREBRAL GIGANTISM

(Sotos' Syndrome)

Large Size, Large Hands and Feet, Poor Coordination

Sotos et al.[1] described five such patients in 1964, and 23 further cases have subsequently been reported.

ABNORMALITIES. Based on 22 cases.[1-4]
Performance. Dull mentality, nonprogressive; I.Q.'s, 18 to 91, with mean about 60. Poor coordination.
Growth. Excessive size, evident at birth. Large hands, feet, and cranium with moderate prognathism. Advanced osseous maturation commensurate with height age.
Other. Relatively thick subcutaneous tissues, sometimes giving coarse facies with full lips. Mild dilation of ventricular system. Occasional nonspecific EEG abnormality, seizures.

NATURAL HISTORY. Full term birth length has varied from 51 to 63.5 cm., usually 52 to 54 cm. Growth is especially rapid in the first three or four years, and final height may not be excessive. Neonatal problems have been frequent, but thereafter general health has been good. The excessive size with dull mentality and poor coordination leads to problems of social adjustment.

ETIOLOGY. Unknown. All cases have been sporadic in the family, and the syndrome has

been reported in one concordant set of identical twins.[3] No consistent endocrine or other metabolic abnormality has been detected, and it is difficult to be certain whether all cases have a common etiology or not. The most plausible hypothesis is a single mutant gene, all cases to date representing fresh mutations. XYY chromosomal abnormality should be considered in males with this pattern of abnormality, at least until the early childhood features of the XYY constitution have been clarified.

REFERENCES

1. Sotos, J. F., Dodge, P. R., Muirhead, D., Crawford, J. D., and Talbot, N. B.: Cerebral gigantism in childhood. A syndrome of excessively rapid growth with acromegalic features and a nonprogressive neurologic disorder. New England J. Med., *271*:109, 1964.
2. Kjellman, B.: Cerebral gigantism. Acta Paediat. Scand., *54*:603, 1965.
3. Hook, E. B., and Reynolds, J. W.: Cerebral gigantism: endocrinological and clinical observations of six patients including a congenital giant, concordant monozygotic twins, and a child who achieved adult gigantic size. J. Pediat., *70*:900, 1967.
4. Stephenson, J. N., Mellinger, R. C., and Manson, G.: Cerebral gigantism. Pediatrics, *41*:130, 1968.

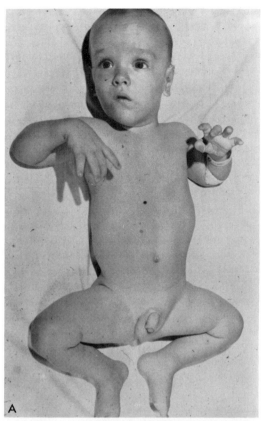

A, Eight and one half month old infant with height age of 21 months and borderline mental deficiency. (From Sotos, J. F., et al.: New England J. Med., *271*:109, 1964.)

B, Twenty five month old with height age of three and one third years and I.Q. of 70.

C, Eleven year old with height of 5 feet, 8 inches and I.Q. of 70. (*B* and *C* are from Hook, E., and Reynolds, J. W.: J. Pediat., *70*:900, 1967.)

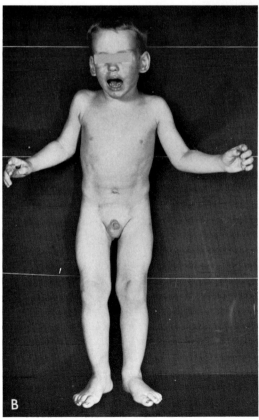

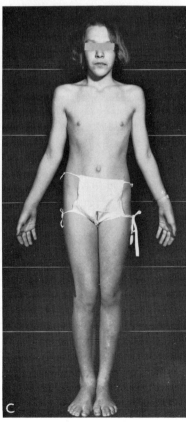

Hamartoses

Syndromes in Which Hamartomata Are a Prominent Feature

Hamartosis implies an organizational defect leading to an abnormal admixture of tissues, often with a tumor-like excess of one or more components of the tissue. Included in this category are such features as hemangiomata, melanomata, irregular skin pigmentation, fibromata, lipomata, osteomata, dental tumors, and adenomata. There are also some strange tissue admixtures which create nosological confusion because the histology of the lesions does not conform to a pathological standard. For example the "adenoma sebaceum" lesions in tuberous sclerosis are not adenoma of sebaceous glands. The very name tuberous sclerosis — potato-like lesions with sclerosis in the brain — emphasizes the nosological problems.

The instability of coordinated growth of particular tissues, a feature of many hamartomata, may allow for local growth toward a tumor, or even metastasis beyond the local site. One advantage in recognizing some of the following patterns of malformation is the enhanced capability of anticipating future problems by knowing the natural history of the disorder. For example, malignant change of a colonic polyp in Gardner's syndrome is sufficiently frequent to justify resection of the colon by the age of 12 in a child who is recognized as having this syndrome with colonic polyps. However, in another syndrome with intestinal polyposis — the Peutz-Jeghers syndrome — the natural history indicates that intestinal malignancy is a rare occurrence, an important fact because the intestinal polyps excised from patients with the Peutz-Jeghers syndrome may be interpreted by the pathologist as potentially malignant.

The "occasional abnormalities" in some of the following syndromes may be "occasional tumors." The physician should be on guard for the occasional rhabdomyoma in tuberous sclerosis, the ovarian tumor in Gardner's syndrome, and the medulloblastoma in the basal cell nevus syndrome.

Hamartomatous lesions are a feature of many syndromes other than those which follow. For example, multiple exostoses represent a hamartomatous process in the diaphyseal portion of the bone, and this condition carries a small but distinct risk toward the development of osteosarcoma. Melanomata are a frequent feature in XO Turner's syndrome. Adrenal carcinoma and Wilms' tumor are occasional complications for individuals with the Wiedemann-Beckwith syndrome. A looser association, in terms of being a distinct syndrome, has been noted in the occurrence of Wilms' tumor in individuals with hemihypertrophy, aniridia, or both. These types of cases emphasize the close relationship which may exist between malformation and neoplasia. The same mutant gene which gives rise to an altered facies in the basal cell nevus syndrome also affects the growth stability of certain cells, allowing for nevi as a usual feature and basal cell carcinoma from such lesions as an occasional feature.

Finally, there would appear to be little value in persisting with the use of the term "phacomatoses" for some of the following conditions. The original "phacomatoses" — Sturge-Weber syndrome, tuberous sclerosis, and neurofibromatosis — may now be viewed as separable entities, clinically distinct from each other, with no apparent etiological relationship.

M. Hamartoses

62. STURGE-WEBER SYNDROME

Flat Facial Hemangiomata, Meningeal Hemangiomata with Seizures

ABNORMALITIES[1, 2]

Facial. Pink to purplish-red nonelevated cutaneous hemangiomata, most commonly in a trigeminal facial distribution, sometimes involving the choroid of the eye with secondary buphthalmos, glaucoma.

Meninges and Central Nervous System. Hemangiomata of arachnoid and pia, especially in occipital and temporal areas with secondary cerebral cortical atrophy, sclerosis, and "double-contour" convolutional calcification. Seizures, paresis, mental deficiency.

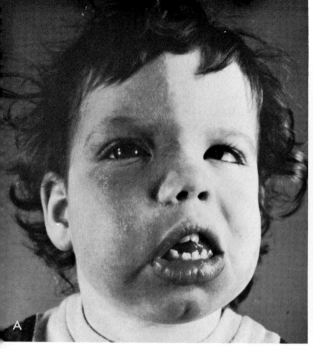
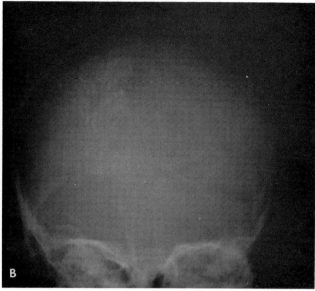

A, Affected child who has had grand mal seizures.
B, Note the fine mineralization (left), which tends to reflect the convolutional pattern of the brain.

OCCASIONAL ABNORMALITIES. Hemangiomatosis in nonfacial areas, central nervous system, other tissues. Cavernous hemangiomata. Colobomata of iris, coarctation, abnormal external ears.

NATURAL HISTORY. The surface cutaneous hemangiomata are usually present at birth and seldom progress. Seizures most commonly begin between two months and seven months of age and are grand mal in type, often asymmetrical. The degree of central nervous system involvement is variable, with 30 per cent having paresis and 56 per cent having seizures; not all patients are mentally deficient. Cerebral calcification is usually not evident by X-ray until latter infancy, the earliest being in a patient 13 months of age.

Medical anticonvulsant treatment is of limited value, and occasionally partial extirpation of affected meninges, brain tissue, or both may be merited in unilateral cases as a measure to control the seizures.

ETIOLOGY. Unknown. Sporadic, with rare exceptions. Occasionally other family members may have hemangiomata of a lesser degree.

REFERENCES

1. Chao, D. H.-C.: Congenital neurocutaneous syndromes of childhood. III. Sturge-Weber disease. J. Pediat., *55*:635, 1959.
2. Butterworth, T., and Strean, L. P.: Clinical Genodermatology. Baltimore, The Williams and Wilkins Co., 1962.

63. VON HIPPEL-LINDAU SYNDROME

Retinal Angiomata, Cerebellar Hemangioblastoma

Lindau,[1] in 1926, recognized this association of angiomatous retina (von Hippel's disease) and angiomatous tumors of the cerebellum and other parts of the central nervous system.

ABNORMALITIES
Eye. Angioma, often peripheral, with "beaded" artery leading into it and tortuous dilated vein from it.
Cerebellum. Hemangioblastoma, sometimes with cyst, most commonly in cortical area of cerebellum, occasionally in spinal cord or elsewhere in brain. May calcify.

OCCASIONAL ABNORMALITIES. Hemangiomata of face, adrenal, lung, liver; multiple cysts of pancreas, kidney; hypernephromata of kidney; pheochromocytoma.

NATURAL HISTORY. Retinal lesions usually not apparent till around 25 years of age with subsequent visual impairment. Cerebellar signs may appear in third decade.

ETIOLOGY. Autosomal dominant with varying expression.

REFERENCES

1. Lindau, A.: Studien über Kleinhirnsystem. Bon Pathogenese und Beziehungen zur Angiomatosis retinae. Acta Path. Microbiol. Scand. Suppl., *1*:1, 1926.
2. Christoferson, L. A., Gustafson, M. B., and Petersen, A. G.: Von Hippel-Lindau's disease. J.A.M.A., *178*:280, 1961.

64. RILEY'S SYNDROME

Macrocephaly, Pseudopapilledema, Hemangiomata

Riley and Smith[1] described this pattern of abnormality in a woman and four of her seven offspring in 1960. Pneumoencephalography disclosed no evidence of hydrocephalus.

ABNORMALITIES
Macrocephaly. The head circumference at birth was 40 and 41 cm. in two of the affected.
Pseudopapilledema.
Hemangiomata. Cutaneous and subcutaneous masses appearing from birth to five years of age.

Note: Three of the five affected individuals had repeated respiratory infections and X-ray evidence of pulmonary fibrosis.

ETIOLOGY. Presumed autosomal dominant.

REFERENCE

1. Riley, H. D., Jr., and Smith, W. R.: Macrocephaly, pseudopapilledema and multiple hemangiomata. A previously undescribed heredofamilial syndrome. Pediatrics, *26*:293, 1960.

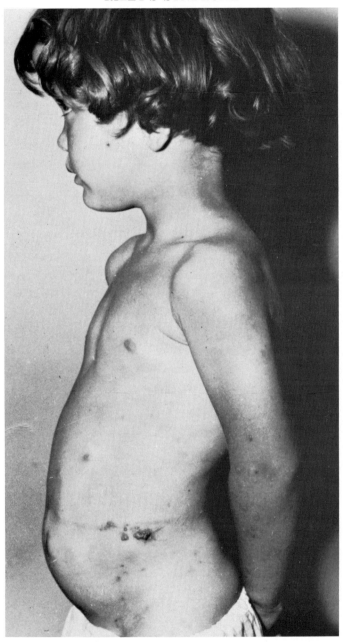

Five year old with 57 cm. head circumference (6 cm. above the mean for age) and brownish-purple skin nodules on abdominal wall. (From Riley, H. D., Jr., and Smith, W. R.: Pediatrics, *26*:293, 1960.)

65. MAFFUCCI'S SYNDROME

Cavernous Hemangiomata, Enchondromatosis

This association of hamartomata was noted by Maffucci in 1881, and subsequently in excess of 60 cases have been documented.

ABNORMALITIES
Hemangiomata. Often cavernous in type, tending to be in similar locale to bone lesions. Phlebectasia, phleboliths, or both may also be a feature.
Endchondromata. Nodular growths in metaphyseal or diaphyseal portion of long bones, sometimes phalanges, and occasionally mandible.

OCCASIONAL ABNORMALITIES
Tumors. Brain tumor, ovarian teratoma, lymphangioma, angiosarcoma, pancreatic adenocarcinoma.
Skin Pigment. Viteligo, areas of hyperpigmentation.

NATURAL HISTORY. The tumors usually become evident in childhood. The enchondromata may grow to a deforming size but are usually static after adolescence, although there is a 19 per cent incidence of chondrosarcoma.

ETIOLOGY. Unknown. All cases have been sporadic.

REFERENCES

1. Maffucci, A. D.: Un caso di encondroma ed angioma multiplo. Movimento Med.-Chir. (2), *3*:399, 1881.
2. Bean, W. B.: Dyschondroplasia and hemangiomata (Maffucci's syndrome. II.) Arch. Int. Med., *102*: 544, 1958.
3. Anderson, I. F.: Maffucci's syndrome. Report of a case with a review of the literature. S. Afr. Med. J., *39*:1066, 1965.

66. TUBEROUS SCLEROSIS

(Adenoma Sebaceum)

Hamartomatous Skin Nodules, Seizures, Phakomata, Bone Lesions

Von Recklinghausen is said to have described this disease over 100 years ago, but Bourneville[1] is usually given credit for its recognition in 1880. Hamartomatous lesions develop in many tissues, especially the skin and brain. About 0.5 per cent of severely mentally defective individuals have this condition.

ABNORMALITIES
Brain and Eye. Glioma-angioma lesions in cortex and white matter with seizures (93 per cent) and mental deficiency (62 per cent) as apparent consequences. Roentgenographic evidence of intracranial mineralization (51 per cent), most commonly in basal ganglia or adjacent area. Phakomata, similar retinal lesions, in 53 per cent.

Skin. Fibrous-angiomatous lesions (83 per cent), varying in color from flesh to pink to yellow to brown, develop in nasolabial fold, cheeks, and elsewhere. Areas of altered pigmentation.
Bone. Cyst-like areas in phalanges (66 per cent) and elsewhere, with areas of periosteal thickening, yielding X-ray evidence of "sclerosis," palpable irregularity, or both.
Kidney. Mixed rhabdomyomatous lesions at autopsy (80 per cent).

OCCASIONAL ABNORMALITIES. Other hamartomata: cutaneous fibromata (especially subungual), lipomata, angiomata, nevi, shagreen patches (goose-flesh-like). Rhabdomyomata and

(Text continued)

TUBEROUS SCLEROSIS

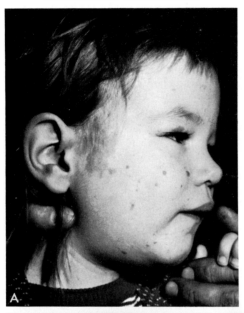

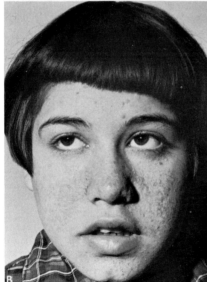

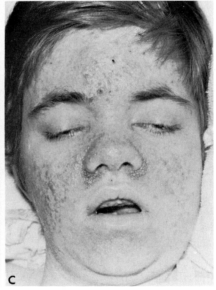

A, Two year old with early pink to red nodular and flat skin lesions and seizures.
B, Girl with mental deficiency and seizures.
C, Young woman with mental deficiency and seizures, on Dilantin therapy.
(B and C courtesy of L. Dobbs, Rainier State Training School, Washington.)

angiomata of heart, cystic changes in lung, hamartomata of liver and pancreas.

NATURAL HISTORY. Hamartomata usually become evident in early childhood and may increase at adolescence. Malignant transformation may occur, and about 6 per cent of patients develop a brain tumor. The seizures, which also tend to develop in early childhood, may initially be myoclonic and later grand mal in type and are difficult to control. EEG abnormality is found in 87 per cent of patients and may be of the grossly disorganized hypsarrhythmic pattern. The seizures and mental defect seem to be related to the extent of hamartomatous change in the brain. For those with mental deficiency 100 per cent have seizures, 88 per cent by five years of age, whereas of those without serious mental deficiency 69 per cent have seizures, 44 per cent by five years of age.

An unknown percentage of patients die prior to 20 years of age as the consequence of status epilepticus, general debility, pneumonia, or tumor. However, it should be appreciated that there is wide variability in expression of the disease; all patients with skin lesions do not develop seizures, mental deficiency, or both, and the earlier-noted pattern of abnormality is biased toward the more severe cases.

ETIOLOGY. Autosomal dominant with at least 25 to 50 per cent of cases representing a fresh mutation.

COMMENT. The reader will note that the term "adenoma sebaceum" is not utilized, and this is because the skin lesions do not directly involve the sebaceous glands. Actually the term tuberous sclerosis (potato-like sclerotic lesions) pertains only to the brain lesions and is a poor eponym for this disease. Such eponyms are indicative of the difficulty in applying descriptive names to these admixed hamartomatous areas of faulty tissue morphogenesis.

REFERENCES

1. Bourneville, D.: Sclereuse tubereuse des circonvolutions cerebrales. Idiote et epilepsie hemiplegique. Arch. Neurol. (Paris), *1*:81, 1880.
2. Bloom, D.: Cutaneous manifestations of systemic genetic diseases. New York J. Med., *63*:3070, 1963.
3. Lagos, J. C., and Gomez, M. R.: Tuberous sclerosis: reappraisal of a clinical entity. Mayo Clin. Proc., *42*:26, 1967.

M. Hamartoses

67. NEUROFIBROMATOSIS

Multiple Neurofibromata, Café au Lait Spots, with or Without Bone Lesions

Von Recklinghausen[1] described this disease in 1882. Crowe et al.[2] estimated the incidence at one in 3000 individuals.

ABNORMALITIES
Skin. Areas of hyper- or hypopigmentation with café au lait spots in 94 per cent, roughly three fourths of affected individuals having six or more spots measuring 1.5 cm. or greater in size, most commonly on trunk. Axillary "freckling" may occur.
Subcutaneous. Dysplastic tumors consisting of connective tissue, neurolemma cells, and/or mast cells; occurring along nerves, in subcutaneous tissues, and sometimes in eye and/or meninges.

OCCASIONAL ABNORMALITIES
Skeletal. Scoliosis, hypoplastic bowing of lower leg with pseudoarthrosis at birth, osseous lesions with localized osteosclerosis, rib fusion, spina bifida, absence of patella, dislocation of radius and ulna, local overgrowth, and scalloping of vertebral bodies with deformed pedicles.
Hamartomata. Cutaneous nevi, lipomata, angiomata.
Neurofibromata in kidney, stomach, heart, tongue.
Fibrosing alveolitis of lung.
Endocrine. Acromegaly, sexual precocity.
Other. Mental deficiency (10 per cent), seizures (12 per cent), syndactyly, glaucoma, corneal opacity.

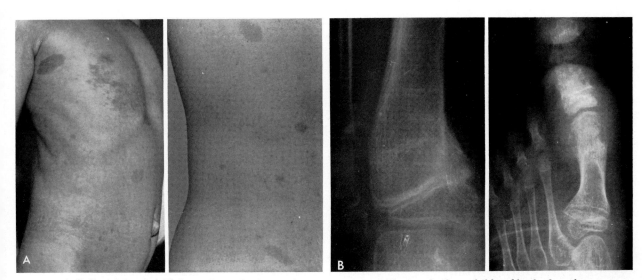

A, Café au lait, ovaloid, irregular and minute pigmentary spots on the trunk of one child and back of another.
B, Pseudofracture of distal tibia and fibula. Hypertrophy of toe, in relation to the hamartomatous process in that area.

NATURAL HISTORY. Often evident in early childhood; 47 per cent of patients develop some neurologic impairment, sometimes secondary to nerve compression as with blindness due to optic nerve pressure. Malignant change occurs in 5 to 10 per cent of cases, most commonly in males.

ETIOLOGY. Autosomal dominant with high penetrance but wide variability in expression. About 50 per cent of patients have a fresh gene mutation, and Crowe et al.[2] calculated the mutation rate per gamete per generation to be 1×10^{-4}, the highest known for the human.

REFERENCES

1. Von Recklinghausen, F.: Ueber die multiplen Fibroma der Haut und ihre Beziehung zu den multiplen Neuromen. Berlin, A. Hirschwald, 1882.
2. Crowe, F. W., Schull, W. J., and Neel, J. V.: Multiple Neurofibromatosis. American Lecture Series No. 281. Springfield, Ill., Charles C Thomas, 1952.
3. Canale, D., Bebin, J., and Knighton, R. S.: Neurologic manifestations of von Recklinghausen's disease of the nervous system. Confin. Neurol., *24*:359, 1964.

163

68. McCUNE-ALBRIGHT SYNDROME

(Osteitis Fibrosa Cystica)

Polyostotic Fibrous Dysplasia, Irregular Skin Pigmentation, Sexual Precocity

McCune[1] and Albright et al.[2] described this condition in 1935 and 1936 respectively. More than 100 cases have been reported. The relative frequency of diagnosis in females vs. males is 3 : 2.

ABNORMALITIES
Bone. Multiple areas of fibrous dysplasia, most commonly in long bones and pelvis; may also include facial bones causing facial asymmetry. May result in deformity, increased thickness of bone, or both.

Skin. Irregular brown pigmentation, most commonly over sacrum, buttocks, upper spine; unilateral in about 50 per cent of cases.

Endocrine. Precocious menarche in female, occasional sexual precocity in male. Occasional instances of basophilic adenoma, acromegaly, hyperthyroidism, hypercalcemia, diabetes mellitus.

NATURAL HISTORY. The pigmentation is usually evident in infancy, and the bone dysplasia may progress during childhood, resulting in deformity, fracture, or both, most commonly in the upper femur. Thickening of bone in the calvarium can lead to cranial nerve compression with such serious consequences as blindness or deafness. The sexual precocity in the female is often unusual in character, with menstruation prior to breast or pubic hair development. The accelerated maturation coincident with sexual precocity may result in early attainment of full stature such that adult height can be relatively short.

ETIOLOGY. The cases have been sporadic occurrences in the families, and the etiology is undetermined.

REFERENCES

1. McCune, D. J.: Osteitis fibrosa cystica. Am. J. Dis. Children, *52*:745, 1936.
2. Albright, F., Butler, A. M., Hampton, A. O., and Smith, P.: Syndrome characterized by osteitis fibrosa disseminata, areas of pigmentation and endocrine dysfunction, with precocious puberty in females. Report of five cases. New England J. Med., *216*:727, 1937.
3. Arlien-Soborg, U., Iversen, T.: Albright's syndrome. A brief survey and report of a case in a seven year old girl. Acta Paediat., *45*:558, 1956.

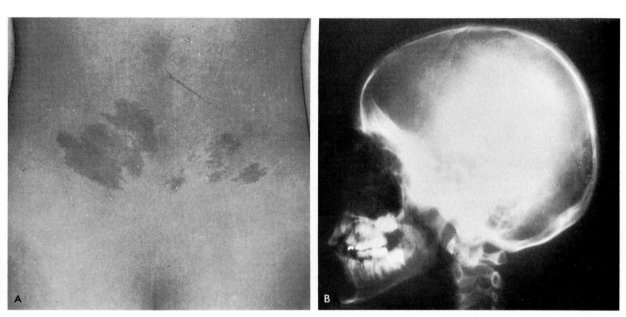

A, Irregular café au lait pigmentation over lower back. *B*, Dense thick bone at the base of the skull. From an older girl who had her menarche at the age of four and one half years.

69. PEUTZ-JEGHERS SYNDROME

Mucocutaneous Pigmentation, Benign Intestinal Polyposis

In 1896 Hutchinson[1] described the pigmentary changes in an individual who later died with intussusception. Peutz[2] clearly set forth the disease in 1921, and Jeghers et al.[3] further established this disease entity in 1949. More than 180 cases have been documented.

ABNORMALITIES

Pigmentation. Vertical bands of epidermal pigment presenting as blue-gray or brownish spots in lips, buccal mucous membrane, perioral area, and sometimes digits and elsewhere.

Polyposis. Hamartomatous benign polyps in jejunum, sometimes in other mucous secreting intestinal mucosa, and occasionally in nasopharynx, bladder, bronchial mucosa.

Other Tumors. Rare (three cases) granulosa cell tumor of ovary.

NATURAL HISTORY.

The pigmentary spots appear from infancy through early childhood and tend to fade in the adult. Seventy per cent of patients have some gastrointestinal problem by age 20 years, most commonly colicky abdominal pain (60 per cent), intestinal bleeding (25 per cent), or both. Intussusception, which may spontaneously recede, is the most serious complication, and iron deficiency anemia may result from chronic blood loss. There is no apparent danger of malignant transformation in the polyps, even though histological evaluation of a polyp may suggest a malignancy. Clubbing of the fingers may occasionally occur in this disease.

ETIOLOGY. Autosomal dominant with a high degree of penetrance.

REFERENCES

1. Hutchinson, J.: Pigmentation of the lips and mouth. Arch. Surg., 7:290, 1896.
2. Peutz, J. L. A.: Very remarkable case of familial polyposis of mucous membrane of intestinal tract and nasopharynx accompanied by peculiar pigmentation of skin and mucous membrane. Nederl. Maanschr. Geneesk., *10*:134, 1921.
3. Jeghers, H., McKusick, V. A., and Katz, K. H.: Generalized intestinal polyposis and melanin spots of the oral mucosa, lips and digits. A syndrome of diagnostic significance. New England J. Med., *241*:993, 1949.
4. Bartholomew, L. G., Moore, C. E., Dahlin, D. C., and Waugh, J. M.: Intestinal polyposis associated with mucocutaneous pigmentation. Surg. Gynec. Obstet., *115*:1, 1962.

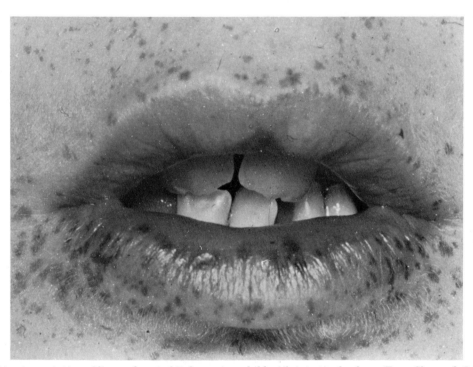

Spotty pigmentation of lips and periorbital area in a child with intestinal polyps. (From Sheward, J. D.: Brit. Med. J., *1*:921, 1962.)

70. GARDNER'S SYNDROME

Polyposis of Colon, Epidermal Cysts, Osteomas

Gardner and Richards[1] set forth a complete evaluation of this disease in 1953. The hamartomatous lesions generally do not become evident until latter childhood.

ABNORMALITIES
Intestine. Adenomatous polyps of colon, rectum, and occasionally stomach and small intestine.
Skin. Epidermal inclusion and/or sebaceous cysts, especially on back, scalp, face. Sometimes fibromas, invasive desmoid, or both.
Bone. Osteomata of calvarium, mandible, face, elsewhere, leading to bone deformation, cortical thickening.

OCCASIONAL ABNORMALITIES.
Other hamartomata, including odontoma, leiomyoma, lipoma, trichoepithelioma, neurofibroma, thyroid carcinoma. Scoliosis.

NATURAL HISTORY.
Hamartomata usually become evident between ten and 20 years of age; thereafter there is grave danger of malignant change in the colonic adenomata, at least 45 per cent of individuals developing carcinoma. The risk is of sufficient magnitude to warrant prophylactic colectomy. Mesenteric fibromatosis and severe adhesions represent potential postoperative problems.

ETIOLOGY.
Autosomal dominant with high degree of penetrance.

REFERENCES

1. Gardner, E. J., and Richards, R. C.: Multiple cutaneous and subcutaneous lesions occurring simultaneously with herditary polyposis and osteomatosis. Am. J. Human Genet., 5:139, 1953.
2. Weary, P. E., Linthicum, A., Cawley, E. P., Coleman, C. C., and Graham, G. F.: Gardner's syndrome. A family group study and review. Arch. Derm., 90:20, 1964.

71. BASAL CELL NEVUS (CARCINOMA) SYNDROME

Basal Cell Nevi, Broad Facies, Rib Anomalies

Though this condition had been previously described, it was not until 1951 that the broad extent of this pattern of altered morphogenesis was set forth by Binkley and Johnson.[1] Subsequently more than 150 cases have been reported.[2, 3]

ABNORMALITIES
Performance. Mild mental deficiency, aberrant behavior.
Craniofacial. Frontoparietal bossing.
  Broad face, mild prognathism.
Dental. Odontogenic cysts of mandible, occasionally maxilla.
  Misshapen and/or carious teeth.
Hands. Short metacarpals, especially the fourth.
Thorax. Ribs bifid, synostotic, and/or partially missing.
Skin. Basal cell nevi over neck, upper arms, trunk and face, prone to become carcinomata. Punctate minute pits on palms and soles. Milia, especially facial.
Ectopic Calcification. Falx cerebri, falx cerebellum.
Ovary. Development of calcified ovarian fibroma.

OCCASIONAL ABNORMALITIES.
Internal strabismus, cataract, coloboma of iris, glaucoma, chalazion, inner canthal folds, hypertelorism;

BASAL CELL NEVUS SYNDROME

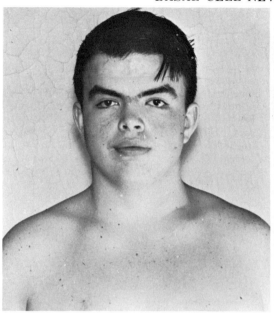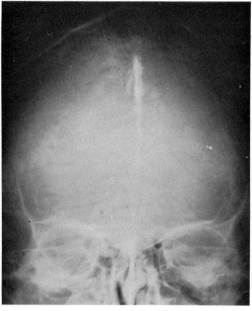

Fifteen year old. Note mineralization in falx cerebri. (From Ferrier, P. E., and Hinrichs, W. L.: Am. J. Dis. Children, *113*:538, 1967.)

bony bridging of sella turcica, scoliosis, cervical and/or thoracic vertebral fusion, arachnodactyly; hydrocephalus, small genitalia, hypogonadism, cryptorchidism. Medulloblastoma, fibromas, lipomas or neurofibromas of skin.

NATURAL HISTORY. The basal cell nevi nodules gradually appear during childhood with increase at adolescence. On the face the nevi may be papillomatous and are likely to occur around the lids. Malignant change is particularly likely after the second decade. The jaw cysts enlarge, especially in latter childhood, and may recur following curettage. A constant vigil must be maintained for malignant transformation of the nevi or other tumors that are a common feature of this syndrome.

ETIOLOGY. Autosomal dominant, full penetrance.

REFERENCES

1. Binkley, G. W., and Johnson, H. H., Jr.: Epithelioma adenoides cysticum: Basal cell nevi, agenesis of the corpus callosum and dental cysts. A clinical and autopsy study. Arch. Derm., *63*:73, 1951.
2. Gorlin, R. J., Vickers, R. A., Kellen, E., and Williamson, J. J.: The multiple basal-cell nevi syndrome. An analysis of a syndrome consisting of multiple nevoid basal-cell carcinoma, jaw cysts, skeletal anomalies, medulloblastoma, and hyporesponsiveness to parathormone. Cancer, *18*:89, 1965.
3. Ferrier, P. E., and Hinrichs, W. L.: Basal-cell carcinoma syndrome. Am. J. Dis. Children, *113*:538, 1967.

169

72. GOLTZ'S SYNDROME

Poikiloderma with Focal Dermal Hypoplasia, Syndactyly, Dental Anomalies

This mesoectodermal disorder was well recognized as a concise entity by Goltz et al.[1] in 1962, although well described cases had been reported prior to that time. At least 17 cases have been documented.

ABNORMALITIES[1-5]

Skin. Linear areas of hypoplasia with altered pigmentation, telangiectasis, lipomatous nodules projecting through localized areas of skin atrophy.

Angiofibromatous nodules around lips and anus.

Nails. Dystrophic nails, narrow and/or hypoplastic.

Teeth. Hypoplasia of teeth, enamel hypoplasia, late eruption, and/or irregular placement.

Extremities. Syndactylism of fingers and/or toes, especially third and fourth fingers.

Eyes. Strabismus, coloboma, and/or microphthalmos.

OCCASIONAL ABNORMALITIES. Moderate short stature, joint hypermotility, mental retardation, microcephaly, bulbar angiofibroma of eye, partial alopecia, congenital heart defects, hernia, skeletal asymmetry, scoliosis, hypoplasia or aplasia of clavicle, failure of pubic bone fusion, polydactyly, adactyly, hypoplasia of digit, cleft hand.

NATURAL HISTORY. The skin lesions are usually present at birth, although the skin lipomata and the lip and anal papillomata may develop later. No effective therapy is known except plastic surgery for the syndactyly and removal of papillomata when indicated.

ETIOLOGY. Wodniansky[4] reported partial expression in the mother and sibling of a patient. All other cases have been sporadic. Only one affected male has been reported. The present hypothesis is that this is a single gene effect, usually lethal in the male, and most cases represent fresh mutations, a similar situation to incontinentia pigmenti. There are many similarities between incontinentia pigmenti and Goltz's syndrome, and it is tempting to consider the possibility that both diseases represent genetic alterations of a similar system.

REFERENCES

1. Goltz, R. W., Peterson, W. C., Gorlin, R. J., and Ravits, H. G.: Focal dermal hypoplasia. Arch. Derm., *86*:708, 1962.
2. Gorlin, R. J., Meskin, L. H., Peterson, W. C., and Goltz, R. W.: Focal dermal hypoplasia syndrome. Acta Dermatovener., *43*:421, 1963.
3. Holden, J. D., and Akers, W. A.: Goltz's syndrome: focal dermal hypoplasia. A combined mesoectodermal dysplasia. Am. J. Dis. Children, *114*:292, 1967.
4. Wodniansky, P.: Über die Formen der congenitalen Poikilodermie. Arch. Klin. Exper. Derm., *205*: 331, 1957.
5. Jenner, M.: Naeviforme, Poikilodermie—artige Hautveränderungen mit Missbildungen (Schwimmhautbildungen an den Fingern, Papillome am Anus). 2 bl. Hautkr., *27*:468, 1928.

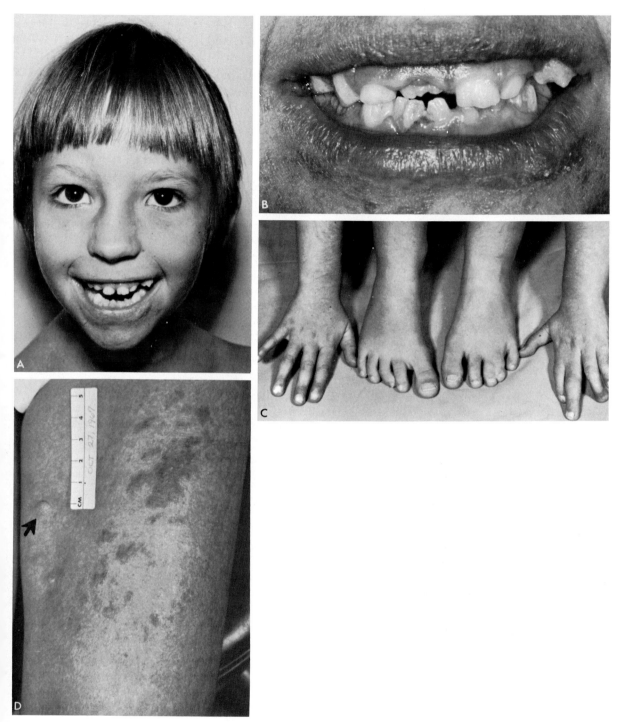

A, Eleven year old girl.

B, Late eruption of teeth with dental hypoplasia and malformation.

C, Note the syndactyly of the left hand and foot.

D, Thigh, showing irregular areas of altered pigmentation and of fatty herniation through loci of focal dermal hypoplasia (arrow).

73. INCONTINENTIA PIGMENTI

Irregular Pigmented Skin Lesions with or Without Dental Anomaly, Patchy Alopecia

Bardach[1] originally described the condition in twin sisters in 1925, and soon thereafter Bloch[2] set forth the term incontinentia pigmenti to depict the unusual skin lesions. More than 200 cases have been described, of which less than 5 per cent have been males.

ABNORMALITIES

Skin. Most consistent feature. Vesiculation, verrucous changes, atrophy, irregular gray-brown pigmentation in fleck, whorl or spidery form, especially on trunk and extremities.

Teeth. Thirty per cent have hypodontia, delayed eruption, and/or conical form.

Hair. Twenty per cent have atrophic patchy alopecia.

Central Nervous System. About one third have mental deficiency, microcephaly, spasticity, and/or seizures.

Eye. About 20 per cent have strabismus, retinal dysplasia, uveitis, keratitis, cataract, retrolental dysplasia, and/or blue sclerae.

Osseous. About 20 per cent have hemivertebrae, extra rib, syndactyly, hemiatrophy, and/or short arms and legs.

OCCASIONAL ABNORMALITIES.
Nail dystrophy, breast hypoplasia, short stature.

NATURAL HISTORY.
Skin lesions are generally present in early infancy and tend to progress from inflammatory or vesicular to pigmented and may fade in childhood. General eosinophilia is often present in infancy and the vesicles contain eosinophils. About half the patients show other features, the most serious being the central nervous system abnormalities.

ETIOLOGY.
Family studies indicate the effect of a single mutant gene, most likely a lethal in affected males because the ratio of females to males in affected sibships is 2 : 1 with half the females affected. Whether the gene is autosomal or X-linked remains to be determined.

COMMENT.
Palmgren,[4] who cultured herpes simplex virus from the vesicular fluid of a patient, has raised the question of whether this viral agent may contribute to the expression of this genetically determined disease.

REFERENCES

1. Bardach, M.: Systematisierte Naevusbildungen bei einem cineiigen Zwillingspaar. Ein Beitrag zur Naevusätiologie. Z. Kinder., *39*:542, 1925.
2. Bloch, B.: Eigentümliche bisher nicht beschreibene Pigmentaffektion (Incontinentia pigmenti). Schweiz. Med. Wschr., *56*:404, 1926.
3. Carney, R. G.: Incontinentia pigmenti. A report of five cases and review of the literature. Arch. Dermat. Syph., *64*:126, 1951.
4. Palmgren, B.: The relationship of dermatitis herpetiformis to incontinentia pigmenti in newborn infants. Pediatrics, *29*:295, 1962.

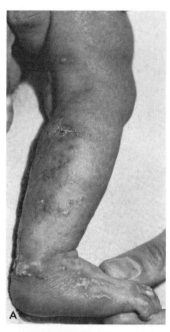
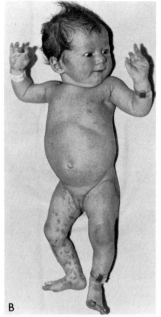
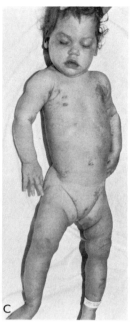

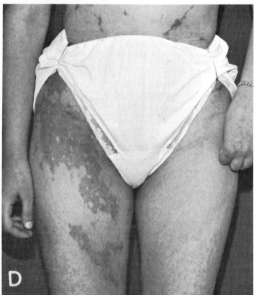

A, Early lesions in the young infant shown in B.

C, Older mentally deficient infant with reticular pigmentation.

D, Mentally deficient woman with spasticity and pseudogliomatous retinal detachment, showing advanced skin pigmentary change.

E, Minor abnormalities of dentition in an affected girl.

(A to E courtesy of J. M. Opitz, University of Wisconsin.)

F, Reticular pigmentation in a three year old mentally deficient girl.

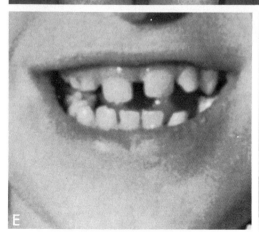
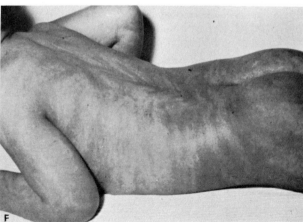

173

74. DYSKERATOSIS CONGENITA SYNDROME

Hyperpigmentation of Skin, Leukoplakia, Nail Dystrophy, Pancytopenia

Cole originally described this condition in 1930 and recently summarized the findings. Only 13 cases have been reported.[1-3]

ABNORMALITIES. Although hyperpigmentation of the skin may be present from birth, most of the abnormalities become apparent between five and 15 years of age. Growth deficit is mentioned, but poorly documented.

Skin. Irregular reticular brownish-gray pigmentation with patchy atrophic areas of hypopigmentation.

Hyperkeratosis and hyperhidrosis of palms and soles.

May have bullae, telangiectasis.

Mucous Membranes. Premalignant leukoplakia may be found on lips, mouth, anus, urethra, conjunctiva.

Eyes. Blepharitis, ectropion, and nasolacrimal obstruction with excessive tearing.

Nails. Dystrophy which may progress to absence of nail.

Teeth. Carious, malaligned.

Hair. Tends to be sparse and fine, occasionally premature graying.

Hematological. Pancytopenia.

Bone. Coarse trabeculation (osteoporosis?) is mentioned, possibly with relative fragility.

Gonad. Testicular hypoplasia.

Other. Partial stenosis of esophagus with dysphagia.

Mental deficiency was noted in two cases.

Hepatic cirrhosis has been detected in at least two cases.

NATURAL HISTORY. The problem in affected tissues tends to become more severe with age, and most patients die before the fourth decade as a consequence of either pancytopenia or malig-

nant transformation in mucous membranes. When present, leukoplakic lesions should be excised as representing premalignant change.

ETIOLOGY. Autosomal recessive determination is implied by a 50 per cent incidence of parental consanguinity and occurrence of affected siblings in three families. Only two of the 13 patients have been females, a finding which is presently unexplained.

COMMENT. The dermatological term dyskeratosis congenita obviously depicts only one feature of this abiotrophic type of disease with hamartomatous features in which the affected individual develop hypoplasia and dysplasia in the skin, mucous membranes, marrow, and other tissues. The sibling of one patient and the niece of another patient died of leukemia, the latter case raising the question of whether there may be an increased likelihood of leukemia in the heterozygote carrying this mutant gene.

Considering the total pattern of abnormality, dyskeratosis congenita is clearly a different entity from Fanconi's syndrome of pancytopenia with congenital malformations.

REFERENCES

1. Cole, H. N., Cole, H. N., Jr., and Lascheid, W. P.: Dyskeratosis congenita. Relationship to poikiloderma atrophicans vasculare and to aplastic anemia of Fanconi. Arch. Derm., 76:712, 1957.
2. Georgouras, K.: Dyskeratosis congenita. Aust. J. Derm., 8:36, 1965.
3. Addison, J., and Rice, M. S.: The association of dyskeratosis congenita and Fanconi's anemia. Med. J. Aust., 1:797, 1965.

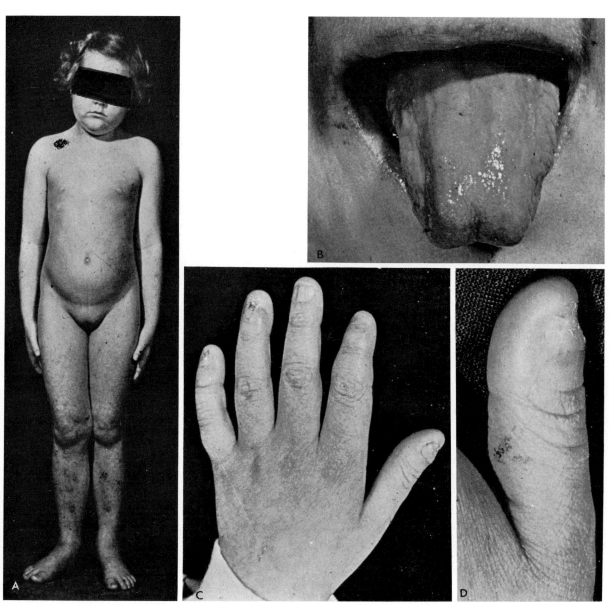

Eight year old patient showing reticulated skin pigmentation (A), smooth tongue without leukoplakia as yet (B), and nail hypoplasia to aplasia (C and D). (Courtesy of K. Georgouras, Sydney, Australia.)

75. ROTHMUND SYNDROME

(Poikiloderma Congenita)

Development of Poikiloderma, Cataract with or Without Other Ectodermal Dysplasia

This condition was first described in 1868 by Rothmund,[1] a Munich ophthalmologist, who discovered multiple cases among an inbred group of people living in the nearby Alps. Over 25 cases have been reported.

ABNORMALITIES. Wide variance in expression, the most usual features being the following:

Skin. Irregular erythema progressing to telangiectasia, scarring, irregular pigmentation and depigmentation, atrophy.

Eyes. Juvenile zonular cataract, occasionally corneal dystrophy.

OCCASIONAL ABNORMALITIES

Skeletal. Small stature, small hands and feet, osteoporosis and/or areas of cystic or sclerotic change.

Facial. Small saddle nose.

Teeth. Microdontia and occasional anodontia.

Nails. Small, dystrophic.

Hair. Sparse, prematurely gray; occasionally alopecia.

Other Skin. Hyperkeratosis of palms and soles.

Other. Mental deficiency, hypogenitalism.

NATURAL HISTORY. Changes in the skin are usually evident between three months and one year of age, and the progression toward irregular "marbled" hypoplasia, termed poikiloderma, is mainly noted in the first few years.

Cataract most commonly becomes evident between two and seven years of age, and the principal problems for affected individuals are skin difficulties, sometimes photosensitivity; visual impairment requiring surgical intervention; and physical appearance, depending on the extent to which stature, hair, teeth, and/or nails are affected.

ETIOLOGY. Autosomal recessive with 70 per cent of affected individuals being female, an unexplained disparity which might not be of significance because the number of reported cases is small.

REFERENCES

1. Rothmund, A.: Ueber Cataracten in Verbindung mit einer eigenthümlichen Hautdegeneration. Arch. Ophth., *14*:159, 1868.
2. Rook, A., Davis, R., and Stevanovic, D.: Poikiloderma congenitale. Rothmund-Thomson Syndrome. Acta Dermatovener., *39*:392, 1959.
3. Francois, J.: Syndromes with congenital cataract. Trans. Am. Acad. Ophth. Otolaryng., *64*:433, 1960.
4. Braun, W., and Unger, C.: Zur Frage des Rothmund-Thomson-Syndromes. Dermat. Wochens., *151*: 1189, 1965.
5. Silver, H. K.: Rothmund-Thomson syndrome: an oculocutaneous disorder. Am. J. Dis. Children, *111*:182, 1966.

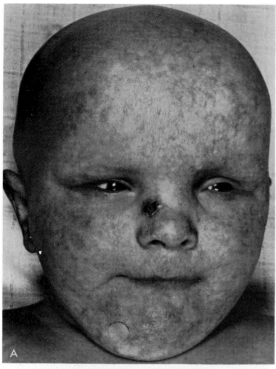

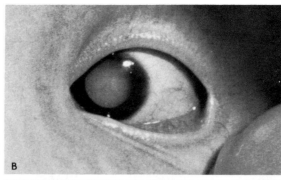

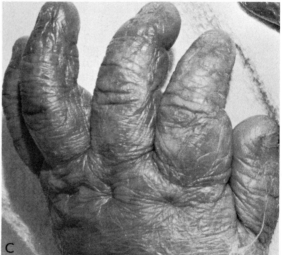

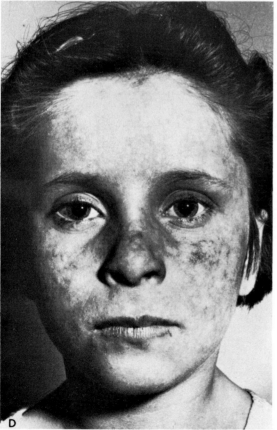

A, Fifteen month old. (From Braun, W., and Unger, C.: Dermat. Wochens., *151*:1189, 1965.)

B, Two and one half year old. Note absence of lashes and mature cataract.

C, Patient shown in *B.* Note severe nail dysplasia. (*B* and *C* from Wahl, J. W., et al.: Am. J. Ophth., *60*:722, 1965).

D, Five year old. (From Rook, A. J., et al.: Acta Dermatovener, *39*:392, 1959.)

76. HYPOHIDROTIC ECTODERMAL DYSPLASIA

Defect in Sweating, Alopecia, Hypodontia

Thurman[1] described this entity in 1848. In 1875, Charles Darwin[2] set forth the following concise commentary about this disease: "I may give an analogous case, communicated to me by Mr. W. Wedderhorn of a Hindoo family in Scinde, in which ten men, in the course of four generations, were furnished, in both jaws taken together, with only four small and weak incisor teeth and with eight posterior molars. The men thus affected have very little hair on the body, and became bald early in life. They also suffer much during hot weather from excessive dryness of the skin. It is remarkable that no instance has occurred of a daughter being thus affected." In 1929, Weech[3] clearly separated this condition from other clinical problems having ectodermal dysplasia as a feature. Over 130 cases had been reported by 1956.

ABNORMALITIES

Skin. Thin and hypoplastic with decreased pigment and tendency toward papular changes on face and thin, wrinkled eyelids.

Skin Appendages. Hair: fine, dry, and hypochromic; sparse to absent.

Sweat glands: hypoplasia to absence of eccrine glands, apocrine glands more normally represented.

Sebaceous glands: hypoplasia to absence.

Mucous Membranes. Hypoplasia with absence of mucous glands in oral and nasal membranes. Mucous glands may also be absent from bronchial mucosa.

Teeth. Hypodontia to adontia. Anterior teeth tend to be conical in shape.

Craniofacial. Low nasal bridge, small nose with hypoplastic alae nasi, full forehead, prominent supraorbital ridges. Prominent lips.

OCCASIONAL ABNORMALITIES.

Hoarse voice, hypoplasia to absence of mammary glands and/or nipples, absence of tears, mild to moderate nail dystrophy, eczematous change in skin, asthmatic symptoms.

NATURAL HISTORY.

Hyperthermia as a consequence of inadequate sweating is not only a serious threat to life, but may be the cause of mental deficiency, which is an occasional feature of this disease. Living in a cool climate and cooling by water when overheated are important measures. The hypoplasia of mucous membranes plus thin nares may require frequent irrigation of the nares to limit the severity of purulent rhinitis. Otitis media and lung infection may also be consequences of the mucous membrane defect. Early roentgen evaluation may reveal the extent of dental deficit, and artificial dentures are usually necessary. Though often hairless at birth, some hair may develop. For cosmetic purposes a wig may merit consideration.

ETIOLOGY.

X-linked. Previous reports indicated that about 10 per cent of presumed heterozygous females show some overt expression. Utilizing direct visualization of dermal ridge sweat pores, Frias and Smith[7] noted a diminished frequency of sweat pores in five of six heterozygous mothers of affected males, the latter having an absence of sweat pores. Therefore the majority of heterozygous females show some expression for the disease.

COMMENT.

This disease can usually be readily distinguished from other disorders having features of ectodermal dysplasia on the basis of the defect of sweat glands, craniofacial anomaly (when expressed), and the lesser likelihood of concomitant nail dystrophy in hypohidrotic ectodermal dysplasia.

REFERENCES

1. Thurman, J.: Two cases in which the skin, hair and teeth were very imperfectly developed. Medico-Chir. Trans., *31*:71, 1848.
2. Darwin, C.: The Variations of Animals and Plants under Domestication. 2nd ed. London, John Murray, 1875.
3. Weech, A. A.: Hereditary ectodermal dysplasia (congenital ectodermal defect). A report of two cases. Am. J. Dis. Children, *37*:766, 1929.
4. Felsher, Z.: Hereditary ectodermal dysplasia. Report of a case, with experimental study. Arch. Dermat. Syph., *49*:410, 1944.
5. Perabo, F., Velasco, J. A., and Prader, A.: Ektodermale Dysplasie vom anhidrotischen Typus Fünf neue Beobachtungen. Helvet. Paediat. Acta, *11*:604, 1956.
6. Lowry, R. B., Robinson, G. C., and Miller, J. R.: Hereditary ectodermal dysplasia. Symptoms, inheritance patterns, differential diagnosis, management. Clin. Pediat., *5*:395, 1966.
7. Frias, J. L., and Smith, D. W.: Diminished sweat pores in hypohidrotic ectodermal dysplasia: A new method for assessment. J. Pediat., *72*:606, 1968.

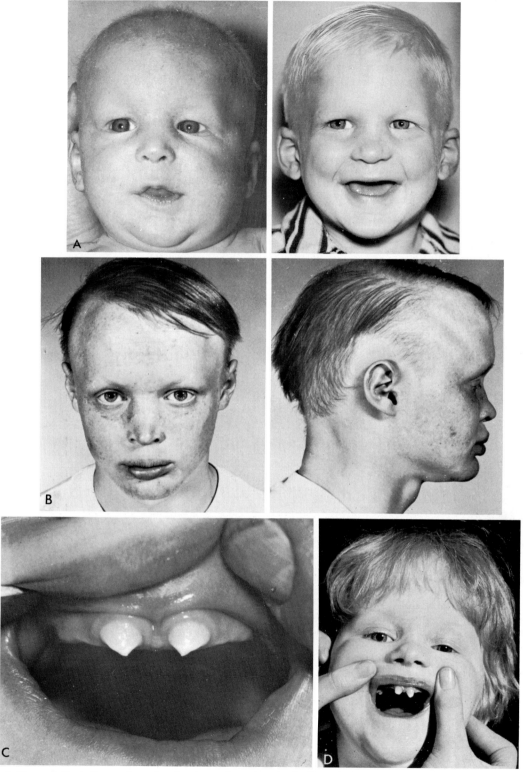

A, Young infant; diagnosis made after hyperthermic episode. Same boy at two years of age.

B, Older boy. The hypoplasia of the skin contributes to the prominent appearance of the lips. Note the mid-facial hypoplasia.

C, Hypoplasia of alveolar ridge in two year old. Hypoplastic conical incisors.

D, Partial expression in a female.

179

77. MARSHALL'S TYPE OF ECTODERMAL DYSPLASIA

Mid-Facial Hypoplasia, Cataract, Deafness

In 1958 Marshall[1] described seven family members in three generations with a specific type of ectodermal dysplasia.

ABNORMALITIES
Facies.   Low nasal bridge with short depressed nose.

Hypoplasia of maxilla and prominent upper teeth.

Thick lips.

Teeth.   Mild deformity.

Eyes.   Congenital or juvenile cataracts, myopia.

Hearing.   Partial deafness (about 50 per cent deficit).

Sweat Glands.   Mild hypohidrosis (about 25 per cent deficit).

NATURAL HISTORY. The cataracts may spontaneously resorb, leading to glaucoma and/or lens dislocation. The mild degree of hypohidrosis generally does not constitute a problem.

ETIOLOGY.   Apparently autosomal dominant.

REFERENCE

1. Marshall, D.: Ectodermal dysplasia. Report of kindred with ocular abnormalities and hearing defect. Am. J. Ophth., 45:143, 1958. (N.B., This is in the supplement to the April issue.)

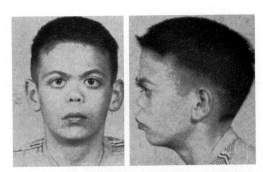

Thirteen year old. (From Marshall, D.: Am. J. Ophth., 45:143, 1958.)

78. ROBINSON-TYPE ECTODERMAL DYSPLASIA

Peg-Shaped Teeth, Nail Dystrophy, Deafness

Robinson et al.[1] described five affected individuals in three generations of a family.

ABNORMALITIES. May have:
Teeth. Pegged shape, partial anodontia.
Nails. Hypoplasia, dystrophy.
Hearing. Moderate sensorineural deafness.

OCCASIONAL ABNORMALITIES. Syndactyly, polydactyly. Note: some of the patients had elevated values for sweat electrolytes.

ETIOLOGY. Autosomal dominant.

REFERENCE

1. Robinson, G. C., Miller, J. R., and Bensimon, J. R.: Familial ectodermal dysplasia with sensorineural deafness and other anomalies. Pediatrics, *30*:797, 1962.

79. FEINMESSER-TYPE ECTODERMAL DYSPLASIA

Deafness and Nail Dystrophy

In 1961 Feinmesser and Zelig[1] described this condition in two siblings of consanguineous parentage.

ABNORMALITIES
Nails. Rudimentary.
Hearing. Nerve deafness.

ETIOLOGY. ? Autosomal recessive.

REFERENCE

1. Feinmesser, M., and Zelig, S.: Congenital deafness with onychodystrophy. Arch. Otolaryng., 74:507, 1961.

80. PILI TORTI AND DEAFNESS

Björnstad[1] noted the association of twisted hair (pili torti) and sensorineural deafness in 1965, five of eight patients with the hair anomaly having deafness from an early age. Further cases have been recognized subsequently. The hair is grooved and flattened at irregular intervals, twisted, and breaks off with ease. The hearing loss, apparently due to cochlear defect, may be profound, and Björnstad noted a relationship between the degree of hair anomaly and the severity of deafness. The family data suggest an autosomal recessive mode of inheritance for this disorder.

REFERENCES

1. Björnstad, R.: Pili torti and sensori-neural loss of hearing. Proceedings, 17th Meeting, Northern Dermatological Society. Copenhagen, May, 1965.
2. Robinson, G. C., and Johnson, M. M.: Pili torti and sensorineural hearing loss. J. Pediat., *70*:621, 1967.

81. CLOUSTON-TYPE ECTODERMAL DYSPLASIA

Nail Dystrophy, Dyskeratotic Palms and Soles, Hair Hypoplasia

Clouston in 1939 described 119 individuals in a French-Canadian family, and over 200 instances have been reported.

ABNORMALITIES. Most usual features:
Skin. Thick dyskeratotic palms and soles. Hyperpigmentation over knuckles, elbows, axillae, areolae, and pubic area.
Hair. Hypoplasia to alopecia (61 per cent).
Nails. Hypoplasia to aplasia, dysplasia.
Eyes. Strabismus.

OCCASIONAL ABNORMALITIES. Cataract, dull mentality, short stature.

ETIOLOGY. Autosomal dominant.

REFERENCES

1. Clouston, H. R.: The major forms of hereditary ectodermal dysplasia (with an autopsy and biopsies on the anhidrotic type). Canad. Med. Assn. J., *40*:1, 1939.
2. Wilkey, W. D., and Stevenson, G. H.: A family with inherited ectodermal dystrophy. Canad. Med. Assn. J., *53*:226, 1945.
3. Joachim, H.: Hereditary dystrophy of the hair and nails in six generations. Ann. Int. Med., *10*:400, 1936.

82. BASAN-TYPE ECTODERMAL DYSPLASIA

Skin Hypoplasia — Nail Dystrophy

Basan[1] described this condition in a family in 1965.

ABNORMALITIES
Skin. Hypoplasia with smooth palms and soles.
Nails. Thin and fragile.
Other. Simian creases.

ETIOLOGY. Autosomal dominant.

REFERENCE

1. Basan, M.: Ektodermale Dysplasie. Fehlendes Papillarmuster, Nagelveränderungen und Vierfingerfurche. Arch. Klin. Exp. Derm., *222*:546, 1965.

83. ENAMEL HYPOPLASIA AND CURLY HAIR

Enamel Hypoplasia, Curly Hair, with or Without Nail Dystrophy

Robinson, Miller, and Worth[1] described this dominantly inherited condition in six family members in 1966.

ABNORMALITIES
Teeth. Severe enamel hypoplasia, microdontia.
Hair. Dry, thick, and tightly curled.

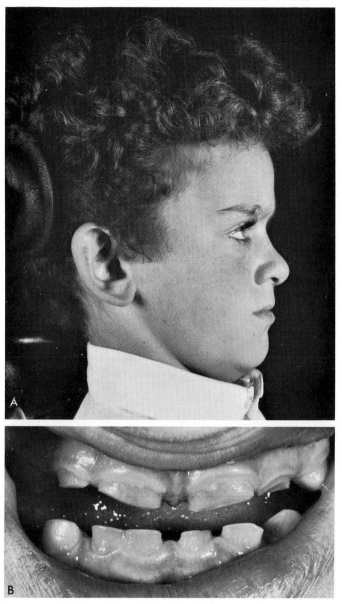

A and *B,* Eleven year old boy. (From Robinson, G. C., et al.: Pediatrics, *37*:498, 1966.)

Nails. Variable flatness, peeling, and fragility.

NATURAL HISTORY. The teeth tend to become worn down, dental abscesses are frequent, and most patients require dentures by adult age.

ETIOLOGY. Apparently autosomal dominant.

REFERENCE

1. Robinson, G. C., Miller, J. R., and Worth, H. M.: Hereditary enamel hypoplasia. Its association with characteristic hair structure. Pediatrics, *37*:498, 1966.

84. PACHYONYCHIA CONGENITA

Thick Nails, Hyperkeratosis, Foot Blisters

Pachyonychia congenita is an ectodermal dysplasia described by Jadassohn and Lewandowsky[1] in which there is excessive keratin and occasionally extra teeth.

ABNORMALITIES

Nail. Progressive thickening of anterior half.

Skin. Patchy to complete hyperkeratosis of palms and soles, callosities of feet which blister easily, and keratosis pilaris with tiny cutaneous horny excrescences.

Epidermal cysts filled with loose keratin on face, neck, and upper chest.

Mucous Membranes. Leukokeratosis of mouth and tongue.

Teeth. Erupted teeth at birth, lost by four to six months.

OCCASIONAL ABNORMALITIES.
Corneal thickening, cataracts, thickening of tympanic membrane, hyperhidrosis. Hair dry and sparse. Osteomata, intestinal diverticuli.

NATURAL HISTORY.
The complications are obvious. Usually the nails are grossly thickened by one year of age. Complete surgical removal of the nails is sometimes merited, although any matrix left behind will reform abnormal nails.

ETIOLOGY.
Autosomal dominant, with wide variability in expression. Predominantly found in Slavs and Jews of Slavonic origin. The basic mechanism of the disease is unknown; however, vacuolization of the cytoplasm of nail matrix cells may be of significance.

REFERENCES

1. Jadassohn, J., and Lewandowsky, F.: Pachyonychia congenita, keratosis disseminata circumscripta (folliculosis): tylomata; leukokeratosis linguae. Ikonographia Dermatologica, Tab., *6*:29, 1906.
2. Joseph, H. L.: Pachyonychia congenita. Arch. Derm., *90*:594, 1964.
3. Soderquist, N. A., and Reed, W. B.: Pachyonychia congenita with epidermal cysts and other congenital dyskeratoses. Arch. Derm., *97*:31, 1968.
4. Butterworth, T., and Strean, L. P.: Clinical Genodermatology. Baltimore, Williams and Wilkins Co., 1962, p. 64.

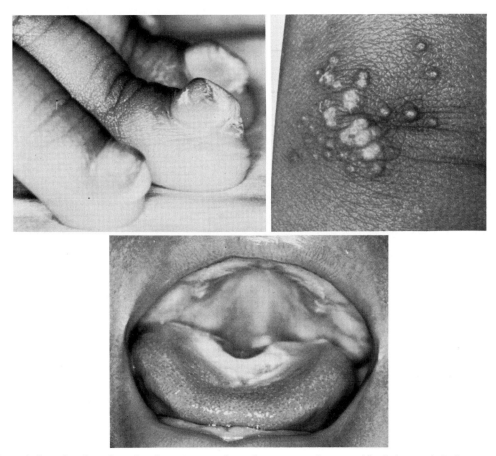

Negro infant showing altered nails, cutaneous hyperkeratoses at knee, and leukokeratotic lesions on tongue and lateral palate.

85. ACHONDROPLASIA

Short Limbs, Low Nasal Bridge, Caudal Narrowing of Spinal Canal

The most common chondrodysplasia, true achondroplasia occurs with a frequency of about one in 10,000.

ABNORMALITIES
Growth. Small stature.
Craniofacial. Megacephaly, small foramen magnum.
   Short cranial base with early spheno-occipital closure.
   Low nasal bridge with prominent forehead.
   Mild mid-facial hypoplasia with narrow nasal passages.
Skeletal. Small cuboid shaped vertebral bodies with short pedicles and progressive narrowing of lumbar interpedicular distance.
   Lumbar lordosis, mild thoracolumbar kyphosis with anterior beaking of first and/or second lumbar vertebrae.
   Small iliac wings with narrow greater sciatic notch.
   Short tubular bones, metaphyseal flare with ball and socket arrangement of epiphysis to metaphysis.
   Short trident hand, fingers being similar in length, with short proximal and mid-phalanges.
   Short femoral neck, incomplete extension of elbow.
Other. Mild hypotonia. Early motor progress is often slow, although eventual intelligence is usually normal.

OCCASIONAL COMPLICATIONS. Hydrocephalus secondary to a narrow foramen magnum may occur, as may cord compression secondary to bony compression or later disc herniation.

NATURAL HISTORY. The physician should be alert to detect any neurological complications due to bony or disc compression. Osteoarthritis is not a usual feature in the adult.

ETIOLOGY. Autosomal dominant, about 90 per cent of the cases representing a fresh mutation. Older paternal age has been a contributing factor in the fresh achondroplasia mutations, which have been estimated to occur once per 12,000 births.[5]

COMMENT. Histologic evaluation at the epiphyseal line discloses shorter cartilage columns which lack the usual linear arrangement, and some cartilage cells appear to be undergoing a mucinoid degeneration.

REFERENCES

1. Caffey, J.: Pediatric X-Ray Diagnosis. 5th ed. Chicago, Year Book Medical Publishers, 1967, p. 819.
2. Maroteaux, P., and Lamy, M.: Achondroplasia in man and animals. Clin. Orthoped., *33*:91, 1964.
3. Shepard, T. H., and Graham, B.: The congenitally malformed. XIII. Achondroplastic dwarfism; diagnosis and management. Northwest Med., *66*: 451, 1967.
•4. Cohen, M. E., Rosenthal, A. D., and Matson, D. D.: Neurological abnormalities in achondroplastic children. J. Pediat., *71*:367, 1967.
5. Mörch, E. T.: Achondroplasia is always hereditary and is inherited dominantly. J. Hered., *31*:439, 1940.

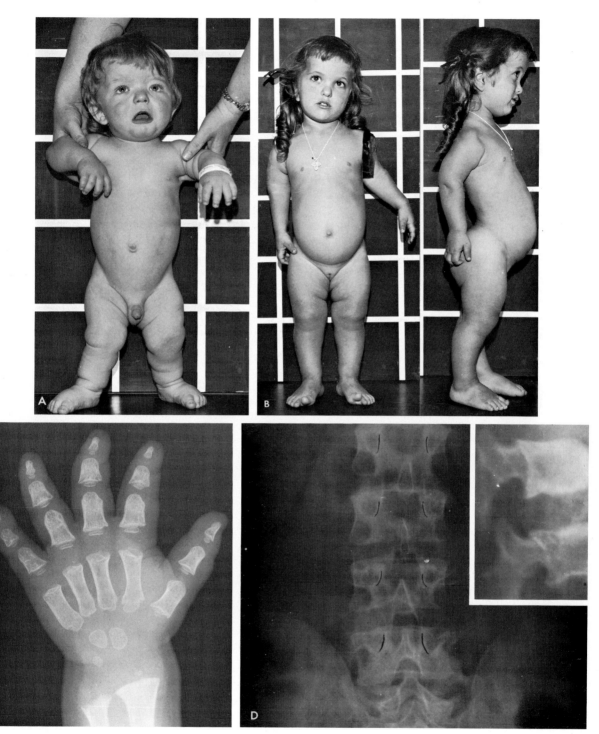

A, One year old with height age of four months. (From Smith, D. W.: J. Pediat., *70*:504, 1967.)
B, Four year old with height age of 20 months.
C, Short "trident" hand with short metacarpals and phalanges.
D, Caudal narrowing of spinal canal (pedicles marked) with short pedicles (upper right).

86. METATROPHIC DWARFISM

Small Thorax, Thoracic Kyphoscoliosis, Metaphyseal Flaring

Maroteaux, Spranger, and Wiedemann[1] set this entity forth with five cases of their own and 12 unrecognized cases from the literature.

ABNORMALITIES.[1]   Small stature, severe.
Skeletal.   Early platyspondyly with progressive kyphosis and scoliosis evident in infancy.
Narrow thorax with short ribs.
Short limbs with metaphyseal flaring and epiphyseal irregularity with hyperplastic trochanters.
Small malformed pelvis.
Partial flexion at knee and hip.

NATURAL HISTORY.   Often evident at birth, the vertebral changes are severe during infancy.

ETIOLOGY.   ? Autosomal recessive.

REFERENCES

1. Maroteaux, P., Spranger, J., and Wiedemann, H. R.: Der metatropische Zwergwuchs. Arch. Kinderh., *173*:211, 1966.
2. Fleury, J., de Menibus, C. H., and Hazard, E.: Un cas singulier de dystrophie ostéo-chondrale congénitale (nanisme métatropique de Maroteaux). Ann. Pédiat., *13*:453, 1966.

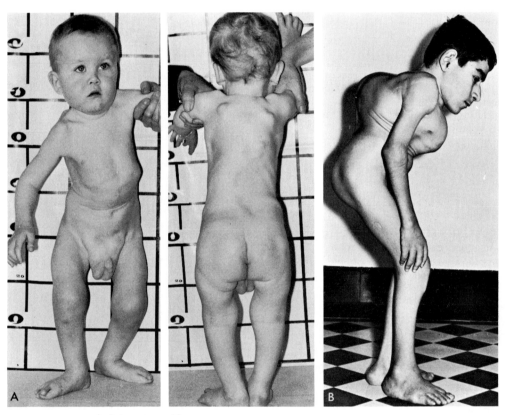

A, A two year old.
B, A 16 year old.
(Courtesy of P. Maroteaux, Hopital des Enfants-Malades, Paris.)

189

87. THORACIC ASPHYXIANT DYSTROPHY

(Jeune's Syndrome, Infantile Thoracic Dystrophy)

Small Thorax, Postnatal Onset of Short Limbs, Limited Elbow Extension

Described by Jeune et al.[1] in 1955, this disorder usually leads to early death as a consequence of the small thorax. More than 20 cases have been reported.

ABNORMALITIES
Growth. Small stature.
Skeletal. Short ribs with irregular costochondral juncture and small thoracic cage.

Irregular epiphyses and metaphyses with relatively short limbs.

Ulnae and fibulae relatively short, limited elbow extension.

Iliac wings hypoplastic.

OCCASIONAL ABNORMALITIES.
Polydactyly, notching of distal end of metacarpal and metatarsal bones, lacunar skull, chronic nephritis.

NATURAL HISTORY.
Early death is usually the consequence of asphyxia with or without pneumonia. Those who survive usually have progressive improvement in the relative growth of the thoracic cage and may have only mild to moderate shortness of stature. Chronic nephritis is a potential feature of the syndrome.

Autopsy has revealed disordered growth at the costochondral juncture with hyperplastic proliferating cartilage and poor progression of enchondral mineralization.

ETIOLOGY.
Presumed autosomal recessive.

REFERENCES

1. Jeune, M., Beraud, C., and Carron, R.: Dystrophie thoracique asphyxiante de caractère familial. Arch. Franç. Pédiat., *12*:886, 1955.
2. Pirnar, T., and Neuhauser, E. B. D.: Asphyxiating thoracic dystrophy of the newborn. Am. J. Roentgenol., *98*:358, 1966.
3. Hanissian, A. S., Riggs, W. W., and Thomas, D. A.: Infantile thoracic dystrophy—a variant of Ellis-van Creveld syndrome. J. Pediat., *71*:855, 1967.

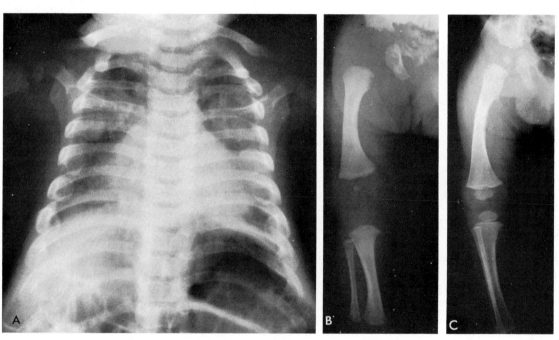

A, Four month old. Note short ribs, high position of clavicles.

B and *C,* Right lower extremity at one month and ten months of age showing improvement in long bones and pelvis, though fibula remains relatively short.

(From Hanissian, A. S., et al.: J. Pediat., *71*:855, 1967.)

88. ELLIS-VAN CREVELD SYNDROME

(Chondroectodermal Dysplasia)

Short Distal Extremities, Polydactyly, Nail Hypoplasia

Ellis and van Creveld[1] set forth this entity in 1940. About 40 cases were reported by 1964 when McKusick et al.[2] added 52 cases from an inbred Amish population.

ABNORMALITIES

Growth. Small stature of prenatal onset.

Skeletal. Disproportionate irregularly short extremities.

Polydactyly of fingers, occasionally of toes.

Fusion of hamate and capitate.

Small thorax.

Hypoplasia of upper lateral tibia with knock knee.

Nails. Hypoplastic.

Teeth. Neonatal teeth, partial anodontia, small teeth, and/or delayed eruption.

Mouth. Short upper lip bound by frenula to alveolar ridge, defects in alveolar ridge with accessory frenula.

Cardiac. About one half of patients have a cardiac defect, most commonly a septal defect.

OCCASIONAL ABNORMALITIES.
Mental retardation, scant or fine hair, cryptorchidism, epispadias, talipes equinovalgus.

NATURAL HISTORY. About half the patients die in early infancy as a consequence of cardiorespiratory problems. The majority of survivors are of normal intelligence. Eventual stature is in the range of 43 to 60 inches. There is usually some limitation in hand function such as inability to form a clenched fist. Dental problems are frequent.

ETIOLOGY. Autosomal recessive.

REFERENCES

1. Ellis, R. W. B., and van Creveld, S.: A syndrome characterized by ectodermal dysplasia, polydactyly, chondro-dysplasia and congenital morbus cordis. Report of three cases. Arch. Dis. Childhood, *15*:65, 1940.
2. McKusick, V. A., Egeland, J. A., Eldridge, R., and Krusen, D. E.: Dwarfism in the Amish. The Ellis-van Creveld syndrome. Bull. Hopkins Hosp., *115*:306, 1964.
3. Feingold, M., Jankoski, J., Johnson, C., Darling, D. B., Kreidberg, M. B., Wilson, D., Cohen, M. M., and Gellis, S. S.: Ellis-van Creveld syndrome. Clin. Pediat., *5*:431, 1966.

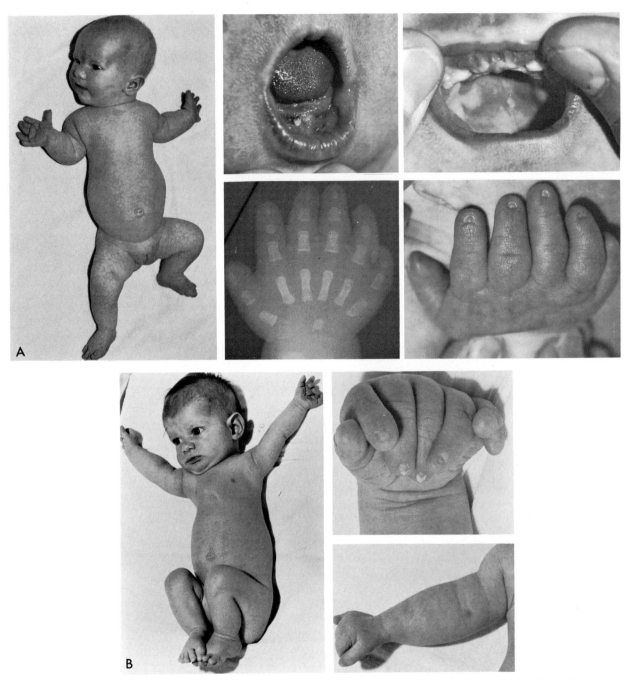

A, Six week old. Note the hypoplasia of the alveolar ridge with frenula and an aberrant tooth. The patient is now doing well at several years of age.

B, Five month old. Note the small thorax. The patient expired as a consequence of a congenital heart defect plus the small thorax. (Courtesy of Professor H. Willi, Kantonsspital, Zurich.)

89. DIASTROPHIC NANISM*

Short Tubular Bones (Especially First Metacarpal), Joint Limitation with Club Foot, and Hypertrophied Auricular Cartilage

The 1960 report of Lamy and Maroteaux[1] concerning three cases of their own and 11 similar cases from the literature established this pattern of malformation as a distinct entity. It is now being recognized with increasing frequency.

ABNORMALITIES
Growth. Short stature of prenatal onset.
Limbs. Varus club foot plus limitation of flexion at proximal phalangeal joints and of extension at elbow, with or without dislocation of hip or knee with weight bearing.

Tubular bones short and thick with development of broad metaphyses and flattened irregular epiphyses that are late in mineralizing. First metacarpal unduly small with proximal thumb.
Spine. Development of scoliosis with or without kyphosis.
Pinna. Soft cystic masses in auricle develop into hypertrophic cartilage.

OCCASIONAL ABNORMALITIES. Thick pectinate strands at root of iris, cleft palate (one fourth), micrognathia, lateral displacement of patellae, subluxation of cervical vertebrae, hyperelasticity of skin, cryptorchidism.

NATURAL HISTORY. Two affected infants with cleft palate and micrognathia, similar in this respect to those with the Pierre Robin malformation, died of respiratory obstruction.[5] Reports of affected young infants have been too few

to indicate the frequency of this complication. General health is usually good and the patients have normal intelligence. Unfortunately the varus club foot and the scoliosis that develop have been rather resistant to corrective orthopedic measures and the functional problem is augmented by the limitation in joint motility. When present, the unusual defect of hypertrophied auricular cartilage may eventually give way to ossification.

ETIOLOGY. Autosomal recessive. The lack of consanguinity suggests that this syndrome may not be extremely rare.

COMMENT. Diastrophic dwarfism can readily be distinguished from other chondrodystrophies and from arthrogryposis multiplex congenita by physical examination alone.

REFERENCES

1. Lamy, M., and Maroteaux, P.: Le nanisme diastrophique. Presse Méd., *68*:1977, 1960.
2. Stover, C. N., Hayes, J. T., and Holt, J. F.: Diastrophic dwarfism. Am. J. Roentgenol., *89*:914, 1963.
3. Rubin, P.: Dynamic Classification of Bone Dysplasias. Chicago, Year Book Medical Publishers, 1964, p. 410.
4. Langer, L. O.: Diastrophic dwarfism in early infancy. Am. J. Roentgenol., *93*:399, 1965.
5. Salle, B., Picot, C., Vauzelle, J. L., Deffrenne, P., Monnet, P., Francois, R., and Robert, J. M.: Le nanisme diastrophique. À propos de trois observations chez le nouveau-né. Pédiatrie, *21*:311, 1966.

*Diastrophic = crooked; nanism = small stature.

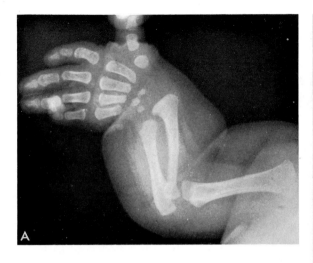

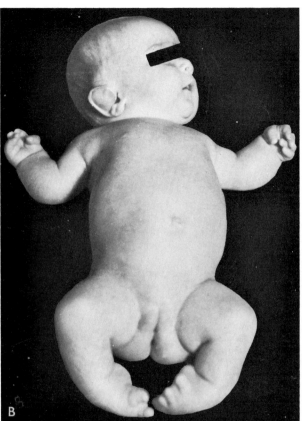

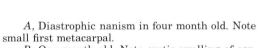

A, Diastrophic nanism in four month old. Note small first metacarpal.

B, One month old. Note cystic swelling of ear. (From Langer, L. O.: Am. J. Radiol., *93*:399, 1965.)

C, Twenty one month old. Note hypertrophy of ear and position of thumbs. (From Smith, D. W.: J. Pediat., *70*:502, 1967.)

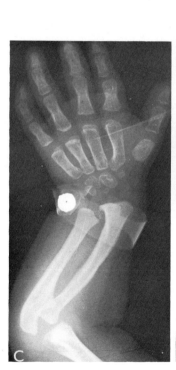

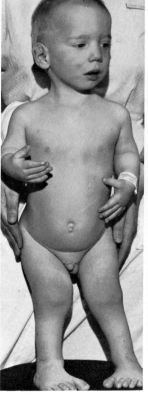

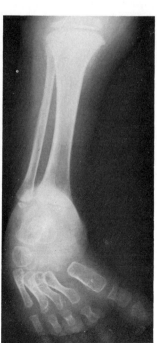

195

90. PSEUDOACHONDROPLASTIC FORM OF SPONDYLOEPIPHYSEAL DYSPLASIA

Small Irregular Epiphyses, Irregular Mushroomed Metaphyses, Flattening and/or Anterior Beaking of Vertebrae, with Normal Craniofacial Appearance

Maroteaux and Lamy[1] described three individuals with this pattern of altered bone morphogenesis in 1963, and subsequently at least four additional cases have been published.[2-4]

ABNORMALITIES

Growth. Apparently postnatal onset of growth deficiency.

Metaphyses. Irregular, mushroomed.

Epiphyses. Small, irregular or "fragmented."

Diaphyses. Short, bowing, especially in lower extremities.

Vertebrae. Variable degrees of flattening, anterior tongue shaped, and short pedicles. Lumbar lordosis and kyphosis.

Ribs. Tend to be spatulate.

OCCASIONAL ABNORMALITIES.
Pelvis: short sacroiliac notch, flaring of iliac crests.

NATURAL HISTORY.
The patients have been described as "normal" at birth, with small size and waddling gait becoming evident between six months and four years of age and final height attainment in the range of 3 to 3½ feet. Bowed lower extremities with waddling gait and scoliosis are the principal orthopedic problems, and there may be some limitation in joint motility. Intelligence is normal.

ETIOLOGY.
Apparently autosomal dominant, Ford et al.[2] having reported a father and his two affected offspring. Most of the cases have been sporadic and presumably represent fresh mutations.

COMMENT.
The postnatal onset and normal craniofacial appearance readily differentiate this entity from true achondroplasia.

REFERENCES

1. Maroteaux, P., and Lamy, M.: Les formes pseudo-achondroplasiques des dysplasies spondylo-épiphysaires. Presse Méd., 67:383, 1959.
2. Ford, N., Silverman, F. N., and Kozlowski, K.: Spondylo-epiphyseal dysplasia (pseudoachondroplastic type). Am. J. Roentgenol., 86:462, 1961.
3. Rubin, P.: Achondroplasia versus pseudoachondroplasia. Radiol. Clin. North America, 1:621, 1963.
4. Lindseth, R. E., Danigelis, J. A., Murray, D. G., and Wray, J. B.: Spondylo-epiphyseal dysplasia (pseudoachondroplastic type). Case report with pathologic and metabolic investigations. Am. J. Dis. Children, 113:721, 1967.

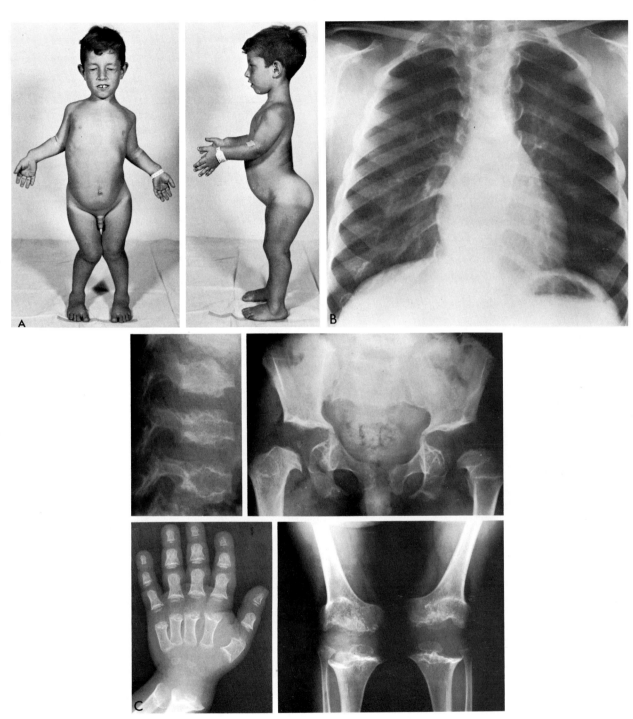

A, Eight year old with height age of three years.

B, Mildly spatulate ribs; scoliosis.

C, Flattened irregular vertebral bodies, hypoplastic abnormal iliac wings, and short tubular bones with irregular "ball-in-socket" epiphyses in relation to metaphyses.

(From Lindseth, R. E., et al.: Am. J. Dis. Children, *113*:721, 1967.)

91. X-LINKED SPONDYLOEPIPHYSEAL DYSPLASIA

Flattened Vertebrae of Mid-Childhood, Small Iliac Wings, Short Femoral Neck

This disorder was recognized in 1939 by Jacobsen.[1]

ABNORMALITIES. Onset between five and ten years of age.
Growth. Short stature; final height, 52 to 62 inches.
Spine. Flattened vertebrae with central hump. Kyphosis, mild scoliosis.
Pelvis. Small iliac wings.
Limbs. Short femoral neck.
Mild epiphyseal irregularity with flattening of femoral head.
Joints. Eventual hip pain and stiffness, back pain.

ETIOLOGY. X-linked recessive.

REFERENCES

1. Jacobsen, A. W.: Hereditary osteochondrodystrophia deformans. A family with twenty members affected in five generations. J.A.M.A., *113*:121, 1939.
2. Maroteaux, P., Lamy, M., and Bernard, J.: La dysplasie spondylo-epiphysaire tardive. Description clinique et radiologique. Presse Méd., *65*:1205, 1957.
3. Langer, L. O.: Spondyloepiphyseal dysplasia tarda. Hereditary chondrodysplasia with characteristic vertebral configuration in the adult. Radiology, *82*:833, 1964.

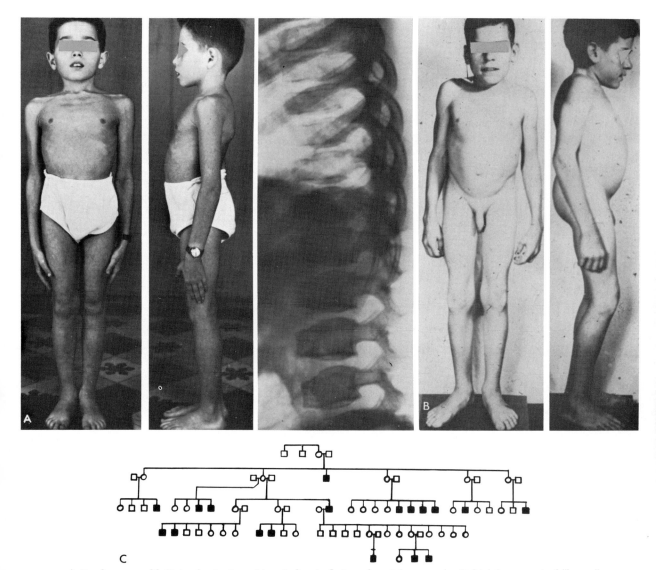

A, Twelve year old. Note shortening of trunk due to flattened vertebrae, each of which has a central "hump" in the area of its epiphyses. (Courtesy of P. Maroteaux, Hospital for Sick Infants, Paris.)

B, Fifteen year old. (From Jacobsen, A. W.: J.A.M.A., *113*:121, 1939.)

C, Pedigree of which patient shown in B is a member, showing evidence of X-linked recessive inheritance. (Courtesy of R. Bannaman, Buffalo General Hospital.)

199

92. MULTIPLE EPIPHYSEAL DYSPLASIA

Small Irregular Epiphyses, Pain and Stiffness in Hips, Short Stature

This condition was described by Fairbank[1] in 1947 and is often difficult to diagnose with assurance.

ABNORMALITIES
Growth. Mild to moderate shortness of stature.

Limbs. Late ossifying, small, irregular, mottled epiphyses with eventual osteoarthritis in many large joints, especially in hips. Short femoral neck.

Mild metaphyseal flare.

Shortness of metacarpals and phalanges.

Spine. Blunted, slightly ovaloid vertebral bodies.

NATURAL HISTORY. Pain and stiffness in joints, particularly the hips, may be a complaint as early as five years, but usually not until 30 to 35 years.

ETIOLOGY. Autosomal dominant with wide variability in expression.

REFERENCES

1. Fairbank, T.: Dysplasia epiphysealis multiplex. Brit. J. Surg., *34*:225, 1947.
2. Maudsley, R. H.: Dysplasia epiphysialis multiplex. A report of fourteen cases in three families. J. Bone Joint Surg., *37B*:228, 1955.
3. Hoefnagel, D., Sycamore, L, K., Russell, S. W., and Bucknall, W. E.: Hereditary multiple epiphysial dysplasia. Ann. Human Genet., *30*:201, 1967.

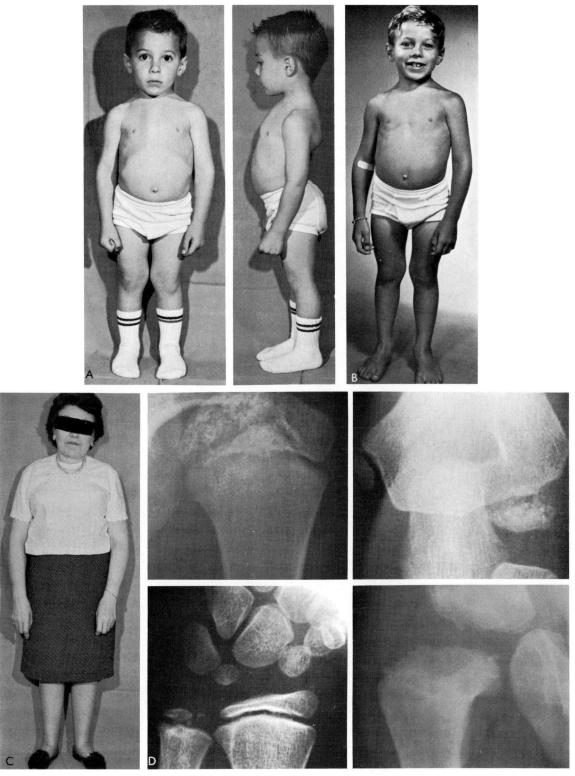

A, Five year old with height age of two and one half years. Patient had occasional aching in legs.

B, Same patient at eight and one half years; height age, four and one half years. He now has ankle and hip discomfort.

C, Affected mother of patient shown in *A* and *B*. She is short of stature and has hip discomfort.

D, Late and irregular mineralization of epiphyses which may be small or aberrant in shape, or both.

201

93. METAPHYSEAL DYSOSTOSIS, JANSEN-TYPE

Wide Irregular Metaphyses, Flexion Joint Deformity, Small Thorax

Since Jansen[1] described this severe type of metaphyseal dysostosis, only a few similar cases have been recorded, as reviewed by Rubin.[2]

ABNORMALITIES

Growth. Severe short stature.

Facies. Small, immature in appearance, with prominent eyes.

Skeletal and Joint. Gross irregular cyst-like areas due to lack of metaphyseal ossification.

Pelvis similarly affected.

Small thoracic cage.

Flexion deformities of joints, especially at knee and hip, yielding a squatting stance.

NATURAL HISTORY. Evident at birth or in early infancy. The defective growth and joint dysfunction are severe. Mental deficiency is mentioned, but not well documented.

REFERENCES

1. Jansen, M.: Über atypische Chondrodystrophie (Achondroplasie) und über eine noch nicht beschriebene angeborne Wachstrumsstörung des Knochensystems: Metaphysäre Dysostosis. 2. Orthop. Chir., *61*:253, 1934.
2. Rubin, P.: Dynamic Classification of Bone Dysplasias. Chicago, Year Book Medical Publishers, 1964, p. 207.

94. METAPHYSEAL DYSOSTOSIS, SCHMID-TYPE

Since the initial description by Schmid[1] in 1949, several large pedigrees of affected individuals have been reported.[2, 3]

ABNORMALITIES

Growth. Mild to moderate shortness of stature.

Skeletal. Splaying of broad irregular metaphyses.

Tibial bowing, especially at ankle.

Waddling gait with coxa vara.

Flare to lower rib cage.

Mild limitation in full extension of fingers.

NATURAL HISTORY. Pain in legs during childhood. Symptomatic and radiographic improvement beginning as early as three years of age with orthopedic measures only indicated for unusual degrees of deformity.

ETIOLOGY. Autosomal dominant with variable expression. Biopsy discloses cartilage hypoplasia.

REFERENCES

1. Schmid, F.: Beitrag zur Dysostosis Enchondralis Metaphysaria. Monats. Kinderh., *97*:393, 1949.
2. Stickler, G. B., Maher, F. T., Hunt, J. C., Burke, E. C., and Rosevear, J. W.: Familial bone disease resembling rickets (hereditary metaphysial dysostosis). Pediatrics, *29*:996, 1962.
3. Rosenbloom, A. L., and Smith, D. W.: The natural history of metaphyseal dysostosis. J. Pediat., *66*:857, 1965.

METAPHYSEAL DYSOSTOSIS, SCHMID-TYPE

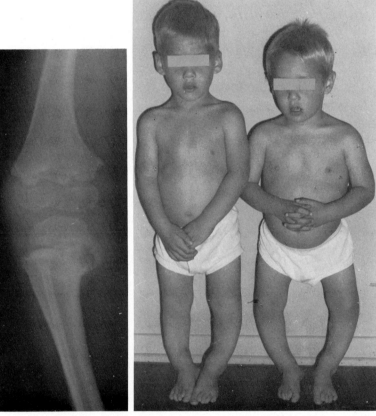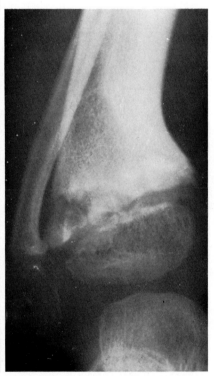

Affected brothers showing bowing of legs, mild changes in thorax, and metaphyseal alterations. (From Rosenbloom, A. L., and Smith, D. W.: J. Pediat., *66*:857, 1965.)

95. CARTILAGE-HAIR HYPOPLASIA

Mild Bowing of Legs, Wide Irregular Metaphyses, Fine Sparse Hair

Discovered by McKusick et al.[1] among an inbred Amish population, this condition has subsequently been detected in non-Amish individuals.

ABNORMALITIES
Growth. Small stature; adult height, 42 to 58 inches.

Skeletal. Irregular scalloped metaphyses. Relatively short limbs, mild bowing of legs.

Short tibia in relation to fibula.

Short hands, fingernails, toenails.

Decreased height of vertebrae.

Incomplete extension of elbow.

Mild flaring of lower rib cage with prominent sternum.

Lumbar lordosis, small pelvic inlet.

Hair. Fine, sparse, light, relatively fragile.

Other. Loose jointed "limp" hands and feet.

Intestinal malabsorption in early childhood.

OCCASIONAL ABNORMALITIES. Severe or fatal response to varicella.

NATURAL HISTORY. The early history is often indicative of an intestinal malabsorption problem, which tends to improve with time. Biopsy of the metaphyseal area reveals diminished cartilage cells forming poorly organized columns.

ETIOLOGY. Autosomal recessive.

REFERENCE

1. McKusick, V. A., Eldridge, R., Hostetler, J. A., Ruangwit, U., and Egeland, J. A.: Dwarfism in the Amish. II. Cartilage-hair hypoplasia. Bull. Hopkins Hosp., *116*:285, 1965.

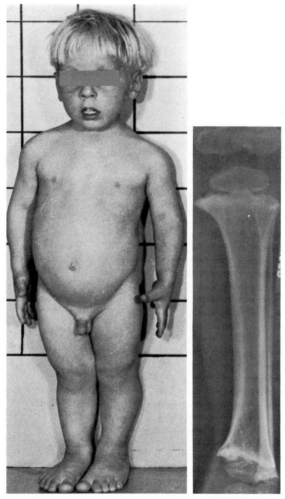

Five and one half year old; height age, 18 months. (From McKusick, V. A., et al.: Bull. Hopkins Hosp., *116*:285, 1965.)

O. Osteochondrodysplasias

96. X-LINKED HYPOPHOSPHATEMIC RICKETS

(Vitamin D Resistant Rickets)

Hypophosphatemia; Rickets, Unresponsive to Usual Dosage of Vitamin D

ABNORMALITIES[1-4]
Metabolic. Hypophosphatemia with diminished renal tubular reabsorption of phosphorus, questionably diminished absorption of phosphorus and calcium from the gastrointestinal tract, and diminished rate of new bone formation.[2] Roentgen evidence of rickets, unresponsive to physiological amounts of vitamin D.

Skeletal. Rickets. Bowing of lower limbs with weight bearing, slow growth, shortness of stature, waddling gait, coxa vara.

OCCASIONAL ABNORMALITIES
Dental.[3] Large pulp chamber with enamel hypoplasia.
 Gingival and periapical infection.
 Delayed eruption of dentition.

Skeletal. Craniosynostosis, dolichocephaly, scoliosis, pseudo-fractures, bony protuberances at the site of major muscle attachments in the adult.

NATURAL HISTORY. Harrison[4] has emphasized that growth is normal in early infancy until the serum phosphorus falls to low values around six months. Although large amounts of vitamin D can improve the X-ray appearance of the bone and limit the amount of deformity, the serum phosphorus usually remains subnormal and the patients continue to grow at a slow pace. The danger of vitamin D in large dosage is potentially a more harmful one than the untreated disease, and therefore such therapy should only be utilized when the serum calcium can be monitored every two to four weeks; normal growth should not be anticipated as a response. Possibly a moderate dosage of vitamin D with excess oral phosphate may be a more efficacious mode of management.

ETIOLOGY. X-linked dominant in terms of hypophosphatemia with lesser severity in affected females.[1] DeLuca et al.[5] administered tritiated vitamin D_3 to two patients and two controls and found a longer half-life of the tritiated D_3 in the hypophosphatemic rickets patients, who had a 20-fold greater amount of aqueous soluble metabolites of D_3 in the serum than did the controls. These data, although inconclusive, suggest an abnormality in degradation of vitamin D in this disorder.

REFERENCES

1. Winters, R. W., Graham, J. B., Williams, T. F., McFalls, V. W., and Burnett, C. H.: A genetic study of familial hypophosphatemia and vitamin D resistant rickets with a review of the literature. Medicine, *37*:97, 1958.
2. Villanueva, A. R., Ilnicki, L., Frost, H. M., and Arstein, R.: Measurement of the bone formation rate in a case of familial hypophosphatemic vitamin D-resistant rickets. J. Lab. Clin. Med., *67*: 973, 1966.
3. Archard, H. O., and Witkop, C. J.: Hereditary hypophosphatemia (vitamin D-resistant rickets) presenting primary dental manifestations. Oral Surg., *22*:184, 1966.
4. Harrison, H. E., Harrison, H. C., Lifshitz, F., and Johnson, A. D.: Growth disturbance in hereditary hypophosphatemia. Am. J. Dis. Children, *112*:290, 1966.
5. DeLuca, H. F., Lund, J., Rosenbloom, A., and Lobeck, C. C.: Metabolism of tritiated vitamin D_3 in familial vitamin D-resistant rickets with hypophosphatemia. J. Pediat., *70*:828, 1967.

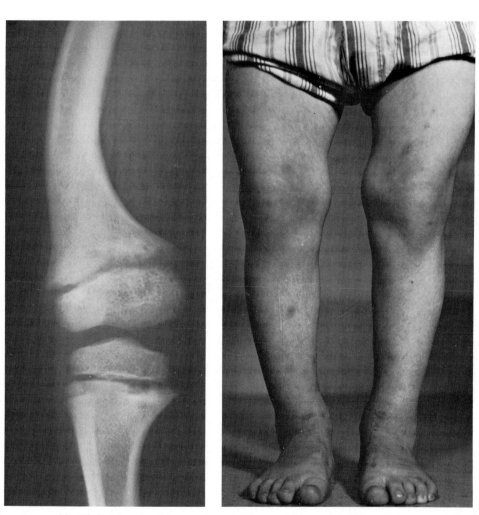

Seven year old with height age of four and one half years. Serum phosphorus, 2.2 mg. per 100 ml.

97. MULTIPLE EXOSTOSES

(Diaphyseal Aclasis, External Chondromatosis)

Diaphyseal Outgrowths Leading to Limb Deformity, with or Without Short Metacarpals

More than 1000 cases have been reported.[1]

ABNORMALITIES[1, 2]

Skeletal. Diaphyseal juxtaepiphyseal outgrowths develop, capped by hyaline cartilage, and tend to grow away from the joint, leading to deformity. Though often present at birth, they are usually not appreciated until early childhood. They are most prominent at ends of long bones, especially at the knee, with variable involvement of pelvis, scapulae, ribs, and vertebrae. Involved bone may be relatively short, especially the ulna, with consequent bowing of the forearm. Shortness of stature is a variable feature.

OCCASIONAL ABNORMALITY. Enchondromata.

NATURAL HISTORY. New outgrowths and enlargement of old exostoses may occur through the age of adolescence. Thereafter no further growth takes place, although there is a 5 to 11 per cent incidence of sarcoma from such lesions in the adult, a risk that does not pertain to childhood.

ETIOLOGY. Autosomal dominant, with 62 per cent of cases being familial.

REFERENCES

1. Solomon, L: Hereditary multiple exostosis. Am. J. Human Genet., *16*:351, 1964.
2. Rubin, P.: Dynamic Classification of Bone Dysplasias. Chicago, Year Book Medical Publishers, 1964, p. 297.

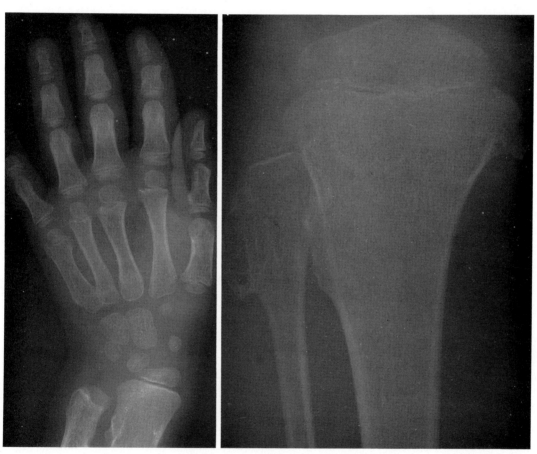

Six year old. Outgrowths from proximal tibia and fibula, less prominently from radius and ulna. Note the short mid-phalanx of the fifth finger and the irregular mid-phalanx of the index finger.

98. CONRADI'S DISEASE

(Chondrodystrophia Calcificans Congenita)

Transient Punctate Mineralization in Developing Cartilage,
Short Proximal Long Bones, Joint Contractures

Though described by Conradi[1] in 1914, this disease has only received broader recognition in the past ten years with more than 115 cases having been reported.

PATTERN OF ABNORMALITY. Percentages are derived from Fritsch and Manzke.[3]

Punctate calcific deposits in infantile cartilaginous skeleton, including epiphyses and cartilage of trachea, larynx, hyoid, vertebral discs, and joint capsules	100%
Short femora and/or humeri, often asymmetrical with dysplasia of the ends	75%
Flexion joint contractures of elbow, knee, and/or hip	56%
Saddle nose secondary to dysplasia of nasal bone	40%
Cataract	26%
Skin and hair: usually hyperkeratosis with erythema in early infancy resolving to follicular atrophoderma, leading to small atrophic cutaneous pits and spotty alopecia, plus sparse coarse hair of uneven diameter in survivors	25%

Shortness of stature is a frequent feature, often evident by birth. Mental deficiency is a variable feature, noted in about half of survivors. Other adverse effects on skeletal morphogenesis are asymmetrical vertebral bodies with or without scoliosis; asymmetrical hypoplasia of metacarpals, metatarsals, and phalanges; large anterior fontanel, craniosynostosis, hypertelorism, micrognathia; syndactyly, polydactyly, clubfoot, dislocation of hip. Congenital heart defect, hernia, and muscle fibrosis are other occasional features.

NATURAL HISTORY. Failure to thrive and infectious episodes, especially pneumonia, limit survival in the more severely affected infants. The punctate areas of mineralization, which histologically occur in foci or mucoid degeneration within the hyaline cartilage, spontaneously resolve during infancy, with epiphyseal mineralization occurring in a near-normal fashion. Spontaneous improvement in joint motility may also occur, and skeletal growth proceeds at an improved rate. Thus the "active" phase of this disease occurs predominantly in prenatal life through infancy, and surviving patients are left with residua from this period of altered morphogenesis. As noted, about half the survivors are left with a residua of mental deficiency.

ETIOLOGY. Autosomal recessive. Frequency of parental consanguinity between 12 per cent and 33 per cent. Rather wide variance in expression.

COMMENT. Probably the alterations in development of bone, joints, lens, and skin in this disease all share a common mode of pathogenesis.

REFERENCES

1. Conradi, E.: Vorzeitiges Auftreten von Knochen- und eigenartigen Verkalkungskernen bei Chondrodystrophia fetalis hypoplastica. Histologische und Röntgenuntersuchungen. J. Kinderh. 80:86, 1914.
2. Allansmith, M., and Senz, E.: Chondrodystrophia congenita punctata (Conradi's disease). Review of literature and report of case with unusual features. Am. J. Dis. Children, *100*:109, 1960.
3. Fritsch, H., and Manzke, H.: Beitrag zur Chondrodystrophia calcificans connata (Conradi-Hünermann-Syndrome). Arch. Kinderh., *169*:235, 1963.
4. Melnick, J. C.: Chondrodystrophia calcificans congenita; chondrodysplasia epiphysialis punctata, stippled epiphyses. Am. J. Dis. Children, *110*: 218, 1965.

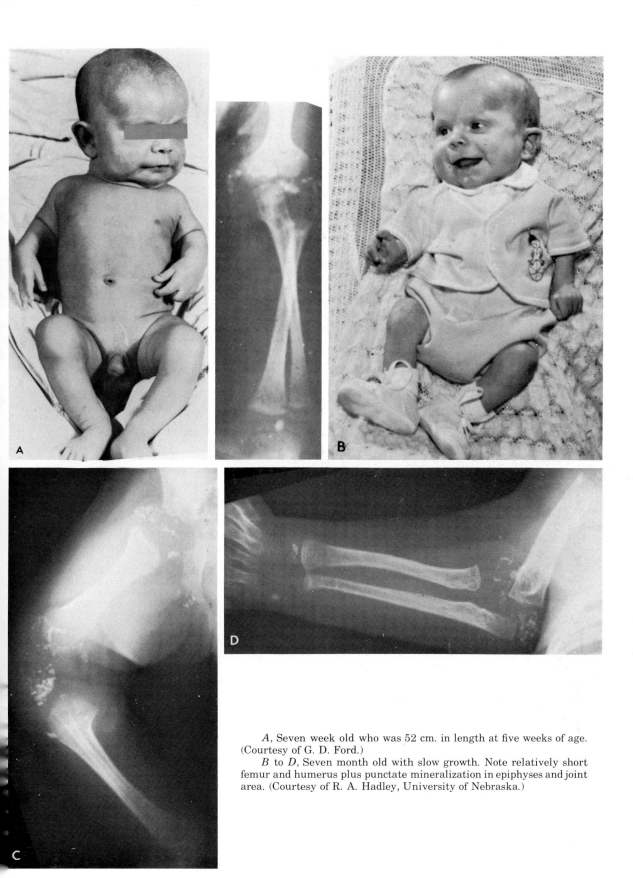

A, Seven week old who was 52 cm. in length at five weeks of age. (Courtesy of G. D. Ford.)

B to D, Seven month old with slow growth. Note relatively short femur and humerus plus punctate mineralization in epiphyses and joint area. (Courtesy of R. A. Hadley, University of Nebraska.)

99. HYPOPHOSPHATASIA

Bow Legs with Irregular Metaphyseal Rarefaction, Early Loss of Deciduous Teeth, Late Closure of Fontanels with or Without Craniosynostosis

Rathbun[1] recognized this disease in 1948, and numerous cases have been documented subsequently.

ABNORMALITIES. There is wide variance in severity.

Growth. Deficiency, variable in degree.

Cranium. Variance from poorly mineralized globular cranium to late closure of wide fontanels with tendency toward craniosynostosis.

Other Skeletal. Varying features include hypoplastic fragile bone of varying density with irregular lack of metaphyseal mineralization, bowed lower extremities with overlying cutaneous dimpling, and short ribs with rachitic rosary and small thoracic cage. Less severely affected patients may have irregular, rachitic appearing incomplete metaphyseal mineralization with bowing of the lower extremities and awkward gait.

Dentition. Defective dentin and cementum with tendency toward premature loss of teeth.

NATURAL HISTORY. Those patients who have the severe type of prenatal defect generally die of respiratory insufficiency during early infancy. Patients with moderately severe cases tend to have early failure to thrive, hypotonia, irritability and occasionally seizures, anemia and/or hypercalcemia, and nephrocalcinosis. The hypercalcemia may be responsive to hydrocortisone analogue therapy. About 50 per cent of the patients die in early infancy. The survivors and those who are more mildly affected may have bone pain, dental problems, and occasionally a fracture; but the osseous abnormalities tend toward improvement with time.

ETIOLOGY. Autosomal recessive. The homozygote has a severe deficiency of tissue and serum alkaline phosphatase and an excessive urinary excretion of phosphoethanolamine. The heterozygote may have a low value for serum alkaline phosphatase.

REFERENCES

1. Rathbun, J. C.: "Hypophosphatasia." A new developmental anomaly. Am. J. Dis. Children, *75*:822, 1948.
2. Rathbun, J. C., MacDonald, J. W., Robinson, H. M. C., and Wanklin, J. M.: Hypophosphatasia: a genetic study. Arch. Dis. Childhood, *36*:540, 1961.
3. Kellsey, D. C.: Hypophosphatasia and congenital bowing of the long bones. J.A.M.A., *179*:187, 1962.

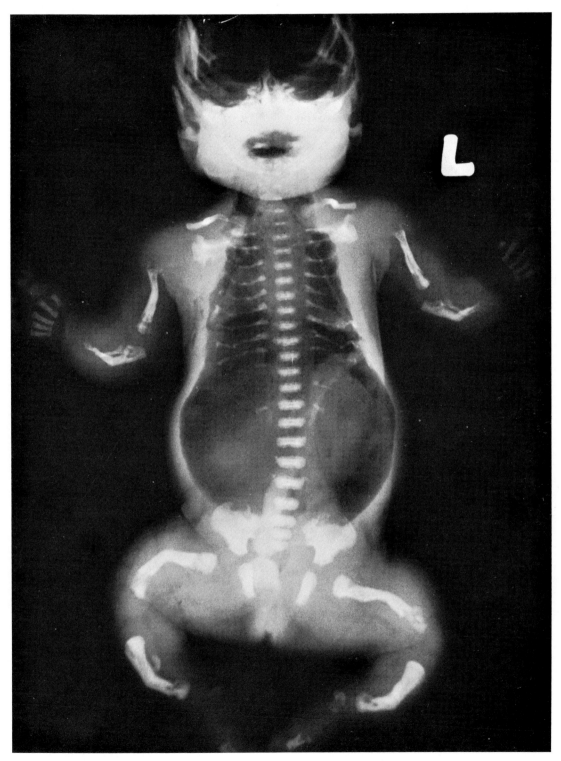

Newborn infant with severe form of hypophosphatasia.

100. KENNY'S SYNDROME

Short Stature, Slim Medullary Cavity, Transient Hypocalcemia, Myopia

Kenny and Linarelli[1] recently described this entity in a mother and her son.

ABNORMALITIES

Growth. Short stature of prenatal onset; the affected woman was 48 inches tall.

Skeleton. Inner cortical thickening of bone with slim medullary cavities.

Late ossification of anterior fontanel.

Eye. Myopia.

Metabolic. Transient hypocalcemia during early infancy in the boy and following surgery in his mother.

ETIOLOGY. Presumed autosomal dominant.

REFERENCES

1. Kenny, F. M., and Linarelli, L.: Dwarfism and cortical thickening of tubular bones. Am. J. Dis. Children, *111*:201, 1966.
2. Caffey, J.: Congenital stenosis of medullary spaces in tubular bones and calvaria in two proportionate dwarfs, mother and son, coupled with transitory hypocalcemic tetany. Am. J. Roentgenol., *100*:1, 1967.

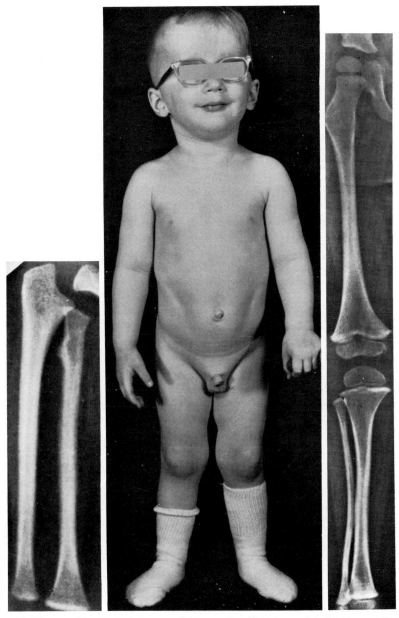

Three and one half year old with height age of 16 months. (Courtesy of F. M. Kenny, Children's Hospital of Pittsburgh.)

101. PYLE'S DISEASE

(Craniometaphyseal Dysplasia)

Bony Wedge over Bridge of Nose, Splayed Metaphyses, Knock Knee

Smith and Jones[1] recorded a skeleton from an archaic Nubian civilization with features resembling those of Pyle's disease. Much later Pyle[2] set forth this entity, and close to 50 cases have been reported.

ABNORMALITIES
Growth. Normal to tall stature.
Craniofacial. Thick, with dense base, cranial vault, facial bones, and mandible. Absence of pneumatization.

Unusual thick bony wedge over bridge of nose and supraorbital area with hypertelorism and relatively small nose. Proptosis of eyes.

Compression of foramina with cranial nerve deficits, headache, and narrow nasal passages with rhinitis.
Dentition. Poor teeth.
Skeletal. Metaphyseal Erlenmeyer splaying with thin cortices and indistinct trabeculae. Knock knee. Wide medial half of clavicles and broad ribs. Loss of normal spinal curvature with mild flattening of vertebral bodies.

NATURAL HISTORY. The disease is evident from infancy, and these individuals may have serious problems from compression of the brain and cranial nerves. They are of normal intelligence. Early in life there may be a striking lack of ossification in the metaphyses.

ETIOLOGY. Both an autosomal recessive and a clearly autosomal dominant type have been described, and at present it is not possible to clearly distinguish between these from a clinical standpoint. The problem in bone morphogenesis is thought to be one of osteoclasis, with defective reabsorption and remodeling of secondary spongiosa.

REFERENCES

1. Smith, G. E., and Jones, F. W.: The archaeological survey of Nubia. Report for 1907–1908. Rep. Human Remains, Cairo, 2:289, 1910.
2. Pyle, E.: A case of unusual bone development. J. Bone Joint Surg., 13:874, 1931.
3. Spranger, J., Paulsen, K., and Lehmann, W.: Die kraniometaphysare Dysplasie (Pyle). Z. Kinderh., 93:64, 1965.
4. Millard, D. R., Jr., Maisels, D. O., Batstone, J. H. F., and Yates, B. W.: Craniofacial surgery in craniometaphyseal dysplasia. Am. J. Surg., 113:615, 1967.

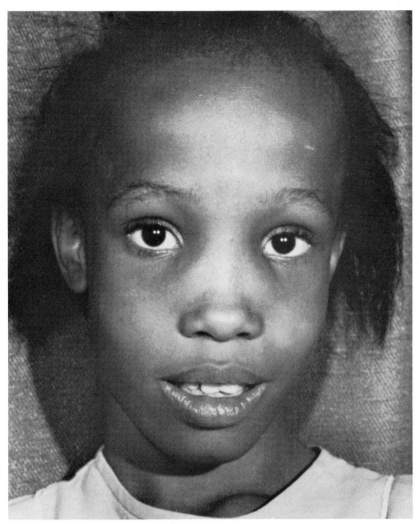

Eleven year old girl with Pyle's disease, inherited as an autosomal dominant. The hyperostosis is already causing the fullness noted in the area of the nasal bridge. Hearing loss began at age nine years. The long bones show the Erlenmeyer flask shape at the metaphyseal area. (Courtesy of D. L. Rimoin, Washington University, St. Louis.)

102. SEVERE OSTEOPETROSIS
(Albers-Schönberg Disease)

Dense, Thick, Fragile Bone; Secondary Pancytopenia, Cranial Nerve Compression

More than 50 cases of this lethal disorder have been reported since the initial description by Albers-Schönberg[1] in 1907.

ABNORMALITIES
Skeleton. Thick, dense, fragile bone with modeling alterations such as obtuse mandibular angle, partial aplasia of distal phalanges, straight femora, blocky "bone within a bone" metacarpals, and macrocephaly with frontal bossing. Marrow compression leads to pancytopenia, and compression of cranial foramina may lead to cranial nerve palsies, blindness, and/or hydrocephalus.

Metabolic. Serum calcium may be low and serum phosphorus elevated.

NATURAL HISTORY. Usually evident at birth with subsequent severe complications and death in infancy or early childhood.

ETIOLOGY. Autosomal recessive. There appears to be defective reabsorption of immature bone. The question has been raised as to whether this disease may represent an abnormality in thyrocalcitonin metabolism, a question which merits close study.

REFERENCES

1. Albers-Schönberg, H.: Eine bisher nicht beschriebene Allgemeinekrankung des Skelettes im Röntgenbilde. Fortschr. Roentgenstr., *11*:261, 1907.
2. Tips, R. L., and Lynch, H. T.: Malignant congenital osteopetrosis resulting from a consanguineous marriage. Acta Paediat., *51*:585, 1962.

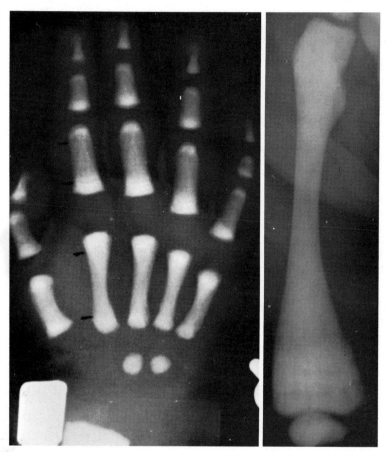

Eight month old. The sclerotic skeleton shows the "bone within a bone" (endobone) appearance, vertical striations at the metaphyseal-diaphyseal juncture, and broad metaphyses.

103. PYKNODYSOSTOSIS OF MAROTEAUX AND LAMY

Osteosclerosis, Short Distal Phalanges, Delayed Closure of Fontanels

Though cleidocranial dysostosis associated with osteosclerosis and bone fragility had been recognized prior to 1962,[1] this condition was not well clarified until Maroteaux and Lamy[2] described it under the eponym of pyknodysostosis (pyknos = dense).

ABNORMALITIES

Growth. Small stature.

Skeletal. Osteosclerosis with tendency toward transverse fracture.

Craniofacial. Frontal and occipital prominence, delayed closure of sutures, wormian bones, lack of frontal sinus. Facial hypoplasia with prominent nose and narrow grooved palate. Obtuse angle to mandible, which may be small.

Teeth. Irregular permanent teeth with or without partial anodontia, delayed eruption.

Clavicle. Dysplasia to loss of acromion end.

Digits. Acro-osteolytic dysplasia of distal phalanges, especially of index finger. Wrinkled skin over dorsum of distal fingers. Flattened nails.

OCCASIONAL ABNORMALITIES. Mental retardation (six of 32).

NATURAL HISTORY. About two thirds of the patients have had fractures, most commonly in the lower extremity, including metatarsals, mandible, and clavicle. There may be a progressive loss in the distal phalanges and outer clavicle and persistent open fontanels, especially the posterior. Special dental care is often indicated.

ETIOLOGY. Consanguinity in seven of 32 families[4] and sibship occurrence from unaffected parents are indicative of an autosomal recessive determination. However, Shuler[3] discovered the syndrome in a maternal uncle of an affected male and therefore raised the question of x-linked recessive in that family.

REFERENCES

1. Thomsen, G., and Guttadauro, M.: Cleidocranial dysostosis associated with osteosclerosis and bone fragility. Acta Radiol., *37*:559, 1952.
2. Maroteaux, P., and Lamy, M.: La pycnodysostose. Presse Méd., *70*:999, 1962.
3. Shuler, S. E.: Pycnodysostosis. Arch. Dis. Childhood, *38*:620, 1963.
4. Elmore, S. M.: Pycnodysostosis: a review. J. Bone Joint Surg., *49-A*:153, 1967.

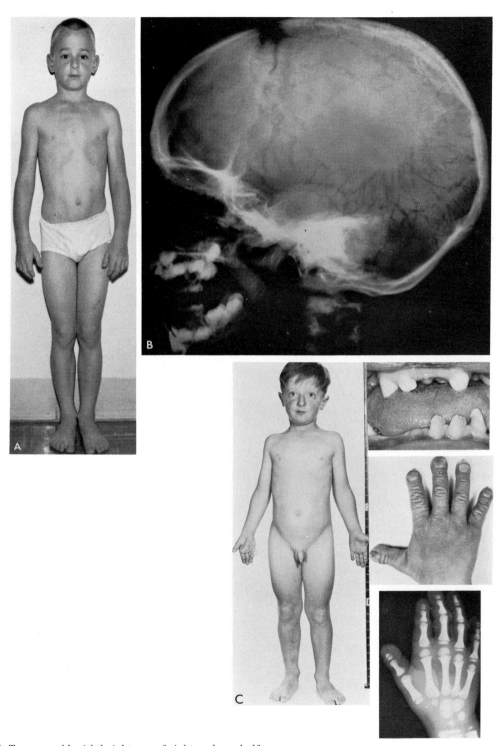

A, Ten year old with height age of eight and one half years.

B, Patient shown in A. Note the open fontanel and lambdoid suture, absence of frontal sinus or mastoid air cells, obtuse angle of mandible, and delay in eruption of permanent dentition.

C, Seven and one half year old with height age of four and one half years. Note the generally dense bone and partial loss of several distal phalanges. (From Shuler, S. E.: Arch. Dis. Childhood, *38*:620, 1963.)

104. CLEIDOCRANIAL DYSOSTOSIS

Defect of Clavicle, Late Ossification of Cranial Sutures, Delayed Eruption of Teeth

A possible example of this rather generalized dysplasia of osseous and dental tissues was detected in the skull of a Neanderthal man.[1] The more obvious features of the defect in clavicle and cranium prompted Marie and Sainton[2] to utilize the term cleidocranial dysostosis for this condition; however, the more generalized dysplasia of bone and teeth has been emphasized, and the term cleidocranial dysostosis only depicts a portion of the abnormal development. Well over 500 cases have been reported.

ABNORMALITIES. The following are frequent but not constant features:

Growth. Mild to moderate shortness of stature.

Craniofacial. Brachycephaly with bossing of frontal, parietal, and occipital bones; late mineralization of sutures; late or incomplete development of accessory sinuses and mastoid air cells; wormian bones; small sphenoid bones.

Mid-facial hypoplasia with low nasal bridge, narrow high-arched palate.

Dentition. Late eruption of dentition, especially the permanent teeth, which are often abnormal with aplasia, malformed roots, retention cysts, enamel hypoplasia, and supernumerary teeth.

Clavicle. Partial to complete aplasia of clavicle with associated muscle defects.

Hands. Hand anomalies including asymmetrical length of fingers with long second metacarpal, short and tapering distal phalanges with or without downcurving nails, accessory proximal metacarpal epiphyses which fuse in childhood, and altered rate of carpal ossification.

Other Skeletal. Delayed mineralization of pubic bone, narrow pelvis, broad femoral head with short femoral neck, with or without coxa vara.

OCCASIONAL ABNORMALITIES. Cervical rib, small scapulae, scoliosis, kyphosis, flat acetabulae, osteosclerosis, increased bone fragility, deafness, cleft palate.

ETIOLOGY. Autosomal dominant with wide variability in expression, but usually showing penetrance. About one-third of the cases represent fresh mutations.

NATURAL HISTORY. Though stature is often reduced, mentality is usually normal. Hearing should be assessed and dental problems should be anticipated. Removal of deciduous teeth does not seem to hasten the eruption of permanent teeth, and the permanent teeth may be difficult to extract because of malformed roots. Narrow pelvis may necessitate cesarian section for delivery of the pregnant female with this condition.

COMMENT. Emphasis should be placed on the rather generalized effect of this mutant gene on the rate and form of development of osseous and dental tissue. The degree of variance in expression includes a lack of defective clavicular development. Many of the radiological signs such as metacarpal pseudoepiphyses and late mineralization of pubic ramus depend on the age of the patient.

REFERENCES

1. Grieg, D. M.: Neanderthal skull presenting features of cleidocranial dysostosis and other peculiarities. Edinburgh Med. J., *40*:407, 1933.
2. Marie, P., and Sainton, P.: Observation d'hydrocephalie héréditaire (père et fils) par vice de developpement du crane et du cerveau. Bull. et Mem. Soc. Med. Hôp. Paris, *14*:706, 1897.
3. Anspach, W. E., and Huepel, R. C.: Familial cleidocranial dysostosis (cleidal dysostosis). A preosseous and dentinal dystrophy. Am. J. Dis. Children, *58*:786, 1939.
4. Lasker, G. W.: The inheritance of cleidocranial dysostosis. Human Biol., *18*:103, 1946.
5. Jackson, W. P. U.: Osteo-dental dysplasia (Cleidocranial dysostosis). The "Arnold head." Acta Med. Scand., *139*:292, 1951.
6. Forland, M.: Cleidocranial dysostosis. A review of the syndrome and report of a sporadic case, with hereditary transmission. Am. J. Med., *33*:792, 1962.

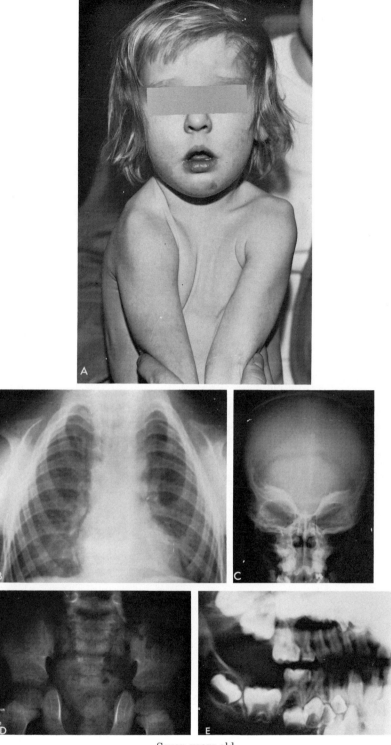

Seven years old

A, Three and one half year old; height age, two and one half years. (From Smith, D. W.: J. Pediat., 70:500, 1967.)

B, Absent clavicles.

C, Poorly mineralized cranial sutures.

D, Hypoplasia of ilia, wide-spread pubic rami.

E, Mandible showing delay in eruption of permanent teeth.

(C and E courtesy of R. Scherz, Madigan General Hospital, Washington.)

105. STANESCO'S DYSOSTOSIS SYNDROME

Thick Cortical Bone, Brachycephalic Thin Skull, Relatively Short Upper Arm, Proportionately Short Fingers

Stanesco et al.[1] studied seven of 11 affected individuals in three generations of one family and reported this condition in 1963. This alteration in bone morphogenesis bears many similarities to the Maroteaux and Lamy type of pyknodysostosis, but differs in several clinical points and in its genetic mode of determination.

ABNORMALITIES. Based on seven cases.[1]
Growth. Small stature.
Craniofacial and Dental. Brachycephalic thin skull, often with depressions at frontoparietal sutures.
  Lack of pneumatization in frontal and sphenoid bone. Shallow orbits with prominent eyes. Narrow maxilla. Small mandible with obtuse angle. Crowded teeth, sometimes small; enamel hypoplasia.
Long Bones. Dense with thick cortices. Relative shortness, especially of upper arm and hand.

OCCASIONAL ABNORMALITIES. Flattened roof of palate, sacralization of S-1, exostoses, fractures.

NATURAL HISTORY. These individuals have been of normal intelligence, with no problems in sexual development or reproduction. The bone tends to become more dense with age. Only one of the 11 affected members of the family was known to have had a fracture.

ETIOLOGY. Autosomal dominant with almost complete expression in all affected individuals.

COMMENT. The lack of defect in the distal phalanges in this disorder appears to be one of the easiest clinical points in distinguishing this disease from the type of pyknodysostosis described by Maroteaux and Lamy.

REFERENCE

1. Stanesco, V., Maximilian, C., Poenaru, S., Florea, I., Stanesco, R., Ionesco, V., and Ioanitiu, D.: Syndrome hereditaire dominant, etc. Rev. Franç. Endocr. Clin., *4*:219, 1963.

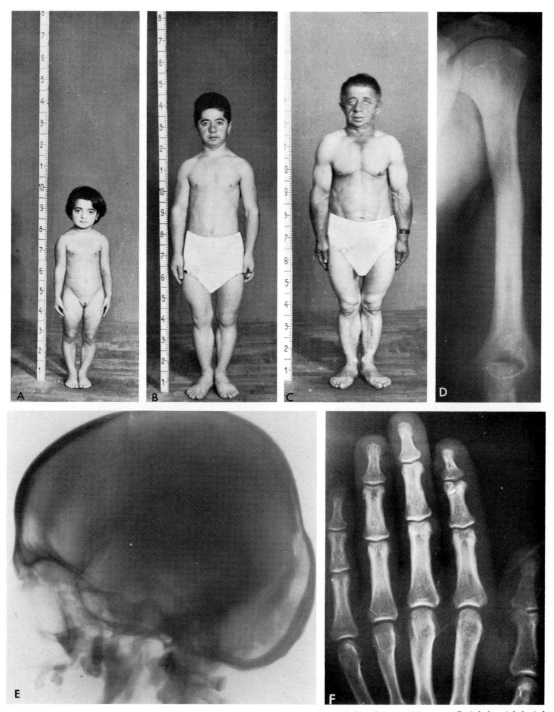

A to *C*: *A*, Nine year old; height age three years. *B*, Sixteen year old; height age, 10 years. *C*, Adult with height of 4 feet, 7 inches.

D, Humerus, showing thick, dense cortices.

E, Adult cranium, relatively dense with shallow sella and obtuse mandibular angle.

F, Adult hand showing minor alterations, but no osteolysis of distal phalanges such as is found in pyknodys-ostosis.

(From Stanesco, V., et al.: Rev. Franç. Endocr. Clin., *4*:219, 1963.)

106. APERT'S SYNDROME

(Acrocephalosyndactyly)

Irregular Craniosynostosis, Midfacial Hypoplasia, Syndactyly, and Broad Distal Phalanx of Thumb and Big Toe

The condition was reported by Wheaton[1] in 1894, in 1906 Apert[2] summarized nine cases, and in 1920 Park and Powers[3] published an exceptional essay on this entity. By 1960 Blank[4] noted the recording of 150 cases.

ABNORMALITIES

Performance. Severe mental deficiency may be present, but normal intelligence has also been observed and the incidence of mental defect is not known.

Craniofacies. Short anterior-posterior diameter with high full forehead and flat occiput.

Irregular craniosynostosis, especially of coronal suture; often late closure of fontanels.

Flat facies, supraorbital horizontal groove, shallow orbits, hypertelorism, strabismus, downslanting of palpebral fissures, small nose, and maxillary hypoplasia.

Narrow palate with median groove with or without cleft palate or bifid uvula.

Limbs. Osseous or cutaneous syndactyly, or both, varying from total fusion to partial fusion; most commonly with complete fusion of second, third, and fourth fingers. Distal phalanges of the thumbs are often broad and malformed. Fingers may be short. Cutaneous syndactyly of all toes with or without osseous syndactyly. Distal hallux may be broad and malformed.

OCCASIONAL ABNORMALITIES.
Other skeletal malformations may include short humerus, synostosis of radius and humerus, and limitation of joint motility.

Other malformations besides the skeletal system have occurred more frequently than expected and include esophageal atresia, pyloric stenosis, ectopic anus, pulmonary aplasia, atrophy of pulmonary arteries, anomalous tracheal cartilage, pulmonic stenosis overriding aorta, ventricular septal defect, endocardial fibroelastosis, polycystic kidney, hydronephrosis, and bicornuate uterus.

NATURAL HISTORY.
There are no adequate data on the long-term follow-up of patients. Early surgery for craniosynostosis, however, would seem indicated when the condition is of sufficient magnitude to give rise to increased intracranial pressure (coronal plus one or more other suture). Though there can be mental deficiency in patients who have no evidence of increased intracranial pressure, mental defect is an irregular occurrence. There should be vigorous early management of the syndrome while waiting to determine whether the infant will be mentally retarded. When the thumb is immobilized, early surgery to allow for a pincer grasp is indicated, with later attempts at further improvement of hand function.

ETIOLOGY.
Autosomal dominant inheritance is indicated with the vast majority of cases representing a fresh mutation.

One factor in the sporadic cases has been older paternal age; the average paternal age at the birth of an infant with Apert's syndrome is 37 years. Older paternal age has also been observed as a factor in sporadic cases of achondroplasia and Marfan's syndrome, two other disorders that are due to a single altered gene.

The recurrence risk for the unaffected parents of a child with Apert's syndrome is negligible, whereas the recurrence risk for the offspring of the affected individual is 50 per cent.

COMMENT.
The osseous developmental pathology appears to be irregular bridging between the early islands of mesenchymal blastema that will become bone, especially in the distal extremities and cranium. This irregular organization presumably has begun before the sixth week of prenatal life. Indications of hypoplasia and abnormal shape of bone are also evident and the mutant gene may adversely affect the organization of other tissues. This is evident in the irregular occurrence of mental deficiency and the greater than expected concurrence of a number of nonskeletal malformations. Therefore, every newborn suspected of having Apert's syndrome deserves a complete evaluation for other malformations.

REFERENCES

1. Wheaton, S. W.: Two specimens of congenital cranial deformity in infants associated with fusion of the fingers and toes. Trans. Path. Soc. London, 45:238, 1894.

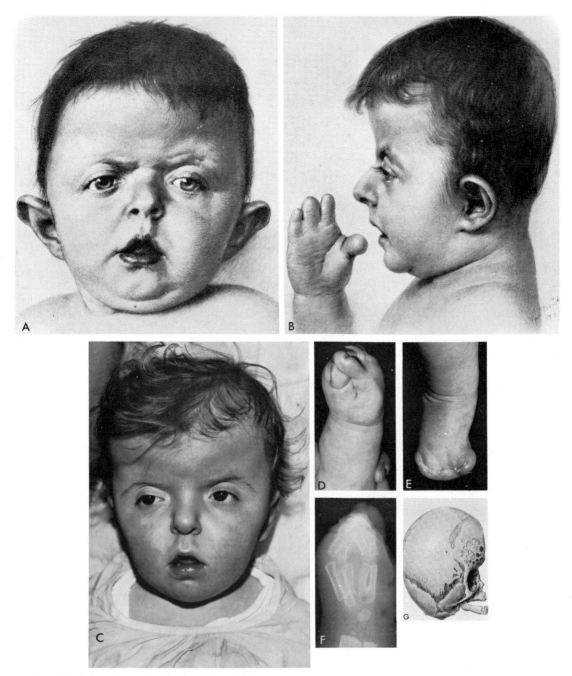

A and *B*, A boy, drawn by the late M. Brödel.

C, Two year old girl, her hand (*D*), foot (*E*), and x-ray of the hand (*F*).

G, The cranium of an infant with Apert's syndrome, showing the irregular synostosis of the coronal suture and the aberrant development in the frontal bone.

(*A, B*, and *G* from Park E. A., and Powers, G. F.: Am. J. Dis. Children, *20*:235, 1920.)

2. Apert, E.: De l'Acrocéphalosyndactylie. Bull. Soc. Med., *23*:1310, 1906.

3. Park, E. A., and Powers, G. F.: Acrocephaly and scaphocephaly with symmetrically distributed malformations of the extremities. A study of the so-called "Acrocephalosyndactylism." Am. J. Dis. Children, *20*:235, 1920.

4. Blank, C. E.: Apert's syndrome (a type of acrocephalosyndactyly) observations on British series of thirty-nine cases. Ann. Hum. Genet., *24*:151, 1960.

5. Weech, A. A.: Combined acrocephaly and syndactylism occurring in mother and daughter. A case report. Bull. Hopkins Hosp., *40*:73, 1927.

107. CARPENTER'S SYNDROME

Acrocephaly, Polydactyly and Syndactyly of Feet, Lateral Displacement of Inner Canthi

Although Carpenter[1] described this condition in 1901, it was not firmly established as an entity until Temtamy's[2] report in 1966. Some of the cases reported in the literature had been mistakenly identified as Apert's syndrome or the Laurence-Moon-Biedl syndrome.

PATTERN OF MALFORMATION. Based on 12 cases.

Mental retardation	9 of 9
Obesity	12 of 12
Acrocephaly	12 of 12
Lateral displacement of inner canthi and/or inner canthal folds	11 of 11
Brachysyndactyly of hands with clinodactyly	12 of 12
Preaxial polydactyly of feet with syndactyly	12 of 12
Hypogenitalism, cryptorchidism	8 of 8

Other less consistently observed or reported features include low-set auricles, congenital heart defect (patent ductus, ventricular septal defect, pulmonic stenosis, transposition), duplication of second phalanx of thumb, metatarsus varus, flat acetabulum, flare to pelvis, coxa valga, genu valgum, lateral displacement of patellae, pilonidal dimple, accessory spleen, abdominal hernias, and generalized aminoaciduria.

ETIOLOGY. The occurrence of this syndrome in both male and female siblings of unaffected parents suggests autosomal recessive inheritance. No chromosomal abnormality was detected by Temtamy.[2]

COMMENT. Presently there are inadequate data upon which to base a natural history for this condition.

REFERENCES

1. Carpenter, G.: Two sisters showing malformations of the skull and other congenital abnormalities. Rep. Soc. Study Dis. Child. Lond., *1*:110, 1901.
2. Temtamy, S. A.: Carpenter's syndrome: Acrocephalo-polysyndactyly, an autosomal recessive syndrome. J. Pediat., *69*:111, 1966.

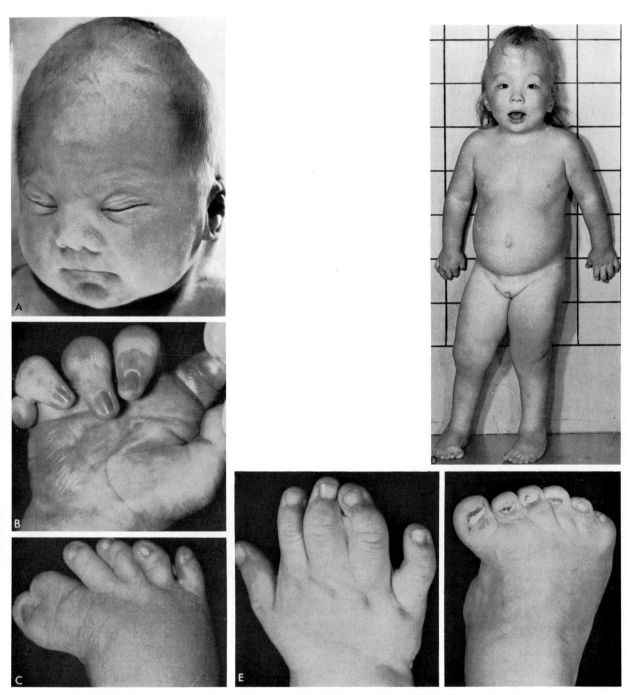

A to *C*, Newborn, necropsy photos. (Courtesy of A. W. Bauer, Group Health Cooperative, Seattle.) *D* and *E*, Three year old. (From Temtamy, S. A.: J. Pediat., *69*:111, 1966.)

108. CRANIOFACIAL DYSOSTOSIS OF CROUZON

Shallow Orbits, Premature Craniosynostosis, Maxillary Hypoplasia

Originally described in 1912 by Crouzon[1] in a mother and her daughter, this condition usually has an adverse effect on craniofacial development alone.

ABNORMALITIES

Craniofacial. Ocular proptosis due to shallow orbits, with or without divergent strabismus, hypertelorism.

Hypoplasia of maxilla with or without curved parrot-like nose, inverted V shape to palate.

Craniosynostosis, especially of coronal, lambdoidal, and sagittal sutures with palpable ridging. Short anterior-posterior and wide lateral dimensions of the cranium may occur with increased intracranial pressure, leading to digital markings on the inner table of the cranium with or without optic nerve alteration and mental deficiency.

OCCASIONAL ABNORMALITIES.
Peg-shaped widely spaced teeth, partial anodontia, large tongue, deviation of nasal septum, atresia of auditory meatus, deafness. Triangular shape to optic foramina.

NATURAL HISTORY.
The degree of craniosynostosis as well as the age of onset is variable. One infant is described who showed no roentgenographic evidence of craniosynostosis at four months but complete closure by 11 months of age. Surgical morcellation procedures to allow for more normal brain development are indicated at an early age when there is increased intracranial pressure. Bertelsen[5] considers synostosis of the coronal suture alone adequate indication for early surgical intervention, because premature closure of this suture appears to be especially deleterious to subsequent enlargement of the cranium. Otherwise, the indications are usually cosmetic and the decision toward surgery is usually mitigated by the severity of the aberrant shape plus the competency of the surgeon who will perform the procedure.

Although craniosynostosis limits the growth of the brain, the cranium can undergo some further enlargement even when all sutures are fused at an early age.[5] This limited growth is apparently from subperiosteal bone growth.

ETIOLOGY.
Autosomal dominant with variable expression, shallow orbits being the most consistent feature. About one quarter of the reported cases have had a negative family history and may represent fresh mutations.

REFERENCES

1. Crouzon, O.: Dysostose cranio-faciale héréditaire. Bull. Mém. Soc. Méd. Hôp. Paris, 33:545, 1912.
2. Dodge, H. W., Jr., Wood, M. W., and Kennedy, R. L. J.: Craniofacial dysostosis: Crouzon's disease. Pediatrics, 23:98, 1959.
3. Gorlin, R. J., and Pindborg, J. J.: Syndromes of the Head and Neck. New York, McGraw-Hill Book Co., 1964, p. 172.
4. Vulliamy, D. G., and Normandale, P. A.: Craniofacial dysostosis in a Dorset family. Arch. Dis. Childhood, 41:375, 1966.
5. Bertelsen, T. I.: The premature synostosis of the cranial sutures. Acta Ophth. supplement 51. Copenhagen, Monksgaard, 1958.

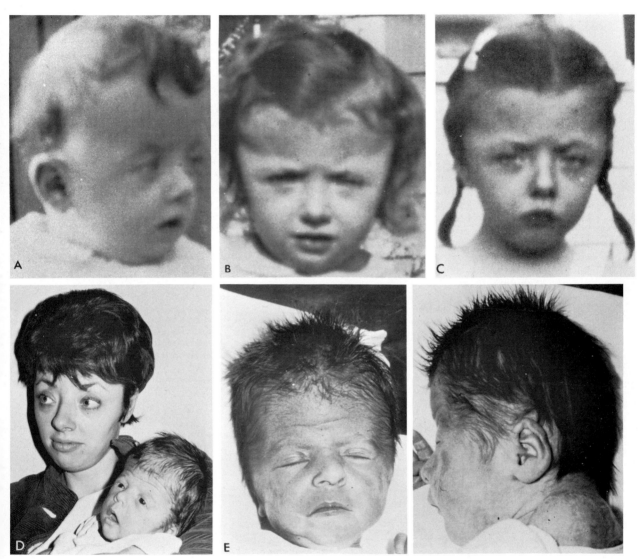

The mother of the patient shown in *E* is shown as a young infant (*A*), at one year of age (*B*), and at three years of age (*C*). No surgical procedure was performed, and *D* shows the mother as an adult of normal intelligence with her affected son who had rather severe synostosis of the coronal suture leading to the short cranium. A surgical morcellation procedure was performed on the son's suture. (Courtesy of R. Luce, Group Health Clinic, Seattle.)

109. AMINOPTERIN-INDUCED SYNDROME

Cranial Dysplasia, Broad Nasal Bridge, Low Set Ears

The folic acid antagonist, aminopterin, has occasionally been utilized as an abortifacient during the first trimester of pregnancy. Thiersch[1] first noted abnormal morphogenesis in three abortuses and one full-term offspring of mothers who received aminopterin from four to nine weeks following the presumed time of conception. Subsequently four other cases have been published and reviewed by Milunsky et al.[2] They reported the birth of a malformed infant, following maternal ingestion of methotrexate, a methyl derivative of aminopterin. The four mothers took 12 to 29 mg. of the folic acid antagonist from four to ten weeks after the presumed time of conception and the gestational duration ranged from 22 to 40 weeks. There was a similar pattern of malformation in these four babies. It consisted of cranial dysplasia, foot anomalies and other less consistent defects, and was predominantly a pattern of skeletal dysplasia.

ABNORMALITIES. Four babies (the number affected is in parentheses).[2]
Craniofacial. Severe hypoplasia of frontal bone (three), parietal bones (two), temporal or occipital bones (one each), wide fontanels (two), and synostosis of lambdoid (two) or coronal sutures (one). Broad nasal bridge (three), prominent eyes (two), micrognathia (three), and cleft palate and low set ears (three), with maxillary hypoplasia and epicanthal folds noted in one.
Feet. Talipes equinovarus (two), hypodactyly (one), and synostosis (one).

OTHER ABNORMALITIES (ONE EACH). Congenital hypoplastic small size, dislocation of hip, retarded ossification of pubis and ischium, rib anomalies, short thumbs, partial syndactyly of third and fourth fingers, single crease on fifth finger, dextroposition of the heart, and hypotonia.

NATURAL HISTORY. Only one affected individual survived past 12 days of age.[2] This baby appeared normal in mental and motor development at 15 months of age, though growth was less than the third percentile for age.

REFERENCES

1. Thiersch, J. B.: Therapeutic abortions with a folic acid antagonist, 4-aminopteroylglutamic acid (4-amino P.G.A.) administered by the oral route. Am. J. Obstet. Gynec., *63*:1298, 1952.
2. Milunsky, A., Graef, J. W., and Gaynor, M. F., Jr.: Methotrexate induced congenital malformations with a review of the literature. J. Pediat., *72*:790, 1968.

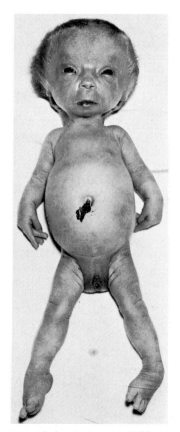

42 weeks' gestation   1280 gm.
(From Warkany et al.: Am. J. Dis. Child., *97*:274, 1959.)

110. NAIL-PATELLA SYNDROME

(Hereditary Osteo-Onychodysplasia)

Nail Dysplasia, Patella Hypoplasia, Iliac Spurs

Little's[1] report in 1897, limited to a presentation of patellar defect, is usually credited as the initial description of this syndrome, whereas this pattern includes multiple other dysplasias of osseous as well as nonosseous mesenchymal tissues. More than 200 cases have ben reported.

ABNORMALITIES. Relative frequency of expression as percentages.

Nail. Hypoplasia, splitting, most commonly of thumbnail — 98%

Knee. Hypoplastic to absent patella, hypoplasia of lateral femoral condyle and small head of fibula — 92%

Elbow. Hypoplastic capitellum, small head of radius — 90%

Ilium. Spur in mid-posterior ilium, 71 per cent palpable — 81%

Scapula. Hypoplasia, convex thick outer border — 44%

Iris. Dark, "clover-leaf" pigmentation at inner margin — 46%

Renal. Proteinuria with or without hematuria, casts, renal insufficiency — 42%

Other Frequent Features. Absence of dorsal distal phalangeal joints, delayed ossification of secondary centers of ossification, valgus of femoral neck, club foot.

OCCASIONAL ABNORMALITIES

Skeletal. Prominent outer clavicle, malformed sternum, spina bifida, scoliosis, enlarged ulnar styloid process, clinodactyly of fifth finger.

Eye. Keratoconus, microcornea, microphakia, cataract, ptosis.

Muscle. Aplasia of pectoralis minor, biceps, triceps, quadriceps.

Central Nervous System. Occasional mental deficiency, psychosis.

NATURAL HISTORY. Patients may have problems owing to limitation of joint motility, dislocation, or both, especially at the elbow and knee where osteoarthritis may eventually limit function. Children should be closely followed for scoliosis. Evidence of renal abnormality may suggest chronic glomerulonephritis, as may the renal histology, but at necropsy the finding of a reticular distribution of interstitial fibrosis may prove to be a more specific renal lesion in this disorder. Renal failure is apparently rare prior to the fourth decade.

ETIOLOGY. Autosomal dominant, always showing some expression. Studies have demonstrated close linkage with the genetic determinants of ABO blood group substances. A closer correlation for the extent of nail dysplasia has been found among affected siblings than between affected parent and offspring. This evidence implies a strong effect of the normal allele (always derived from the unaffected parent) on the expression of the mutant allele for the nail-patella syndrome.

COMMENT. The osseous abnormality consists of specific regions of hypoplasia such as the lateral knee and elbow, and other specific regions of hyperplasia such as the iliac spurs. The latter defect, as yet unknown in any animal or in other diseases of man, appears to be pathognomonic as an expression of this mutant gene.

REFERENCES

1. Little, E. M.: Congenital absence or delayed development of the patella. Lancet, 2:781, 1897.
2. Carbonara, P., and Alpert, M.: Hereditary osteo-onycho-dysplasia (Hood). Am. J. Med. Sci., *248:* 139, 1964.
3. Lucas, G. L., and Opitz, J. M.: The nail-patella syndrome. Clinical and genetic aspects of 5 kindreds with 38 affected family members. J. Pediat., *68:*273, 1966.
4. Darlington, D., and Hawkins, C. F.: Nail-patella syndrome with iliac horns and hereditary nephropathy. Necropsy report and anatomical dissection. J. Bone Joint Surg. (Brit.), *49-B:*164, 1967.
5. Renwick, J. H., and Izatt, M. M.: Some genetical parameters of the nail-patella locus. Ann. Human Genet., *28:*369, 1965.

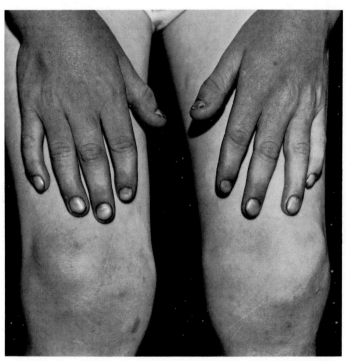

Adolescent male showing nail hypoplasia, most evident for thumbs, and displacement of small patellae. (Courtesy of J. M. Opitz, University of Wisconsin.)

111. DYSCHONDROSTEOSIS OF LERI-WEILL

Short Forearms with Madelung Deformity, with or Without Short Lower Leg

Leri and Weill[1] described this condition in 1929, and more than 30 cases have been reported subsequently. Most patients previously categorized as having Madelung's deformity are examples of this entity.

ABNORMALITIES

Growth. Variable, moderate shortness of stature.

Extremities. Short forearm with bowing of radius, widened gap between radius and ulna and altered osseous alignment at wrist. May have partial dislocation of ulna at wrist, elbow, or both, with limitation of movement. Short lower leg.

OCCASIONAL ABNORMALITIES. Short hands and feet with metaphyseal flaring in metacarpal and metatarsal bones, curvature of tibia, exostoses from proximal tibia and/or fibula, abnormal femoral neck, coxa valga, abnormal tuberosity of humerus.

NATURAL HISTORY. Becker[3] has noted associated paramyotonia in affected individuals in one family; it remains to be determined whether or not this is a frequent feature. Otherwise the only usual problems are moderate shortness of stature and limitation of joint mobility at the wrist, elbow, or both.

ETIOLOGY. Autosomal dominant with an excess of affected females in the recorded cases.

REFERENCES

1. Leri, A., and Weill, J.: Une affection congenitale et symetrique du developpement osseus: la dyschondrosteose. Bull. Mém. Soc. Méd. Hôp. Paris, *45*:1491, 1929.
2. Herdman, R. C., Langer, L. O., Good, R. A.: Dyschondrosteosis. The most common cause of Madelung's deformity. J. Pediat., *68*:432, 1966.
3. Becker, P. E.: Ein weiterer Fall von Dyschondrosteose (Leri-Weill). Humangenetik, *1*:563, 1965.

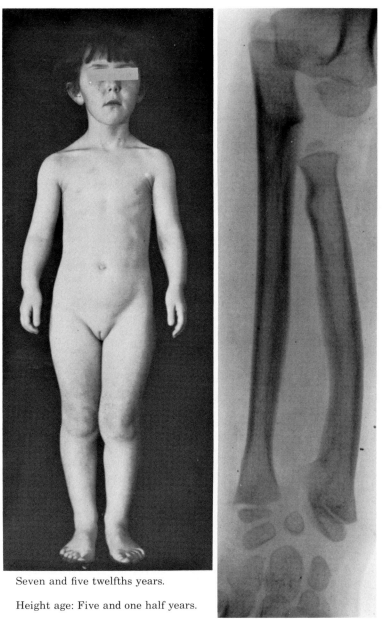

Seven and five twelfths years.

Height age: Five and one half years.

(From Lamy and Maroteaux: Les chondrodystrophies génotypiques. Paris, L'Expansion Scientifique Française, 1960.)

237

112. ALBRIGHT'S HEREDITARY OSTEODYSTROPHY

(Pseudohypoparathyroidism; Pseudopseudohypoparathyroidism)

Short Metacarpal, Rounded Facies, with or Without Hypocalcemia and/or Vicarious Mineralization

Albright[1] described this condition in 1942 and referred to it as pseudohypoparathyroidism because of hypocalcemia and hyperphosphatemia that were unresponsive to parathormone. Subsequently patients were detected with a comparable phenotype but with normocalcemia, even in the same family as a patient with hypocalcemia. The term pseudopseudohypoparathyroidism was utilized to designate such instances. Because it is now obvious that hypocalcemia is a variable expression in this hereditable disease, the term Albright's hereditary osteodystrophy seems preferable. More than 100 cases have been reported.

ABNORMALITIES

Growth. Small stature; final height, 54 inches to 5 feet; occasionally taller. Obesity, moderate.

Performance. Mental deficiency, intelligence quotient of 20 to 99, mean I.Q. about 60; occasionally normal.

Facies. Rounded, low nasal bridge.

Dentition. Delayed dental eruption, aplasia, and/or enamel hypoplasia.

Extremities. Short metacarpals and metatarsals, especially the fourth and fifth.

Extra Skeletal Calcification. Areas of mineralization in subcutaneous tissues, basal ganglia.

Calcium and Phosphorus. Hypocalcemia and hyperphosphatemia.

OCCASIONAL ABNORMALITIES.

Distal palmar axial triradii, osteochondromata, thick calvarium, short ulna, epiphyseal dysplasia, genu valgum, hypothyroidism, hypogonadism with or without gonadal dysgenesis, peripheral lenticular opacities.

NATURAL HISTORY.

Hypocalcemia, when present, usually becomes evident in childhood, seizures being the most common presenting symptom. Cautious vitamin D therapy in dosage of 25,000 to 100,000 units per day may be necessary; however, the therapy should be discontinued every few years to reassess the situation, because spontaneous amelioration of the hypocalcemia may occur with time.

GENETICS.

The family data are indicative of a single mutant gene giving rise to this syndrome. The findings of a 2 : 1 female to male sex incidence have favored an X-linked dominant mode of determination, but autosomal dominant with more severe expression in females also seems a possibility, especially considering two instances of male to male transmission.[5]

REFERENCES

1. Albright, F., Burnett, C. H., Smith, P. H., and Parson, W.: Pseudohypoparathyroidism—an example of 'Seabright-bantam syndrome.' Report of three cases. Endocrinology, *30*:922, 1942.
2. Mann, J. B., Alterman, S., and Hills, A. G.: Albright's hereditary osteodystrophy comprising pseudohypoparathyroidism and pseudopseudohypoparathyroidism. With a report of two cases representing the complete syndrome occurring in successive generations. Ann. Int. Med., *56*: 315, 1962.
3. Miller, J. Q., Rostafiniski, M. J., and Hyde, M. S.: Gonadal dysgenesis and brachymetacarpal dwarfism (pseudopseudohypoparathyroidism). Arch. Int. Med., *116*:940, 1965.
4. Christiaen, L., Gontaine, G., Farriaux, J. P., and Biserte, G.: Le pseudohypoparathyroidisme chronique. À propos de trois cas familiaux. Acta Paediat. Belg., *21*:5, 1967.
5. Spranger, J.: Personal communication.

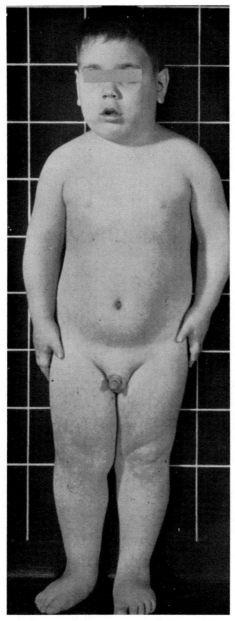

Five year old with height age of three and one half years and bone age of five years. Hypocalcemia and hyperphosphatemia were first detected at one year of age.

113. BRACHYDACTYLY, TYPE E

Short Metacarpals (Third and Fifth), Brachydactyly, Mild to Moderate Short Stature

McKusick and Milch[1] described a dominantly inherited syndrome consisting of moderate shortness of stature and brachydactyly with unusually small third and fifth metacarpal bones. X-linked inheritance was excluded by two instances of male to male transmission. The lack of mental retardation, hypocalcemia, or vicarious mineralization in any affected individual tended to exclude the diagnosis of Albright's hereditary osteodystrophy. Similar phenotypic and genetic findings are set forth in at least two reports on "pseudopseudohypoparathyroidism"[2, 3] which leads to some confusion in the literature on Albright's hereditary osteodystrophy. Obviously shortness of the third and fifth metacarpals is not pathognomonic for any specific disease.

REFERENCES

1. McKusick, V. A., and Milch, R. A.: The clinical behavior of genetic disease. Selected aspects. Clin. Orthop., *33*:22, 1964.
2. Brailsford, J. F.: Familial brachydactyly. Brit. J. Radiol., *18*:167, 1945.
3. Goeminne, L.: Albright's hereditary poly-osteochondrodystrophy. Acta Genet. Med. Gem., *14*:226, 1965.

114. WEILL-MARCHESANI SYNDROME

(Brachydactyly-Spherophakia)

Brachydactyly, Small Spherical Lens, Short Stature

More than 18 instances of this condition have been described since the initial recognition by Weill in 1932 and the broader description by Marchesani in 1939.

ABNORMALITIES
Growth. Small stature.
Craniofacial. Broad skull, small shallow orbits, mild maxillary hypoplasia with narrow palate.
Eye. Small spherical lens, myopia with or without glaucoma, ectopia lentis in half of cases, blindness in one third.
Teeth. Malformed and malaligned.
Limbs. Brachydactyly with broad metacarpals and phalanges, with or without late ossification of epiphyses.

OCCASIONAL ABNORMALITY. Cardiac anomaly.

NATURAL HISTORY. The mean age of recognition of an ocular problem in this disorder is 7.5 years, the youngest recorded age being nine months. Dilatation of the pupil is often necessary to appreciate the lens defect. Intelligence is usually not affected.

ETIOLOGY. Unknown; either autosomal dominant with variable expression or autosomal recessive with partial expression in heterozygotes. More than one etiological entity may be represented. More studies of affected families are merited.

REFERENCES

1. Weill, G.: Ectopie du cristallin et malformations generales. Ann. Ocul., *169*:21, 1932.
2. Marchesani, O.: Brachydaktylie und angeborene Kugellinse als Systemerkrankung. Klin. Monatsbl. Augenh., *103*:392, 1939.
3. Zabriskie, J., and Reisman, M.: Marchesani syndrome. J. Pediat., *52*:158, 1958.
4. Feinberg, S. B.: Congenital mesodermal dysmorphodystrophy (brachymorphic type). Radiology, *74*:218, 1960.

WEILL-MARCHESANI SYNDROME

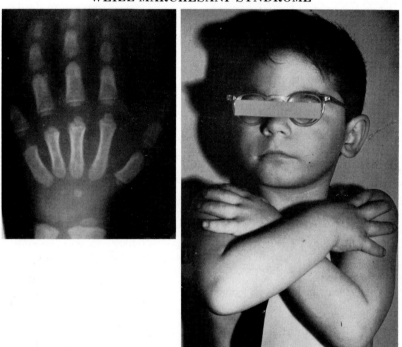

Nine year old with height age of five and one half years. Small lens and myopia. (From Zabriskie, J., and Reisman, M.: J. Pediat., *52*:158, 1958.)

115. GENERALIZED GANGLIOSIDOSIS

(Caffey's Pseudo-Hurler's Syndrome, Familial Neurovisceral Lipidosis)

Coarse Facies, Joint Limitation and Kyphosis in Early Infancy

In 1951, Caffey[1] described two neonates who had many of the features of Hurler's syndrome, but of prenatal onset. Landing et al.[2] reported pathological studies in similar cases showing foamy histiocytes in liver and spleen, swollen neurons, and vacuoles in the glomerular epithelium. They interpreted the storage material as a glycolipid and set forth the name "familial neurovisceral lipidosis," which was changed to "generalized gangliosidosis" by O'Brien et al.[3] on the basis of finding elevated levels of ganglioside in liver, spleen, and brain tissue from such a patient. Finally Scott et al.[4] identified mucopolysaccharide in the glomerular epithelium from a patient and suggested that the disease belongs in the group of mucopolysaccharidoses.

ABNORMALITIES[5]

Growth. Growth deficiency with relatively low birth weight and severe postnatal deficit in growth.

Performance. Severe early defect in developmental performance with hypotonia, poor coordination, and later spasticity. Neuronal lipidosis with swollen neurons at necropsy.

Orofacial. Coarse features with low nasal bridge, broad nose, flaring alae nasi, frontal bossing, hypertrophied alveolar ridges with prominent maxilla and mild macroglossia. Hirsutism.

Eyes. Cherry-red macular spot in about one half of patients.

Skeletal. Moderate joint limitation with thick wrists and development of claw hand. Early roentgenograms show poorly mineralized, coarsely trabeculated long bones with medullary mid-shaft broadening and a "cloak" of subperiosteal new bone formation, especially evident in the humerus. Some metaphyseal cupping and epiphyseal irregularity are usually present. With time the bones appear more like those of Hurler's syndrome, including kyphosis with anterior bullet wedging of vertebrae. Ribs are thick, legs may be bowed, and club foot may be present.

Viscera. Variable hepatomegaly with some foamy histiocytes. Vacuolization in glomerular epithelial cells containing swollen lysosomes.

Leukocytes. Vacuolization within cytoplasm of leukocytes and foam cells in marrow.

Urinary Excretion. Mucopolysaccharide normal or slightly elevated.

NATURAL HISTORY. Severe developmental lag, feeding problems with failure to thrive, and frequent infections usually culminate in death during early infancy. Deterioration of cerebral function is rapid if the patient survives the first year, leading to a decerebrate status with seizures and death prior to two years of age. The mean age of survival for 17 patients was 13.5 months, with a range from 3.5 to 25 months. No form of therapy other than life-supportive tube-feeding and antibiotic management of infections has been effective. Considering the natural history of this disorder, the author favors discussion with the parents followed by the withholding of life-supportive medical treatment if this course of management is acceptable to the parents.

ETIOLOGY. Autosomal recessive. O'Brien[5] has detected a severe deficit (one twentieth of normal) of the lysosomal enzyme galactosidase in liver from these patients. The presumed developmental pathology of the disease is as follows: (1) inability to cleave the terminal galactose from ganglioside and mucopolysaccharide, (2) accumulation of these products within lysosomes where they would normally be degraded, and (3) the storage disease.

REFERENCES

1. Caffey, J.: Gargoylism (Hunter-Hurler disease, dysostosis multiplex, lipochondrodystrophy); prenatal and neonatal bone lesions and their early postnatal evolution. Bull. Hosp. Joint Dis., 12: 38, 1951.
2. Landing, B. H., Silverman, F. N., Craig, J. M., Jacoby, M. D., and Chadwick, D. L: Familial neurovisceral lipidosis. An analysis of eight cases of a syndrome previously reported as "Hurler-variant," "Pseudo-Hurler disease," and "Tay-Sachs disease with visceral involvement." Am. J. Dis. Children, 108:503, 1964.
3. O'Brien, J. S., Stern, M. B., Landing, B. H., O'Brien, J. K., and Donnell, G. N.: Generalized gangliosidosis. Another inborn error of ganglioside metabolism? Am. J. Dis. Children, 109:338, 1965.
4. Scott, C. R., Lagunoff, D., and Trump, B. F.: Familial neurovisceral lipidosis. J. Pediat., 71:357, 1967.
5. O'Brien, J.: Generalized gangliosidosis. The First Conference on the Clinical Delineation of Birth Defects. D. S. Bergsma, Editor. Part IV, The National Foundation (in press).

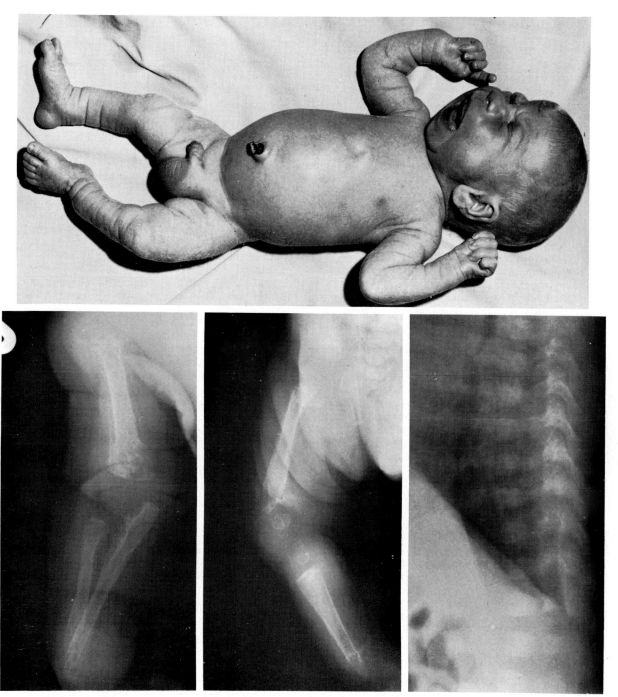

Two week old with x-rays of the arm, leg, and thoracolumbar vertebrae. Note the coarse facies, hypertrophied alveolar ridges, broad wrists, periosteal cloaking with thin cortices, altered shape of head of humerus and femur, and hypoplastic vertebrae. (From Scott, R., et al.: J. Pediat., 71:357, 1967.)

116. HURLER'S SYNDROME

(Mucopolysaccharidosis I)

Coarse Facies, Stiff Joints, Mental Deterioration, Cloudy Cornea by One to Two Years

Hurler[1] set forth this entity in 1919, two years after the Hunter syndrome was described. O'Brien[2] has recently attributed the cellular accumulation of mucopolysaccharide and ganglioside to the diminished (one fifth of normal) degradative lysosomal enzyme β-galactosidase found in these patients.

ABNORMALITIES.[3, 4]   Onset by one to two years of age.

Growth.   Deficiency, becoming severe.

Performance.   Mental regression toward severe apathetic deficiency.

Craniofacial and Eye.   Scaphocephalic cranial enlargement, coarse facies with full lips, flared nostrils, low nasal bridge and tendency toward hypertelorism.
Cloudy corneas, retinal pigmentation.

Mouth.   Hypertrophied alveolar ridge and gum with small malaligned teeth. Enlarged tongue.

Skeletal and Joints.   Diaphyseal broadening of short misshapen bones and joint limitation yield the claw hand and other joint deformities. Flaring of the rib cage. Kyphosis and thoracolumbar gibbus secondary to anterior vertebral wedging.

Cardiac.   Murmurs; cardiac failure may be due to intimal thickening in the coronary vessels or the cardiac valves.

Other.   Hirsutism, hepatosplenomegaly, inguinal hernia, dislocation of hip, mucoid rhinitis, deafness.

Urinary Excretion.   Dermatan sulfate and heparan sulfate.

OCCASIONAL ABNORMALITIES.   Hydrocephalus, presumably due to meningeal involvement.

NATURAL HISTORY.   Growth during the first year may actually be more rapid than usual with subsequent deterioration. Subtle changes in the facies with development of a gibbus, cloudy cornea, and slowing in developmental progress may be evident prior to one year. The mental deterioration is severe. Death usually occurs in childhood secondary to respiratory or cardiac complications, and survival past ten years of age is unusual.

ETIOLOGY.   Autosomal recessive. The asymptomatic carriers may be recognized by abnormal lysosomal accumulation of mucopolysaccharide in their cultured fibroblast cells, a phenomenon which is more striking in the homozygote.

REFERENCES

1. Hurler, G.: Ueber einen Typ multipler Abartungen, vorwiegend am Skelettsystem. Z. Kinderh., *24*: 220, 1919.
2. O'Brien, J.: Personal communication.
3. McKusick, V.: Heritable Disorders of Connective Tissue. 3rd ed. St. Louis, C. V. Mosby Co., 1966, p. 328.
4. Leroy, J. G., and Crocker, A. C.: Clinical definition of the Hurler-Hunter phenotypes. A review of 50 patients. Am. J. Dis. Children, *112*:518, 1966.

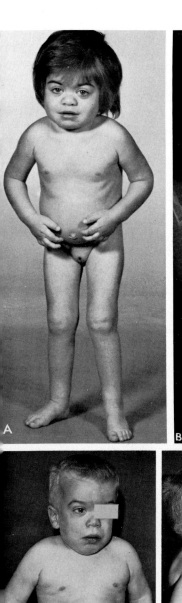
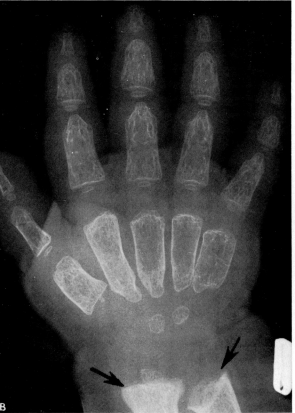
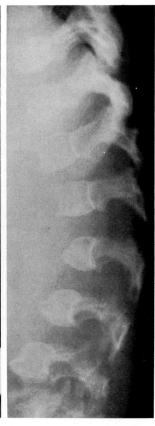
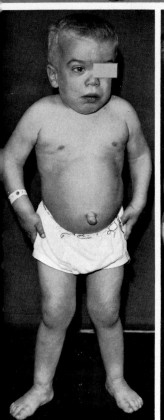
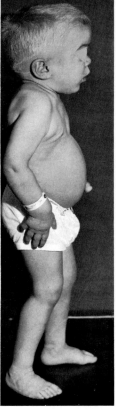

A, Two year old who sat at one year and walked at 21 months. Height age at six months was ten months; at one year, 16 months; and at two years, two years.

B, Broad irregular bone, especially at metaphyses. Thoracic and lumbar vertebrae are short with anterior wedging.

C, Five year old with height age of three years.

117. MAROTEAUX-LAMY SYNDROME

(Mucopolysaccharidosis VI)

Coarse Facies, Stiff Joints, Cloudy Cornea in Infancy, Without Mental Deterioration

Maroteaux et al.[1] recognized this disorder as being distinct from Hurler's syndrome, in that mental deterioration did *not* occur during early childhood and the only mucopolysaccharide found in the urine was dermatan sulfate. However, Fallis et al.[3] reported heparan sulfate as well as dermatan sulfate in the urine of such a patient.

ABNORMALITIES. Onset by one to three years of age.
Growth. Deficiency, usually evident between two and three years.
Craniofacial. Coarse facies with large nose and thick lips.
Eye. Fine corneal opacity.
Skeletal and Joints. Mild stiffness of joints.
  Metaphyses slightly broad and irregular.
  Epiphyseal irregularity, especially femoral epiphysis.
  Vertebrae flattened with anterior wedging of T-12 and L-1.
  Ribs broad.
  Sella turcica elongated.
  Lumbar kyphosis, genu valgum.
Other. Umbilical hernia.
  Hepatosplenomegaly.
  Varying degrees of deafness.
  Cytoplasmic granules in leukocytes.

NATURAL HISTORY. The age of onset of growth deficiency is usually a little later than in Hurler's disease; the extent of skeletal broadening, joint limitation, hepatosplenomegaly, and corneal opacification is generally less than with Hurler's disease, and cerebral deterioration has not been noted during childhood. The data on prognosis after ten years of age are presently inadequate.

ETIOLOGY. Presumed autosomal recessive.

REFERENCES

1. Maroteaux, P., Levêque, B., Marie, J., and Lamy, M.: Une nouvelle dysostose avec élimination urinaire de chondroitine-sulfate B. Presse Méd., *71*:1849, 1963.
2. Maroteaux, P., and Lamy, M.: Hurler's disease, Morquio's disease, and related mucopolysaccharidoses. J. Pediat., *67*:312, 1965.
3. Fallis, N., Barnes, F. L., II, and di Ferrante, N.: A case of polydystrophic dwarfism with urinary excretion of dermatan sulfate and heparan sulfate. J. Clin. Endocr., *28*:26, 1968.

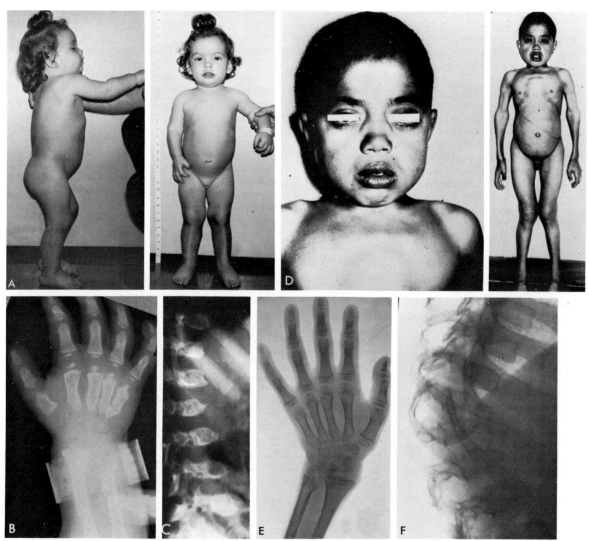

A to C, Eighteen month old; height age, 16 months. (Courtesy of R. Summitt, University of Tennessee.) D to F, Older boy, short of stature, with normal intelligence. (Courtesy of P. Maroteaux, Hôpital des Enfants-Malades, Paris.)

118. HUNTER'S SYNDROME

(Mucopolysaccharidosis II)

Coarse Facies, Growth Deficiency, Stiff Joints by Two to Four Years, Clear Cornea

Hunter[1] described this condition in 1917 in two brothers.

ABNORMALITIES.[2,3] Onset around two to four years.

Growth. Growth deficiency.

Performance. Mental deficiency.

Facies. Coarsening of facial features, full lips.

Joint and Skeletal. Stiff partial contracture of joints, claw hand. Broadening of bone.

Other. Hepatosplenomegaly, hypertrichosis, inguinal hernias, mucoid nasal discharge, progressive deafness.

Urinary Excretion. Dermatan sulfate and heparan sulfate.

OCCASIONAL ABNORMALITIES. Diarrhea, nodular skin lesions over scapular area and on arms, kyphosis, pes cavus, osteoarthritis of head of femur, retinal pigmentation, congestive heart failure, coronary occlusion.

IMPORTANT NEGATIVES IN CONTRAST TO HURLER'S SYNDROME. (1) Clear corneas. (2) No gibbus. (3) No affected females.

NATURAL HISTORY. Gradual decline in growth rate and mental development from two to six years, often reaching a plateau in mental capabilities around six years. These patients tend to be more noisy and obstreperous than those with the Hurler syndrome. Cardiac complications not uncommonly lead to death prior to 20 years; however, survival to 60 years has been recorded.

ETIOLOGY. X-linked, with no overt expression in the heterozygous female who may be recognized by the fact that cultured fibroblasts show cytoplasmic accumulation of mucopolysaccharide, though to a lesser extent than those of the hemizygous male.

REFERENCES

1. Hunter, C.: A rare disease in two brothers. Proc. Roy. Soc. Med., *10*:104, 1917.
2. McKusick, V.: Heritable Disorders of Connective Tissue. 3rd ed. St. Louis, The C. V. Mosby Co., 1966, p. 346.
3. Leroy, J. G., and Crocker, A. C.: Clinical definition of the Hurler-Hunter phenotypes. A review of 50 patients. Am. J. Dis. Children, *112*:518, 1966.

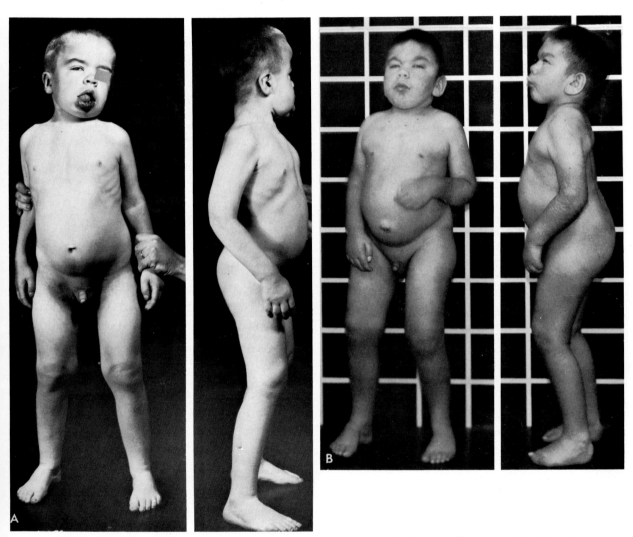

A, Nine and one half year old with height age of seven and two thirds years. (Courtesy of A. C. Crocker, Boston Children's Hospital.)

B, Thirteen and one half year old with height age of seven years.

249

119. MORQUIO'S SYNDROME

(Mucopolysaccharidosis IV)

*Onset at One to Three Years of Age, Mild Coarse Facies,
Severe Kyphosis and Knock Knee, Late Cloudy Cornea*

Mistakenly interpreted by Osler[1] in 1898, this condition was described by Morquio[2] in 1929; it was only recently recognized as a mucopolysaccharidosis.[3]

ABNORMALITIES. Onset between one and three years.

Growth. Severe limitation with cessation by latter childhood.

Craniofacial. Mild coarsening of facial features with broad mouth and short nose.

Eye. Cloudy cornea, usually after five to ten years of age.

Skeletal and Joint. Marked platyspondyly with vertebrae changing to ovaloid, ovaloid with anterior projection, to flattened form with short neck and trunk plus kyphoscoliosis.

Early flaring of rib cage progressing to bulging sternum.

Short curved long bones with irregular tubulation, widened metaphyses, abnormal femoral neck, flattening of femoral head, knock knee with medial spur of tibial metaphysis, conical bases of widened metacarpals, irregular epiphyseal form, osteoporosis.

Joint laxity, most evident at wrist.

Mouth. Widely spaced teeth with thin enamel.

Cardiac. Late onset of aortic regurgitation, frequency unknown.

Other. Hearing loss. Inguinal hernia.

Urinary Excretion. Keratosulfate.

NATURAL HISTORY. The earliest recognized indication of the disease has been flaring of the lower rib cage. Severe defect of vertebrae may result in cord compression or respiratory insufficiency. These and cardiac complications usually result in death prior to 20 years, although later survival has occurred. Mentality is usually normal.

ETIOLOGY. Autosomal recessive.

REFERENCES

1. Osler, W.: Sporadic cretinism in America. Trans. Cong. Am. Phys., 4:169, 1897.
2. Morquio, L.: Sur une forme de dystrophie osseuse familiale. Arch. Med. Enf., 32:129, 1929.
3. Robins, M. M., Stevens, H. F., and Linker, A.: Morquio's disease: an abnormality of mucopolysaccharide metabolism. J. Pediat., 62:881, 1963.
4. Langer, L. O., and Carey, L. S.: The roentgenographic features of the ks mucopolysaccharidosis of Morquio (Morquio-Brailsford's disease). Am. J. Roentgenol., 97:1, 1966.
5. McKusick, V.: Heritable Disorders of Connective Tissue. 3rd ed. St. Louis, C. V. Mosby Co., 1966, p. 361.

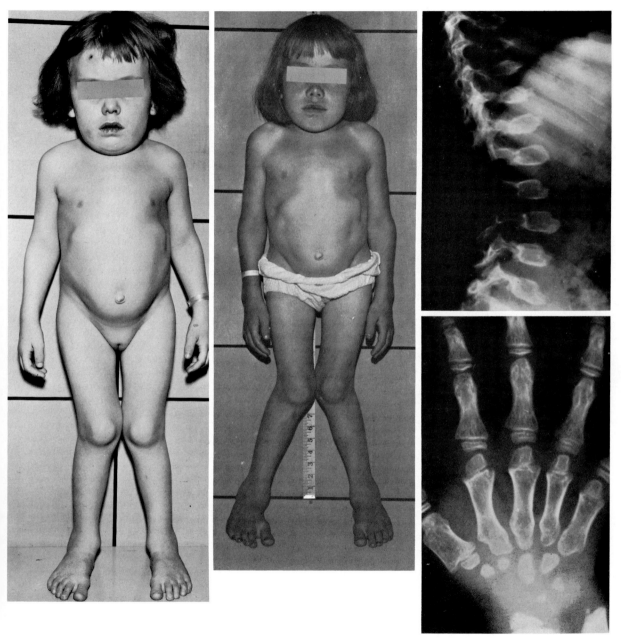

Left, three and one half years; height age, two and three fourths years. Center, same patient at seven years; height age, two and three fourths years. Right, x-rays of patient at seven years. (From Robins, M. M., et al.: J. Pediat., *62*:881, 1963.)

120. SANFILIPPO'S SYNDROME

(Mucopolysaccharidosis III)

Mild Coarse Facies, Mild Stiff Joints, Mental Deficiency

This disorder was recognized by Sanfilippo et al.[1] in 1963; the excess mucopolysaccharide urinary excretion is heparitin sulfate alone. These individuals usually have clear corneas.

ABNORMALITIES. Onset in early childhood.
Growth. Mild to moderate shortness of stature.
Performance. Progressive mental deterioration, usually to idiocy in later childhood.
Facies. Mild coarsening of features.
Skeletal and Joint. Mild limitation of joint motility.
Dense calvarium, thickened ribs, ovoid vertebral bodies, mild pelvic dysplasia.
Lymphocytes. Toluidine blue metachromasia, coarse and sparse granules.
Urinary Excretion. Heparitin sulfate.

NATURAL HISTORY. Compatible with long survival as a severely mentally defective strong individual with little physical impairment.

ETIOLOGY. Autosomal recessive.

REFERENCES

1. Sanfilippo, S. J., Podosin, R., Langer, L. O., Jr., and Good, R. A.: Mental retardation associated with acid mucopolysacchariduria (heparitin sulfate type). J. Pediat., *63*:837, 1963.
2. McKusick, V.: Heritable Disorders of Connective Tissue. 3rd ed. St. Louis, C. V. Mosby Co., 1966, p. 357.
3. Spranger, J., Teller, W., Kosenow, W., Murken, J., Eckert-Husemann, E.: Die HS-Mucopolysaccharidose von Sanfilippo (Polydystrophe Oligophrenie). Bericht über 10 Patienten. Z. Kinderh., *101*:71, 1967.

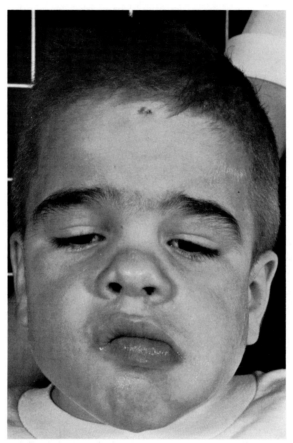

A seven year old with the height age of five and three fourths years. His capabilities have been regressing and his present intelligence quotient is about 50. A sibling is similarly affected. (Courtesy of R. Scott, University of Washington Medical School.)

121. SCHEIE'S SYNDROME

(Mucopolysaccharidosis V)

Broad Mouth with Full Lips, Early Corneal Opacity, Normal Mentality

This disorder was originally described by Scheie et al.[1] in 1962. Only a few cases have been recognized, and there have been no necropsy observations.

ABNORMALITIES.[1-3]
General. Little, if any, impairment of intelligence.
Facies. Broad mouth with full lips by five to eight years of age.
Cornea. Early clouding of cornea, becoming most dense in periphery.
Limbs. Joint limitation leading to claw hand, small carpal bones, femoral head dysplasia.
Cardiac. Presumed aortic valvular defect.
Other. Body hirsutism. Retinal pigmentation.
Urinary Excretion. Proportionately more dermatan sulfate than usual.

OCCASIONAL ABNORMALITIES. Carpal tunnel narrowing may cause median nerve compression. Psychosis and possible mental deterioration may occur. Mild impairment of growth. Hearing loss.

ETIOLOGY. Autosomal recessive, with excess urinary excretion of dermatan sulfate.

REFERENCES

1. Scheie, H. G., Hambrick, G. W., Jr., and Barness, L. A.: A newly recognized forme fruste of Hurler's disease (gargoylism). Am. J. Ophth., *53*:753, 1962.
2. Emerit, I., Maroteaux, P., and Vernant, P.: Deux observations de mucopolysaccharidose avec atteinte cardio-vasculaire. Arch. Franç. Pédiat., *23*:1075, 1966.
3. McKusick, V.: Heritable Disorders of Connective Tissue. 3rd ed. St. Louis, C. V. Mosby Co., 1966.

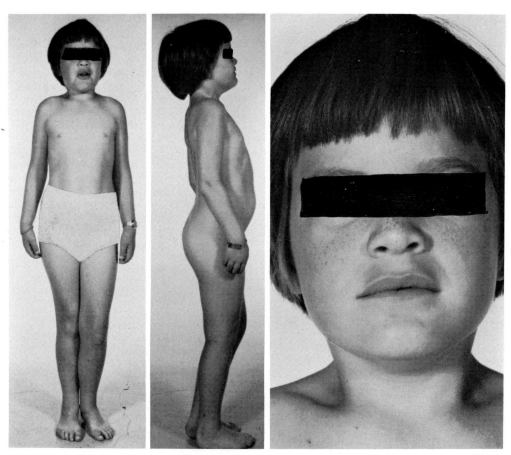

Nine and three fourths year old with height age of nine years and I.Q. of 102. Mild to moderate limitation of shoulder, elbow, and hand movement. Mild corneal opacity. (Courtesy of R. Scott, University of Washington.)

122. LEROY'S SYNDROME

(I [Inclusion] Cell Disease)

Early Alveolar Ridge Hypertrophy, Joint Limitation, Thick Tight Skin in Early Infancy

This disorder was recognized by Leroy,[1] when he noted unusual cytoplasmic inclusions in the cultured fibroblasts of a girl who had been considered to have Hurler's syndrome, despite the fact that she did not have cloudy corneas or excessive acid mucopolysaccharide in the urine.

ABNORMALITIES. Based on two cases.[4]

Growth. Birth weight less than 5½ pounds. Marked growth deficiency with lack of linear growth after infancy.

Performance. Slow progress from early infancy, reaching a plateau around 18 months with no apparent deterioration by seven years.

Craniofacial. High narrow forehead with metopic ridge.

Inner epicanthic folds, clear corneas.

Low nasal bridge, anteverted nostrils.

Mouth. Hypertrophy of alveolar ridges.

Skeletal and Joints. Moderate joint limitation in flexion, especially hips.

Dorsolumbar kyphosis.

Broadening of wrists and fingers.

X-ray findings similar to those of Hurler's disease.

Skin. Thick, relatively tight skin during early infancy.

Cavernous hemangiomata.

Other. Minimal hepatosplenomegaly.

Diastasis recti.

Inguinal hernia (one case).

Note. No metachromatic granules noted in leukocytes.

Urinary mucopolysaccharides normal to mildly increased.

NATURAL HISTORY. Both patients[2] are now beyond six years of age. One cannot sit with support; the other is able to move about with a walker. Neither has intelligible speech, but they are socially responsive and pleasant, and one mother stated that "despite the very low I.Q. she is very responsive to people." Ear infections have been frequent during early childhood, and mucous nasal discharge has been a minor problem.

ETIOLOGY. Autosomal recessive. The material which swells the lysosomes and thereby gives rise to the cytoplasmic inclusions noted in cultured fibroblasts has not been identified. There is accumulation of acid mucopolysaccharide and glycolipids, and the optically dense granular inclusions stain with Sudan black B and para-aminosalicylic acid. The lysosomal enzyme activity is altered, with excessive acid phosphatase (five times normal) and reduced β-glucuronidase. Further studies are in progress to more distinctly differentiate this condition from other lipomucopolysaccharidoses. Similar but less frequent cytoplasmic inclusions were noted in the fibroblast cells of the otherwise normal parents, a presumed heterozygous expression.

REFERENCES

1. Leroy, J. G., and DeMars, R. I.: Mutant enzymatic and cytological phenotypes in cultured human fibroblasts. Science, *157*:804, 1967.
2. Wiedemann, H. R., and Spranger, J.: Lipomucopolysaccharidosis. Lancet, *1*:861, 1968.
3. Matalon, R., Cifonelli, J. A., Zellweger, H., and Dorfman, A.: Lipid abnormalities in a variant of the Hurler syndrome. Proc. Nat. Acad. Sci., *59*:1097, 1968.
4. Leroy, J. G., DeMars, R. I., and Opitz, J. M.: "I-cell" disease. The First Conference on the Clinical Delineation of Birth Defects. D. S. Bergsma, Editor. Part IV, The National Foundation (in press).

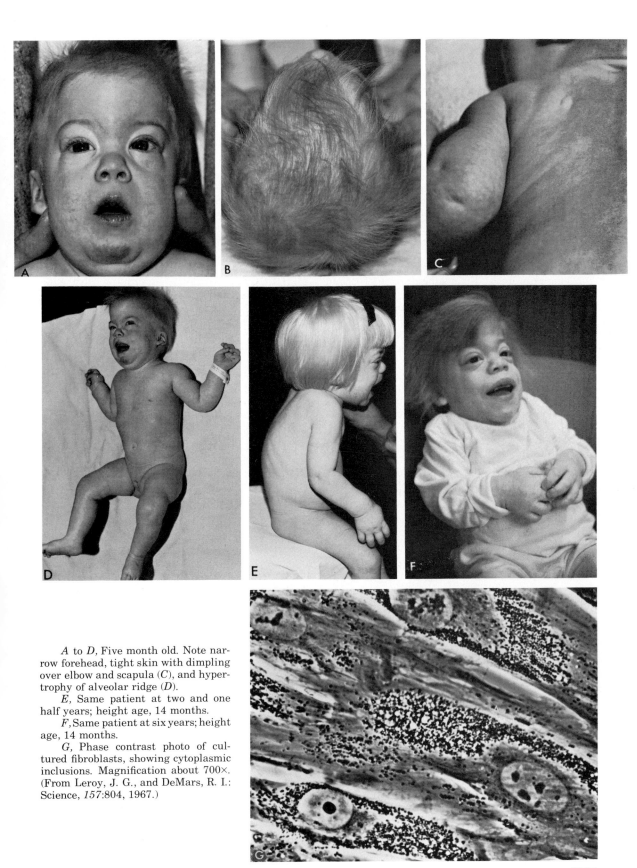

A to *D,* Five month old. Note narrow forehead, tight skin with dimpling over elbow and scapula (*C*), and hypertrophy of alveolar ridge (*D*).

E, Same patient at two and one half years; height age, 14 months.

F, Same patient at six years; height age, 14 months.

G, Phase contrast photo of cultured fibroblasts, showing cytoplasmic inclusions. Magnification about 700×. (From Leroy, J. G., and DeMars, R. I.: Science, *157*:804, 1967.)

123. MARFAN'S SYNDROME

Arachnodactyly with Hyperextensibility, Lens Subluxation, Aortic Dilatation

Described as dolichostenomelia in the initial report of Marfan,[1] this disorder has been extensively studied and recognized as a connective tissue disorder by McKusick.[2]

ABNORMALITIES[2]
Skeletal. Tendency toward tall stature with long slim limbs, little subcutaneous fat, and muscle hypotonia.
Joint laxity with scoliosis and kyphosis.
Pectus excavatum or carinatum.
Narrow facies with narrow palate.
Eye. Lens subluxation with defect in suspensory ligament.
Myopia. Bluish sclerae.
Cardiovascular. Dilatation with or without dissecting aneurysm of ascending aorta, less commonly of thoracic or abdominal aorta or pulmonary artery.
Secondary aortic regurgitation.
Other. Inguinal, femoral hernias.

OCCASIONAL ABNORMALITIES.
Large ears, retinal detachment, striae in pectoral or deltoid area, diaphragmatic hernia, pulmonary malformation contributing toward spontaneous pneumothorax and/or emphysema with an increased susceptibility to respiratory infection. Hemivertebrae, colobomata of iris, cleft palate, incomplete rotation of colon.

NATURAL HISTORY.
During childhood and adolescence special care should be devoted toward prevention of scoliosis. The serious vascular complications may develop anytime from fetal life through old age and are the chief cause of death. The mean age of survival is 43 for men and 46 for women. These individuals are of normal intelligence.

ETIOLOGY.
Autosomal dominant with sufficiently wide variability in expression that diagnosis is often tenuous in sporadic nonfamilial cases. Cases occur without ectopia lentis and without pronounced arachnodactyly. The basic defect in connective tissue has not been determined; however, accumulation of mucopolysaccharide has been noted within cells of the aorta from an affected individual, and the cultured fibroblast cells from individuals with Marfan's syndrome show cytoplasmic metachromatic inclusion.

REFERENCES

1. Marfan, A. B.: Un cas de déformation congénitale des quatre membres plus prononcée aux extrémites charactérisée par l'allongement des os avec un certain degré d'amincissement. Bull. Mém. Soc. Méd. Hôp. Paris, *13*:220, 1896.
2. McKusick, V.: Heritable Disorders of Connective Tissue. 3rd ed. St. Louis, C. V. Mosby Co., 1966, p. 38.

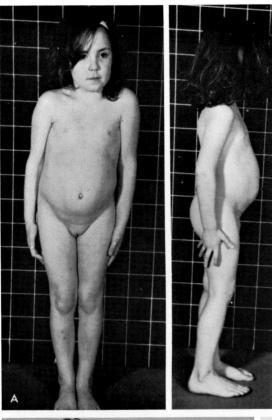

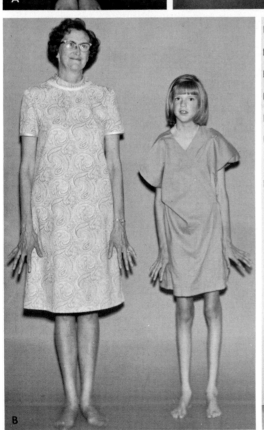

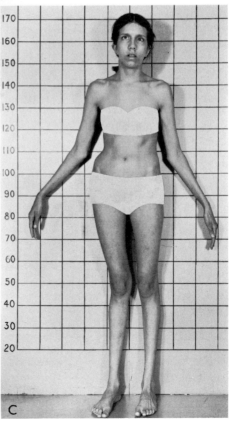

A, Three and one half year old, with height age of five years, who has lens dislocation, mild arachnodactyly of the hands and feet, unusually soft skin, and narrow palate. The family history of Marfan's syndrome in the mother and grandfather tend to confirm the diagnosis in this case.

B, Nine and one fourth year old girl with height age of twelve and one fourth years and her mother. Both have arachnodactyly, but only the mother has dislocation of the lenses.

C, Sixteen year old with arachnodactyly, hyperextensible hands and knees, limitation of extension at elbow, scoliosis, systolic and diastolic murmurs, superiorly dislocated lenses, glaucoma, and retinal detachments despite numerous surgical procedures. She represents a fresh mutation, no other family members being affected. (Courtesy of Drs. Victor McKusick and Judith Hall, the Johns Hopkins Hospital.)

124. HOMOCYSTINURIA

Subluxation of Lens, Malar Flush, Osteoporosis

Urinary aminoacid screening of mentally defective patients resulted in the independent discovery of this entity by Carson et al.[1] and Gerritsen and Waisman[2] in 1963. Mudd[3] and co-workers found a lack of cystathionine synthetase activity in the liver of affected individuals, and this enzyme defect apparently leads to the accumulation of homocystine and methionine with a deficiency of cystathionine and cystine. The more appropriate name for the condition would therefore be cystathionine synthetase deficiency. This inborn error often results in mental defect as well as defective development in blood vessels and of connective tissues, resembling Marfan's syndrome in the latter regard.

ABNORMALITIES
General. Mental defect in 58 per cent of 38 cases in McKusick's study.[5]
Eye. Subluxation of lens by the age of ten years, the earliest instance noted being two years. Myopia.
Skeletal. Slim skeletal build resembling arachnodactyly with pectus excavatum or carinatum, genu valgum, pes cavus, everted feet with or without kyphoscoliosis. Osteoporosis.
Vasculature. Medial degeneration of aorta and elastic arteries with internal hyperplasia and fibrosis leading to pads and ridges within the vessels. Both arterial and venous thromboses are frequent.
Skin. Malar flush with tendency to patchy erythematous blotches elsewhere.
Hair. Tends to be fine, sparse, dry, and light in color.

OCCASIONAL ABNORMALITIES.
Cataracts, glaucoma, optic atrophy, cystic retinal degeneration or detachment, irregular crowded teeth, high arched palate, hernias, and hepatomegaly with fatty liver.

NATURAL HISTORY.
Seizures with onset from six months to five years of age have been noted, and the electroencephalographic pattern is usually abnormal. Excessive nervousness may be a feature, occasionally with schizophrenic behavior. Neurological defect, especially spasticity, may be present and is often asymmetrical — presumably the consequence of vascular thrombosis which can be arterial or venous and not infrequently involves the coronary arteries. Venipuncture or surgical procedures may be followed by excessive vascular thrombosis and should be avoided when possible. Thromboembolic phenomena constitute the most life-threatening feature of this disease. Another problem, osteoporosis, frequently leads to partial collapse of vertebrae, and there is an increased likelihood of fractures.

Failure to thrive has been a feature of some cases with severe mental defect. However, normal to tall stature is the more usual growth pattern.

Because the degree of mental defect and the age and severity of complications vary considerably, it is not possible to state the prognosis with assurance for an affected individual.

ETIOLOGY.
Autosomal recessive. Decreased cystathionine synthetase activity has been found in the liver of the parents of homocystinuric individuals, supporting the contention that they are heterozygotes.

COMMENT.
The urinary cyanide nitroprusside test may not always yield a positive result in patients with homocystinuria, and specific amino acid studies therefore constitute the most important diagnostic measure. A completely successful mode of therapy has not yet been demonstrated. A low methionine, high cystine diet is being tried; unfortunately cystathionine is too expensive to warrant dietary replacement.

REFERENCES

1. Carson, N. A. J., Cusworth, D. C., Dent, C. E., Field, C. M. B., Neill, D. W., and Westall, R. G.: Homocystinuria: a new inborn error of metabolism associated with mental deficiency. Arch. Dis. Childhood, *38*:425, 1963.
2. Gerritsen, T., and Waisman, H. A.: Homocystinuria, an error in the metabolism of methionine. Pediatrics, *33*:413, 1964.
3. Finkelstein, J. D., Mudd, S. H., Irreverre, F., and Laster, L.: Homocystinuria due to cystathionine synthetase deficiency: the mode of inheritance. Science, *146*:785, 1964.
4. White, H. H., Thompson, H. L., Rowland, L. P., Cowen, D., and Araki, S.: Homocystinuria. Trans. Am. Neurol. Assn., *89*:24, 1964.
5. McKusick, V.: Heritable Disorders of Connective Tissue. 3rd ed. St. Louis, C. V. Mosby Co., 1966, p. 150.

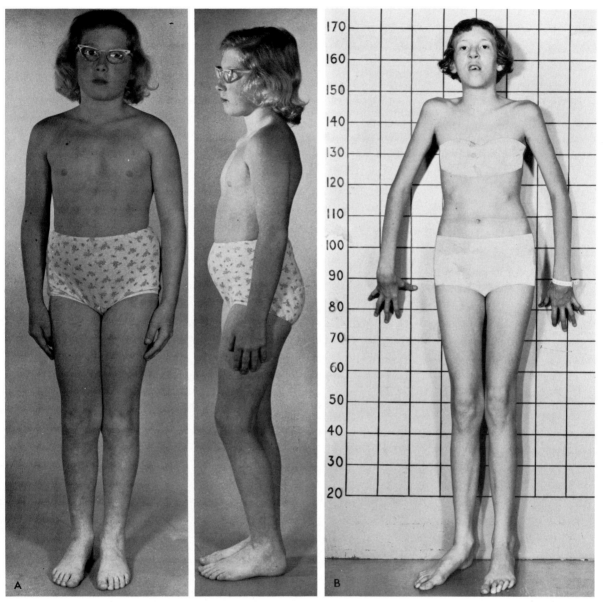

A, Ten year old girl with homocystinuria who presented with lens subluxation which was first noted at four years of age. Her early developmental progress was within normal limits, but she has been receiving special schooling and her intelligence quotient is 67.

B, Twelve year old girl with arachnodactyly, "tight" joints, and inferiorly and nasally dislocated lenses. She is of low normal intelligence with a "schizoid personality" and has had two episodes of gastrointestinal bleeding, one documented as being secondary to a gastric infarct. (Courtesy of Drs. Victor McKusick and Judith Hall, Johns Hopkins Hospital.)

125. EHLERS-DANLOS SYNDROME

Hyperextensibility of Joints, Hyperextensibility of Skin,
Poor Wound Healing with Thin Scar

Originally described Van Meekeren[1] in 1682, this condition was further clarified by Ehlers[2] in 1901 and Danlos in 1908.[3] More than 100 cases have been described, the most complete review being that of McKusick.[4] The possibility has been raised that the celebrated violinist Paganini may have had Ehlers-Danlos syndrome, thus accounting for his unusual dexterity and reach.

ABNORMALITIES. Most consistent features:
Face. Narrow maxilla.
Auricles. Hypermobile with tendency toward "lop ears."
Skin. Velvety, hyperextensible, and fragile with poor wound healing leaving parchment-thin scars. Small movable subcutaneous spherules contain either mucinous material or adipose.
Joints. Hyperextensibility with liability toward dislocation at hip, shoulder, elbow, knee, or clavicle. Pes planus.
Blood Vessels. Easy bruisability.

OCCASIONAL ABNORMALITIES

Eyes and Facies. Wide nasal bridge. Epicanthic folds, blue sclerae, myopia, microcornea, keratoconus, glaucoma, ectopia lentis, retinal detachment.
Skeletal. Small stature, kyphoscoliosis, long neck, slim skeletal build, downsloping ribs, club foot, overlapping toes.
Dentition. Small, irregular placement, partial anodontia.
Blood Vessels. Dissecting aneurysm, intracranial aneurysm, hemorrhage.
Gastrointestinal. Inguinal hernia, diaphragmatic hernia, ectasia of intestine and intestinal diverticuli.
Renal. Ureteropelvic anomaly, renal tubular acidosis.
Other. Mental deficiency. Anomalies of mitral valve.

NATURAL HISTORY. Barabas[5] discovered that most patients with Ehlers-Danlos syndrome are born prematurely following premature rupture of the membranes, possibly the first obvious indication of relative friability of tissues in these individuals. The integrity of tissues is easily disturbed as evidenced by the fragility of skin and blood vessels. Wound healing is delayed with relatively inadequate scar tissue, and prolonged hemorrhage may occur following trauma. Both these factors plus the tendency of sutures to tear out mitigate against unnecessary surgical procedures. These patients should be cautioned to avoid traumatic situations. Gastrointestinal hemorrhage or hemoptysis may be a problem, the poor integrity of vessels may occasionally lead to a dissecting aneurysm, and affected women are liable to postpartum hemorrhage. Whether or not the tendency to chilblains and acrocyanosis is secondary to vascular alterations is undetermined.

The peculiar fat or mucinoid containing subcutaneous spherules, most commonly found in areas of frequent mild trauma, may mineralize and thereby be evident on roentgenograms.

ETIOLOGY. Autosomal dominant with wide variance in expression.

COMMENT. The basic problem is presumably a defect in connective tissue, the basic nature of which is undetermined. Electron microscopy and quantitative measures of elastin have revealed no definite abnormality.

REFERENCES

1. Van Meekeren, J. A.: De dilatabilitate extraordinaria cutis. Chapter 32 in Observations Medicochirogicae. Amsterdam, 1682.
2. Ehlers, E.: Cutis laxa, Neigung zu Harmorrhagien in der Haut, Lockerung mehrer Artikulationen. Dermat. Ztschr., 8:173, 1901.
3. Danlos, H.: Un cas de cutis laxa avec tumeurs par contusion chronique des coudes et des genoux (santhome juvenile pseudodiabetique de MM. Hallopeau et Mace de Lepinay). Bull. Soc. Franç., Dermat. Syph., 19:70, 1908.
4. McKusick, V. A.: Heritable Disorders of Connective Tissue. 3rd ed. St. Louis, C. V. Mosby Co., 1966, p. 179.
5. Barabas, A. P.: Ehlers-Danlos syndrome: associated with prematurity and premature rupture of foetal membranes; possible increase in incidence. Brit. Med. J., 2:682, 1966.
6. Wechsler, H. L., and Fisher, E. R.: Ehlers-Danlos syndrome. Pathologic, histochemical, and electron microscopic observations. Arch. Path., 77: 613, 1964.

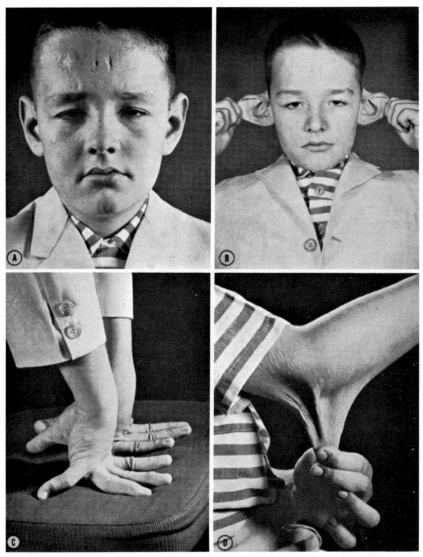

Twelve year old boy showing thin persisting scars on forehead (A), hyperelasticity of auricles and skin (B and D), and hyperextensibility of joints (C). (From Rees, T. D., et al.: Plastic & Recon. Surg., *32*:39, 1963.)

126. OSTEOGENESIS IMPERFECTA

Fragile Bone, Blue Sclerae, Hyperextensibility, and/or Odontogenesis Imperfecta

This rather generalized disorder of connective tissue occurs with a frequency of about one in 25,000 individuals. There is wide individual variability in the manifestations of the disease, and the following individual defects occur in roughly 25 to 60 per cent of patients, with no alteration being a consistent feature.

ABNORMALITIES

Growth. Small stature in severe cases, sometimes with unduly short extremities.

Bones. Thin cortices and sparse trabeculae with fragility leading to bowing of leg bones in severe cases. Occasionally thin calvarium with wide fontanels and wormian bones; biconcave flattening of vertebrae; pectus carinatum or excavatum.

Joints and Ligaments. Hyperextensible, sometimes leading to kyphoscoliosis, flat feet, and in extreme cases joint dislocation.

Dentition. Hypoplasia of dentin and pulp with translucency of teeth and propensity to caries, irregular placement, and late eruption.

Sclerae and Skin. The skin and sclerae tend to be thin and translucent, with partial visualization of the choroid, giving the sclerae a blue appearance.

Hearing. Deafness is usually secondary to otosclerosis and is seldom present until adult life.

Other. Inguinal and/or umbilical hernia. Poor muscle development.

OCCASIONAL ABNORMALITIES

Eye. Embryotoxon (opacity in the peripheral cornea), keratoconus, megalocornea.

Other. Syndactyly.

NATURAL HISTORY. There is wide individual variability with early mortality among severely affected infants, chiefly related to bronchopneumonia. Beyond infancy the outlook for survival is good, and the chief problems are orthopedic deformity and otosclerosis. The long leg bones are the most frequent site of breakage with the peak ages for fractures being two to three years and ten to 15 years. After adolescence the likelihood of fracture diminishes, although inactivity, pregnancy, or lactation can apparently enhance the likelihood of fracture. Intramedullary support by metal rods should be considered for treatment of the serious multiple fracture cases, and optimal orthopedic management is merited because many of these patients make a surprisingly good life adaptation. By 30 to 39 years of age, 35 per cent of patients have deafness; it occurs in 50 per cent by 60 years of age.

ETIOLOGY. Apparently the vast majority of cases are due to a single autosomal mutant gene (autosomal dominant). The majority of severe cases represent a sporadic occurrence within the family, presumably a fresh gene mutation, for which the parents need have little concern for recurrence. However, there have been rare reports of multiple affected siblings from normal parents, and the distinct possibility exists of a minor proportion of osteogenesis imperfecta cases being autosomal recessive. Ibsen,[4] reviewing the literature, found 12 families in which normal parents had multiple affected offspring, all with the severe type, with early mortality. The consanguinity rate was more than 66 per cent, and the frequency of affected sibs was 24 per cent, both indicating autosomal recessive inheritance in these latter families.

REFERENCES

1. McKusick, V. A.: Heritable Disorders of Connective Tissue. 3rd ed. St. Louis, C. V. Mosby Co., 1966.
2. Herndon, C. N.: Osteogenesis imperfecta: some clinical and genetic considerations. Clin. Orthop., 8:132, 1956.
3. Freda, V. J., Vosburgh, G. J., and Di Liberti, C: Osteogenesis imperfecta congenita. A presentation of 16 cases and review of the literature. Obstet. Gynec., 18:535, 1961.
4. Ibsen, K. H.: Personal communication.
5. Smars, G.: Osteogenesis Imperfecta in Sweden. Clinical, Genetic, Epidemiological, and Socio-Medical Aspects. Stockholm, Scandinavian University Books, 1961.
6. Schroder, G.: Osteogenesis imperfecta. Eine klinischerbiologische Untersuchung des Krankengutes in Westfalen. Schatzung der Mutationsraten für den Regierungsbezirk Munster (Westfalen). Z. Menschl. Vererb. Konstit. Lehre, 37: 632, 1964.

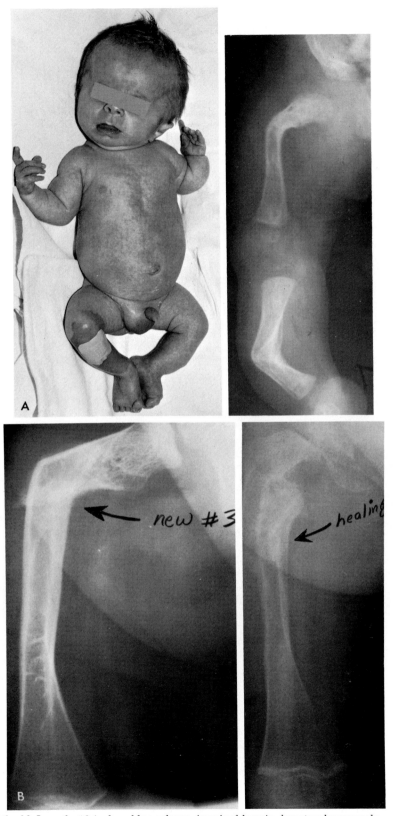

A, Two month old. Length, 19 inches; blue sclerae, inguinal hernia, hepatosplenomegaly.

B, Seventeen month old with a third fracture which was healing well by 18 months. Note the thin cortices and the ground glass "washed-out" appearance of the bone.

127. FIBRODYSPLASIA OSSIFICANS CONGENITA

Short Hallux, Fibrous Dysplasia Leading to Ossification in Muscles and Subcutaneous Tissues

This condition, described in a letter by Guy Patin in 1692, was extensively reviewed by Rosenstirn in 1918.[1] Fibroplasia ossificans congenita is the terminology utilized by McKusick[2] because myositis ossificans congenita is basically a misnomer. More than 350 cases have been reported.

ABNORMALITIES[1-3]
Digits. Short hallux, often with synostosis. Less frequently, short thumb.
Fibrous Tissues. Swellings, sometimes with pain and fever, in aponeuroses, fasciae, and tendons leading to ossification in muscles and fibrous tissues; most prominent in neck, dorsal trunk and proximal limbs with sternocleidomastoid frequently involved.

OCCASIONAL ABNORMALITIES. Short phalanges other than hallux or thumb, clinodactyly of fifth finger, short femoral neck, hernia.

NATURAL HISTORY. The unusual fibrodysplasia leading to ossification may have become evident during fetal life or as late as 25 years, most patients experiencing onset in early childhood. Ossification is usually evident within two to eight months of the time swelling occurred. Although some affected individuals never express the fibrodysplasia and others survive to late adult life with severe disability, the majority who have fibrodysplasia within the first five years succumb to the consequences of severe immobilization prior to 15 years of age. No effective treatment has been discovered, although symptomatic relief of pain may be achieved by salicylates or hydrocortisone analogue therapy. The natural history tends toward exacerbation and remission, and therefore the results of therapy should be interpreted with caution. Another matter for caution is the interpretation of biopsies from affected tissues. The pathological interpretation may be osteogenic sarcoma, although such a malignant growth is not a feature of this disease.

ETIOLOGY.[3] Autosomal dominant with almost full penetrance for short hallux and varying expression for the fibrodysplasia. About 90 per cent of cases represent fresh mutations for which older paternal age has been noted as a factor.

COMMENT. Although the fundamental defect in fibrous tissue is unknown, it is obvious that it allows for ossification to normal appearing bone in tissues in which ossification would normally not occur.

REFERENCES

1. Rosenstirn, J.: A contribution to the study of myositis ossificans progressiva. Ann. Surg., *68*:485, 1918.
2. McKusick, V.: Heritable Disorders of Connective Tissue. 3rd ed. St. Louis, C. V. Mosby Co., 1966, p. 400.
3. Tünte, W., Becker, P. E., v. Knorr, G.: Zur Genetik der Myositis ossificans progressiva. Humangenetik, *4*:320, 1967.

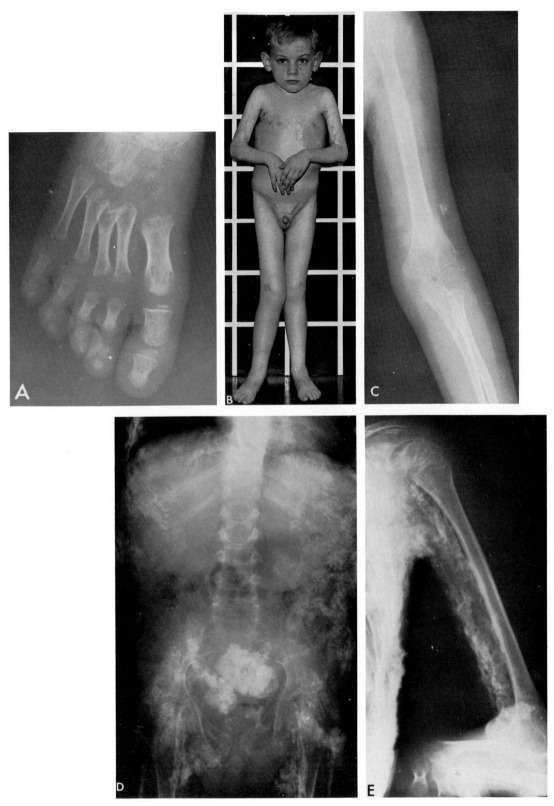

A, Borderline increased breadth of proximal phalanx of big toe.

B, Patient with limitation of joint motility.

C, Early soft tissue mineralization in left arm.

D and *E*, Several years after the changes shown in *A* to *C*, the soft tissue mineralization has become more extensive. (From the University of Wisconsin; courtesy of R. Summitt.)

128. PSEUDOXANTHOMA ELASTICUM

*Thickened Yellowish Flexural Skin, Angioid Retinal Streaks,
Medial Arterial Degeneration with Hemorrhagic Tendency*

This disease, so aptly described by McKusick,[1] appears to be the consequence of degeneration in the collagenous-elastic tissue with accumulation of elastic-appearing fibers, many in fragmented form.

ABNORMALITIES
Skin. Thick, grooved, lax yellowish skin in flexures and other areas of wear, often involving oral mucous membranes.
Eye. Retinal breaks with angioid streaks and degeneration.
Cardiovascular. Arterial medial thickening with secondary vascular insufficiency leading to diminished or absent pulses, intermittent claudication, and angina pectoris.
Vascular hemorrhagic tendency with bleeding into gastrointestinal tract and many other sites.
Thickening of endocardium including valve leaflets.

Calcification. Within degenerating tissues, i.e., subcutaneous, vascular, and falx cerebri.

NATURAL HISTORY. Skin changes, though they may be present from early in life, are usually not recognized until the second decade or later. Visual impairment is frequent, and hemorrhagic episodes can be severe. The frequent psychic and neurological problems are possibly secondary to central nervous system hemorrhages, vascular insufficiency, or both.

ETIOLOGY. Autosomal recessive.

REFERENCE

1. McKusick, V. A.: Heritable Disorders of Connective Tissue. 3rd ed. St. Louis, C. V. Mosby Co., 1966.

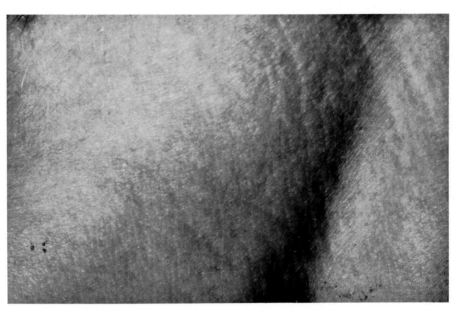

Posterior-oblique view of neck of an adolescent female showing thickened and grooved skin which had a yellowish-pink coloration.

129. X-LINKED HYDROCEPHALUS

Hydrocephalus, Short Flexed Thumb, Mental Deficiency

Bickers and Adams[1] first described this entity in 1949, and subsequently at least 47 cases have been reported.

ABNORMALITIES
Performance.   Mental deficiency and spasticity, especially of lower extremities.
Brain.   Aqueductal stenosis with hydrocephalus.
Hand.   Thumb flexed over palm (cortical thumb) with short first metacarpal.

OCCASIONAL ABNORMALITIES.   Asymmetry of somewhat coarse facies, brain defects such as fusion of thalami, small pons, absence of septum pellucidum, hypoplasia of corticospinal tracts, porencephalic cyst.

NATURAL HISTORY.   Prenatal hydrocephalus may be severe enough to impede delivery.

However, an occasional patient has no hydrocephalus, and such individuals often have a narrow scaphocephalic cranium with an intelligence quotient in the range of 30. The electroencephalogram may show diffuse abnormality, and the patient may have seizures.

ETIOLOGY.   X-linked recessive.

REFERENCES

1. Bickers, D. S., and Adams, R. D.: Hereditary stenosis of the aqueduct of Sylvius as a cause of congenital hydrocephalus. Brain, *72*:246, 1949.
2. Edwards, J. H.: The syndrome of sex-linked hydrocephalus. Arch. Dis. Childhood, *36*:486, 1961.

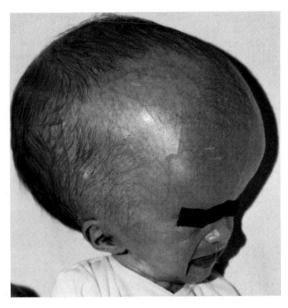

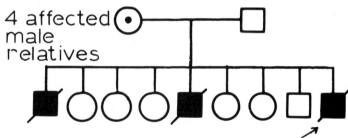

Male infant who later died and who was shown to have aqueductal stenosis as the cause for hydrocephalus. Note the family pedigree showing other affected males for whom this X-linked condition was lethal. (Courtesy of J. M. Opitz, University of Wisconsin.)

130. FABRY'S DISEASE

(Angiokeratoma Corporis Diffusum)

Dark Nodular Angiectases, Attacks of Burning Pain, Renal Insufficiency

This disease was originally described by Fabry.[1] Its basis has recently been recognized as the cellular accumulation of ceramidetrihexoside as a consequence of the deficiency of ceramidetrihexosidase, the enzyme that normally degrades this neutral glycolipid.[2]

ABNORMALITIES IN AFFECTED MALES[3]

General. Attacks of burning pain in hands and feet.

Cutaneous. Minute dark nodular angiectases in clusters around umbilicus, on genitalia, knees, hips, mucous membranes, etc.

Eye. Superficial corneal opacities.

Renal. Proteinuria; variable red cells, white cells, and casts in urine; progressive renal insufficiency.

Central Nervous System. May have seizures, hemiplegia, other presumed reactions to cerebrovascular disease.

OCCASIONAL ABNORMALITIES.

Diarrhea, epistaxes, hemoptysis, anemia secondary to blood loss, saccular retinal vessels, coronary disease, varicosities, edema of ankles, hands, and face, hypohidrosis.

NATURAL HISTORY.

The skin angiectases, though often present in earlier childhood, are usually not noted until after ten years of age. The burning pain, sometimes associated with fever, may start in childhood; it occurs in attacks precipitated by heat, cold, exercise, or fever. Renal insufficiency progresses to a fixed specific gravity of the urine, and the mean age of survival is 42 years. No effective therapy has yet been devised.

ETIOLOGY.

X-linked with full penetrance in the hemizygous male and variable mild expressivity in the heterozygous female who may show mild corneal opacities and has a value of ceramidetrihexosidase which is intermediary between that of the affected male and the normal.

REFERENCES

1. Fabry, J.: Ein Beitrag zur Purpura haemorrhagica nodularis. Arch. Derm. Syph., *43*:187, 1898.
2. Brady, R. O., Gal, A. E., Bradley, R. M., Martensson, E., Warshaw, A. L., and Laster, L.: Enzymatic defect in Fabry's disease. Ceramidetrihexosidase deficiency. New England J. Med., *276*:1163, 1967.
3. Opitz, J. M., Stiles, F. C., Wise, D., Race, R. R., Sanger, R., von Gemmingen, G. R., Kierland, R. R., Cross, E. G., and De Groot, W. P.: The genetics of angiokeratoma corporis diffusum (Fabry's disease) and its linkage relations with the Xg locus. Am. J. Hum. Genet., *17*:325, 1965.

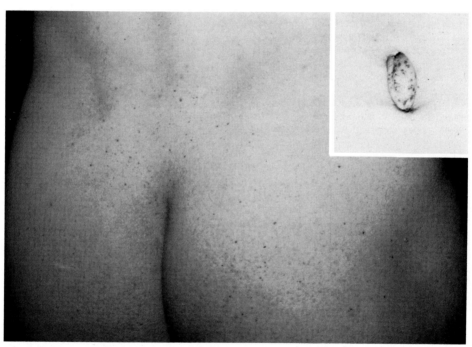

Lower back and buttock area of older child showing small dark nodular lesions, which are especially prominent in the umbilicus (inset). (From R. Summitt, University of Tennessee Medical School.)

131. OSLER'S HEMORRHAGIC TELANGIECTASIA

Epistaxes, Multiple Telangiectases

This entity was set forth in 1901 by Osler.[1] The telangiectases contain dilated vessels having only an endothelial wall with no elastic tissue. Over 264 affected families have been reported, and the incidence is about 1 : 50,000.

ABNORMALITIES
Vessels. Pinpoint, spider, and/or nodular telangiectases most commonly on tongue, mucosa of lips, face, conjunctiva, ears, fingertips, nail beds, and nasal mucous membrane; occasionally in gastrointestinal tract, bladder, vagina, uterus, lungs, liver, and/or brain.

OCCASIONAL ABNORMALITIES. Arteriovenous fistulas in lung, cirrhosis of liver, cavernous angiomata, port wine stain, aneurysms.

NATURAL HISTORY. Epistaxes often occur in childhood, and the telangiectases become apparent in latter childhood and tend to enlarge, giving rise to increased frequency of hemorrhage. Generally aggravated by pregnancy.

ETIOLOGY. Autosomal dominant with varying expression.

REFERENCES
1. Osler, W.: On a family form of recurring epistaxis, associated with multiple telangiectases of skin and mucous membrane. Bull. Hopkins Hosp., *12*:333, 1901.
2. Bird, R. M., Hammarsten, J. F., Marshall, R. A., and Robinson, R. R.: Family reunion: study of hereditary hemorrhagic telangiectasia. New England J. Med., *257*:105, 1957.

132. RILEY-DAY SYNDROME

(Familial Dysautonomia)

Dysautonomia, Poor Coordination, Lack of Tearing

Multiple indications of autonomic dysfunction were first noted in this condition by Riley, Day and others.[1] McKusick et al.[2] recently reported on 200 patients.

ABNORMALITIES
Evidences of Dysautonomia. Swallowing difficulty in infancy, aspiration, cyclic vomiting, diarrhea.
Emotional lability, breath holding.
Skin blotching, hyperhidrosis.
Insensitivity to pain; may develop Charcot neuropathic knee joint.
Lack of tearing; may develop corneal ulcer.
Taste deficiency, decreased fungiform and circumvallate papillae.
Unstable temperature, unexplained bouts of fever.

Labile blood pressure.
Urinary frequency.
Absent deep tendon reflexes.
Poor coordination; scoliosis often develops at eight to ten years.
Absence of flare response to cutaneous histamine.
Exaggerated response to norepinephrine.
Other. Small stature is a variable feature. Mental deficiency occurs in 55 per cent and seizures in 50 per cent.

OCCASIONAL ABNORMALITIES. Microcephaly, hydrocephalus, craniofacial disproportion (small face), congenital heart defect, dislocation of hip, pes cavus, megacolon, megaesophagus.

NATURAL HISTORY. Failure to thrive is the rule in infancy, with aspiration and pneumonia being the chief causes of death. One fourth die before ten years of age and one half before 22 years.

ETIOLOGY. Autosomal recessive, especially in Ashkenazic Jews. Hypoplasia of autonomic ganglia with cytological changes in hypothalamus, brain stem, and autonomic ganglia.

REFERENCES

1. Riley, C. M., Day, R. L., Greeley, D. McL., and Langford, W. S.: Central autonomic dysfunction with defective lacrimation. I. Report of five cases. Pediatrics, 3:468, 1949.
2. McKusick, V. A., Norum, R. A., Farkas, H. J., Brunt, P. W., and Mahloudji, M.: The Riley-Day syndrome — observations on genetics and survivorship. An interim report. Israel J. Med. Sci., 3:372, 1967.

U. Miscellaneous Syndromes

133. SCHWACHMAN'S SYNDROME

Lack of Exocrine Pancreas, Leukopenia

In 1963 Schwachman et al.[1] described five children with evidence of pancreatic insufficiency and leukopenia, none of whom had cystic fibrosis of the pancreas. A total of at least 39 cases have been documented.

ABNORMALITIES. Lack of exocrine pancreas, which is replaced by adipose tissue. Pancreatic trypsin, lipase, and amylase are absent.

Leukopenia, variable in degree.

OCCASIONAL ABNORMALITIES. Anemia, thrombocytopenia, eczema, metaphyseal dysostosis,[3] trace galactosuria; one patient developed leukemia.

NATURAL HISTORY. Failure to thrive with diarrhea is the most common presenting situation at two to ten months of age. Of interest is the observation that there is no steatorrhea; presumably the intestinal lipases are adequate in the absence of pancreatic lipase. Viscosity of duodenal secretions is also normal in contrast to cystic fibrosis of the pancreas which can be readily excluded by sweat electrolyte studies. The diarrhea tends to improve with age even without pancreatic replacement therapy. The latter therapy is followed by dramatic response in some patients but not in others. The leukopenia is variable from time to time and may be accompanied by a high frequency of bacterial infections.

ETIOLOGY. Presumed autosomal recessive.

COMMENT. The exocrine pancreas is replaced by adipose tissue, whereas the islet cells of Langerhans are intact. Both are derived from a common endodermal outpouching from the foregut, and therefore it is assumed that the exocrine pancreatic cells are lost early in life and replaced by fat. One possibility is a defect in the integrity of the lysozymes in these cells, allowing the cells to be destroyed by the very enzymes they produce.

REFERENCES

1. Schwachman, H., Diamond, L. K., Oski, F. A., and Khaw, K.-T.: Pancreatic insufficiency and bone marrow dysfunction. A new clinical entity. J. Pediat., 63:835, 1963.
2. Bodian, M., Sheldon, W., and Lightwood, R.: Congenital hypoplasia of the exocrine pancreas. Acta Paediat., 53:282, 1964.
3. Burke, V., Colebatch, J. H., Anderson, C. M., and Simons, M. J.: Association of pancreatic insufficiency and chronic neutropenia in childhood. Arch. Dis. Childhood, 42:147, 1967.

134. WISKOTT-ALDRICH SYNDROME

Thrombocytopenia, Eczema, Immunological Deficiency

Wiskott[1] described three brothers in 1937 with eczema, thrombocytopenia, and frequent infections, a similar pattern to that noted 17 years later by Aldrich et al.[2] who recognized the X-linked mode of inheritance of this condition. It has been reported in at least 57 boys.[3]

ABNORMALITIES. Thrombocytopenia from early infancy causing melena and purpura. Megalokaryocytes usually diminished.

Immunological deficiency with frequent infections, especially of skin, middle ear, sinuses, and lung. Often hypoplastic thymus, diminished lymphocytes, low gamma M with elevated gamma A, and low isoagglutinins.

Eczema, especially in infancy.

OCCASIONAL ABNORMALITIES. Eosinophilia, leukocytosis with myeloid hyperplasia, anemia, hypoaminoaciduria, joint effusions, and development of malignancy such as reticuloendotheliosis, reticulum cell sarcoma, astrocytoma, malignant lymphoma, or myelogenous leukemia.

NATURAL HISTORY. Most patients die in infancy or childhood from the consequences of bleeding, infection, or malignant neoplasia. Therapeutic endeavors with splenectomy, hydrocortisone analogue, or gamma globulin have been met with no appreciable improvement. The oldest survivor is 14 years.[3]

ETIOLOGY. X-linked recessive.

REFERENCES

1. Wiskott, A.: Familiärer angeborener Morbus Werlhofii? Mschr. Kinderh., 68:212, 1937.
2. Aldrich, R. A., Steinberg, A. G., and Campbell, D. C.: Pedigree demonstrating a sex-linked recessive condition characterized by draining ears, eczematoid dermatitis and bloody diarrhea. Pediatrics, 13:133, 1954.
3. Wolff, J. A.: Wiskott-Aldrich syndrome: clinical, immunologic, and pathologic observations. J. Pediat., 70:221, 1967.

135. CHEDIAK-HIGASHI SYNDROME

Partial Albinism, Neutropenia with Cytoplasmic Inclusions

César[1] originally described this disorder in 1943, and later Chediak[2] and Higashi each independently recognized the disease. More than 40 cases have been reported.

ABNORMALITIES
Partial Albinism. Gray sheen to light-colored hair, diminished uveal and retinal pigmentation with photophobia and nystagmus.
Hematological and Reticuloendothelial. Neutropenia with tendency toward lymphocytosis, anemia, and thrombocytopenia. Large cytoplasmic inclusions in leukocytes, promyeloblasts, and myeloblasts. Lymphoidhistiocytic cell infiltration with variable hepatosplenomegaly and lymphadenopathy.

OCCASIONAL ABNORMALITIES. Mental deficiency, seizures, peripheral neuropathy; corneal opacity; hyperhidrosis; buccal ulcerations; neonatal icterus; hyperlipemia.

NATURAL HISTORY. The majority of affected individuals die in early childhood as the result of recurring infection or a peculiar malignant lymphoma. Survival to adulthood can occur, but is unusual.

ETIOLOGY. Autosomal recessive with high frequency of consanguinity. The heterozygote may show enlarged cytoplasmic inclusions in leukocytes.

COMMENT. Electron microscopy has provided evidence for the leukocyte cytoplasmic granules being swollen lysosomes; the melanocytes contain giant melanosomes, which may explain the partial albinism. Windhorst et al.[3] have interpreted this evidence as being indicative of a disease of limiting membranes.

REFERENCES

1. César, A. B.: Neutropenia crónica maligna familiar con granulaciones atípicas de los leucocitos. Bol. Soc. Cub. Ped., *15*:900, 1943.
2. Chediak, M.: Nouvelle anomalie leucocytaire de caractère constitutionnel et familial. Rev. Hémat., *7*:362, 1952.
3. Windhorst, D. B., Zelickson, A. S., and Good, R. A.: Chediak-Higashi syndrome: hereditary gigantism of cytoplasmic organelles. Science, *151*:81, 1966.
4. Barkve, H.: Chediak-Higashi-Steinbrinck syndrome. Acta Paediat. Scand., *56*:105, 1967.

INDIVIDUAL ANOMALIES

The following tables were developed from the foregoing text. For each anomaly are listed the syndromes in which this defect is a frequent feature, as well as those syndromes in which it is an occasional feature. The number following each syndrome refers to its listing in the section on dysmorphic syndromes (pp. 33-277).

The anomalies are set forth under the following headings:

1. Cranium
2. Ocular Region
3. Eye
4. Nose
5. Facies
6. Maxilla and Mandible
7. Oral Region
8. Mouth
9. External Ears
10. Neck, Thorax, and Vertebrae
11. Limbs
12. Limbs; Nails, Creases, Dermatoglyphics
13. Limbs; Joint Anomalies
14. Skin and Hair
15. Central Nervous System
16. Deafness
17. Cardiac Anomaly
18. Abdominal Anomalies
19. Renal Anomalies
20. Genital Anomalies
21. Endocrine and Metabolic Dysfunction
22. Hematology-Oncology

1. CRANIUM

Microcephaly

Frequent in

Cornelia de Lange S.	13
Cri-du-Chat S.	6
Rubella S.	56
Seckel's S.	17
Smith-Lemli-Opitz S.	52
13 Trisomy S.	4
No. 18 Long Arm Deletion S.	7

Occasional in

Fanconi's S.	49
Goltz's S.	72
Incontinentia Pigmenti	73
Myotonic Dystrophy	31
Riley-Day S.	132
XXXXY S.	2
18 Trisomy S.	3

Macrocephaly

Frequent in

Achondroplasia	85
Cerebral Gigantism	61
Hurler's S.	116
Osteopetrosis, Severe	102
Riley's S.	64

Occasional in

Generalized Gangliosidosis	115
Wiedemann-Beckwith S.	60

Hydrocephalus

Frequent in

Osteopetrosis, Severe	102
X-Linked Hydrocephalus	129

Occasional in

Achondroplasia	85
Basal Cell Nevus S.	71
Hurler's S.	116
Oral-Facial-Digital S.	44
Riley-Day S.	132
13 Trisomy S.	4
18 Trisomy S.	3

Craniosynostosis

Frequent in

Apert's S.	106
Carpenter's S.	107
Crouzon's S.	108

Occasional in

Aminopterin-Induced S.	109
Conradi's S.	98
Hallerman-Streiff S.	18
Hypercalcemia–Peculiar Facies– Supravalvular Aortic Stenosis	59
Hypophosphatasia	99
Hypophosphatemic Rickets	96
Lowe's S.	29

Occiput, Flat or Prominent

Frequent in

Apert's S. (flat)	106
Carpenter's S. (flat)	107
Down's S. (flat)	1
Oto-Palato-Digital S. (prominent)	48
18 Trisomy S. (prominent)	3

Occasional in

XXXXY S. (flat)	2

Delayed Closure of Fontanels

Frequent in

Aminopterin-Induced S.	109
Cerebro-Hepato-Renal S.	28
Cleidocranial Dysostosis S.	104
Down's S.	1
Hallerman-Strieff S.	18
Hypophosphatasia	99
Kenny's S.	100
Progeria	19
Pyknodysostosis, Lamy and Maroteaux Type	103
Stanesco's Dysostosis S.	105
13 Trisomy S.	4
18 Trisomy S.	3

Occasional in

Conradi's S.	98
Oto-Palato-Digital S.	48
Rubinstein-Taybi S.	14

Frontal Bossing or Prominent Central Forehead

Frequent in

Basal Cell Nevus S. 71
Generalized Gangliosidosis 115
Hallerman-Streiff S. 18
Leroy's I-Cell S. 122
Osteopetrosis, Severe 102
Oto-Palato-Digital S. 48
Riley's S. 64
Rubinstein-Taybi S. 14
Silver's S. 15

Occasional in

Oral-Facial-Digital S. 44

2. OCULAR REGION

Hypertelorism, Relative to Facial Breadth

Frequent in

Aminopterin-Induced S. 109
Apert's S. 106
Hypertelorism-Hypospadias S. 54
Oto-Palato-Digital S. 48
Pyle's Disease 101

Occasional in

Basal Cell Nevus S. 71
Cleidocranial Dysostosis S. 104
Coloboma of Iris–Anal Atresia–Small
  Extra Chromosome S. 9
Conradi's S. 98
Cri-du-Chat S. 6
Crouzon's S. 108
Fraser S. 53
Hurler's S. 116
Hypercalcemia–Peculiar Facies–
  Supravalvular Aortic Stenosis 59
Sjögren-Larsson S. 37
Turner-like S. 12
XXXXX S. 10
XXXXY S. 2
13 Trisomy S. 4
No. 18 Long Arm Deletion S. 7

Short Palpebral Fissure, Lateral Displacement of Inner Canthi

Frequent in

Blepharophimosis, Familial 41
Carpenter's S. 107
Mohr S. 45
Oral-Facial-Digital S. 44
Waardenburg's S. 55
18 Trisomy S. 3

Occasional in

Oculodentodigital S. 47

Inner Epicanthal Fold

Frequent in

Blepharophimosis, Familial 41
Cerebro-Hepato-Renal S. 28
Cri-du-Chat S. 6
Down's S. 1

Freeman-Sheldon S. 32
Hypercalcemia–Peculiar Facies–
  Supravalvular Aortic Stenosis 59
Leroy's S. 122
Rubinstein-Taybi S. 14
Smith-Lemli-Opitz S. 52
Turner-like S. 12
XO S. 11
XXXXX S. 10
XXXXY S. 2
No. 4 Short Arm Deletion S. 5

Occasional in

Aminopterin-Induced S. 109
Basal Cell Nevus S. 71
Ehlers-Danlos S. 125
Oculodentodigital S. 47
18 Trisomy S. 3
No. 18 Long Arm Deletion S. 7

Slanted Palpebral Fissures

Frequent in

Apert's S. (down) 106
Coloboma of Iris–Anal Atresia–Small
  Extra Chromosome (down) 9
Cri-du-Chat S. (up or down) 6
Down's S. (up) 1
Leri's Pleonosteosis (up) 23
Rubinstein-Taybi S. (down) 14
Treacher Collins S. 39
XXXXX S. (up) 10
XXXXY S. (up) 2

Occasional in

Hallerman-Streiff S. 18
Prader-Willi S. (up) 26
XXXXY S. 2
13 Trisomy S. 4
18 Trisomy S. 3
No. 18 Long Arm Deletion S. 7

Shallow Orbital Ridges

Frequent in

Aminopterin-Induced S. 109
Apert's S. 106
Cerebro-Hepato-Renal S. 28
Crouzon's S. 108
Stanesco's Dysostosis S. 105
18 Trisomy S. 3

Occasional in

13 Trisomy S. 4

Prominent Eyes

Frequent in

Aminopterin-Induced S. 109
Apert's S. 106
Leprechaunism 57
Metaphyseal Dysostosis; Jansen-type 93
Pyle's Disease 101
Wiedemann-Beckwith S. 60

Eyebrows Extending to Midline

Frequent in

Cornelia De Lange S. 13
Waardenburg's S. 55

Occasional in

Basal Cell Nevus S.	71
13 Trisomy S.	4
No. 4 Short Arm Deletion S.	5

Ptosis of Eyelid

Frequent in

Blepharophimosis, Familial	41
Freeman-Sheldon S.	32
Schwartz's S.	33
Smith-Lemli-Opitz S.	52
Steinert's S.	31

Occasional in

Fanconi's S.	49
Rubinstein-Taybi S.	14
Turner-like S.	12
XO S.	11
18 Trisomy S.	3

3. EYE

Strabismus

Frequent in

Apert's S.	106
Clouson-type Ectodermal Dysplasia	81
Cri-du-Chat S.	6
Freeman-Sheldon S.	32
Goltz's S.	72
Incontinentia Pigmenti	73
Mieten's S.	46
Prader-Willi S.	26
Rubinstein-Taybi S.	14
Smith-Lemli-Opitz S.	52
XO S.	11
XXXXY S.	2
18 Trisomy S.	3
No. 4 Short Arm Deletion S.	5

Occasional in

Basal Cell Nevus S.	71
Blepharophimosis, Familial	41
Cornelia De Lange S.	13
Down's S.	1
Fanconi's S.	49
Hallerman-Streiff S.	18
Hypercalcemia–Peculiar Facies–Supravalvular Aortic Stenosis	59
Laurence-Moon-Biedl S.	25
Marinesco-Sjögren S.	34
Radial Aplasia-Thrombocytopenia	50
Seckel's S.	17

Nystagmus

Frequent in

Chediak-Higashi S.	135
Marinesco-Sjögren S.	34
No. 18 Long Arm Deletion S.	7

Occasional in

Blepharophimosis, Familial	41
Cockayne's S.	21
Down's S.	1
Fanconi's S.	49
Hallerman-Streiff S.	18
Laurence-Moon-Biedl S.	25

Myopia

Frequent in

Homocystinuria	124
Kenny's S.	100
Marfan's S.	123
Marshall S.	77
Schwartz's S.	33
Stickler's S.	24
Weill-Marchesani S.	114

Occasional in

Cornelia De Lange S.	13
Ehlers-Danlos S.	125
XXXXY S.	2

Blue Sclerae

Frequent in

Osteogenesis Imperfecta	126

Occasional in

Ehlers-Danlos S.	125
Hallerman-Streiff S.	18
Incontinentia Pigmenti	73
Marfan's S.	123
18 Trisomy S.	3

Microphthalmos

Frequent in

Goltz's S.	72
Hallerman-Streiff S.	18
Oculodentodigital S.	47
13 Trisomy S.	4
No. 4 Short Arm Deletion S.	5

Occasional in

Fanconi's S.	49
Goldenhar's S.	40
Treacher Collins S.	39
18 Trisomy S.	3
No. 18 Long Arm Deletion S.	7

Colobomata of Iris

Frequent in

Coloboma of Iris–Anal Atresia–Small Extra Chromosome	9
Goltz's S.	72
Rieger's S.	30
13 Trisomy S.	4
No. 4 Short Arm Deletion S.	5

Occasional in

Basal Cell Nevus S.	71
Goldenhar's S.	40
Marfan's S.	123
Rubinstein-Taybi S.	14
Sturge-Weber S.	62
XXXXX S.	10
18 Trisomy S.	3

Glaucoma

Frequent in

Stickler's S.	24
Weill-Marchesani S.	114

Occasional in

Basal Cell Nevus S.	71
Cerebro-Hepato-Renal S.	28

Keratocornea, Microcornea

Corneal Opacity

Cataract, Lenticular Opacities

Lens Dislocation

Retinal Pigmentation

4. NOSE

Low Nasal Bridge

Small Nose, with or without Anteverted Nostrils

5. FACIES

6. MAXILLA AND MANDIBLE

Maxillary Hypoplasia, Often with a Narrow Palate

Frequent in

Occasional in

Micrognathia

Frequent in

Occasional in

Prognathism

Frequent in

7. ORAL REGION

Cleft Lip with or without Cleft Palate

Frequent in

Occasional in

Abnormal Philtrum

Frequent in

Prominent Full Lips

Frequent in

Lower Lip Pits

Frequent in

Occasional in

Downturning Corners of Mouth

Frequent in

Microstomia

Frequent in

Occasional in

Macrostomia

Frequent in

Occasional in

8. MOUTH

Cleft Palate or Bifid Uvula Without Cleft in Lip

Oral Frenula (Webs)

Cleft Tongue

Macroglossia

Hypertrophied Alveolar Ridges

Dental Defect

9. EXTERNAL EARS

Low Set Ears

Treacher Collins S. 39
18 Trisomy S. 3

Occasional in
Carpenter's S. 107
Cri-du-Chat S. 6
Down's S. 1
Goldenhar's S. 40
Schwartz's S. 33
XXXXX S. 10
XXXXY S. 2
13 Trisomy S. 4
No. 4 Short Arm Deletion S. 5
No. 18 Long Arm Deletion S. 7

Malformed Auricles

Frequent in
Diastrophic Nanism (hypertrophied
    cartilage) 89
Down's S. (small) 1
Ehlers-Danlos S. (hypermobile) 125
Fraser S. 53
Goldenhar's S. 40
Rubinstein-Taybi S. 14
Seckel's S. 17
Smith-Lemli-Opitz S. 52
Treacher Collins S. 39
Turner-like S. 12
Wiedemann-Beckwith S. (linear fissure
    lobuli) 60
XO S. (prominent) 11
XXXXY S. 2
13 Trisomy S. 4
18 Trisomy S. 3
No. 18 Long Arm Deletion S. (prominent
    antihelix, antitragus) 7
No. 21 Long Arm Deletion S. (large) 8

Occasional in
Bloom's S. (prominent) 16
Cerebro-Hepato-Renal S. 28
Coloboma of Iris–Anal Atresia–Small
    Extra Chromosome 9
Cri-du-Chat S. (preauricular skin tag) 6
Fanconi's S. 49
Hypercalcemia–Peculiar Facies–
    Supravalvular Aortic Stenosis
    (prominent) 59
Hypertelorism-Hypospadias S. 54
Oral-Facial-Digital S. (milia in skin of
    auricle) 44
Prader-Willi S. 26

10. NECK, THORAX, AND VERTEBRAE

Web Neck

Frequent in
Turner-like S. 12
XO S. 11

Occasional in
Down's S. 1
XXXXY S. 2
18 Trisomy S. 3

Nipple Anomaly

Frequent in
Cornelia De Lange S. (small) 13

XO S. (widely spaced, small) 11
18 Trisomy S. (small, occasionally wide
    spaced) 3

Occasional in
Fraser S. (wide spaced) 53
Smith-Lemli-Opitz S. 52
Turner-like S. (wide spacing) 12
No. 18 Long Arm Deletion S. 7

Hypoplasia of Clavicles

Frequent in
Cleidocranial Dysostosis S. 104
Goltz's S. 72
Holt-Oram S. 51

Occasional in
Progeria 19

Pectus Excavatum or Carinatum

Frequent in
Cartilage-Hair Hypoplasia 95
Homocystinuria 124
Marfan's S. 123
Morquio's S. 119
Osteogenesis Imperfecta 126
Oto-Palato-Digital S. 48
Schwartz's S. 33
Turner-like S. 12
XO S. 11

Occasional in
Down's S. 1
Hallerman-Streiff S. 18
Mietens' S. 46
Mohr S. 45
Oculo-Cerebro-Renal S. 29
XXXXY S. 2

Small Thoracic Cage

Frequent in
Ellis-van Creveld S. 88
Metaphyseal Dysostosis; Jansen-type 93
Metatrophic Dwarfism 86
Thoracic Asphyxiant Dystrophy 87

Occasional in
Achondroplasia 85
Diastrophic Nanism 89
Osteogenesis Imperfecta 126
Pseudoachondroplastic Form of
    Spondyloepiphyseal Dysplasia 90

Rib Defects Other Than Small Thorax

Frequent in
Basal Cell Nevus S. (bifid, synostoses,
    hypoplasia) 71
Generalized Gangliosidosis (thick) 115
Hunter's S. (thick) 118
Hurler's S. (thick) 116
Incontinentia Pigmenti (extra rib) 73
Morquio's S. 119
Pyle's S. 101
Sanfilippo's S. (thick) 120
Seckel's S. 17
13 Trisomy S. 4

Occasional in

Aminopterin-Induced S.	109
Down's S.	1
Neurofibromatosis (rib fusion)	67
XO S.	11
18 Trisomy S.	3
No. 18 Long Arm Deletion	7

Vertebral Defects

Frequent in

Achondroplasia	85
Cartilage-Hair Hypoplasia	95
Cockayne's S. (biconvex flattening)	21
Generalized Gangliosidosis	115
Hurler's S.	116
Leroy's S.	122
Maroteaux-Lamy S.	117
Metaphyseal Dysostosis; Jansen-type	93
Metatrophic Dwarfism	86
Morquio's S.	119
Multiple Epiphyseal Dysplasia	92
Oto-Palato-Digital S.	48
Progeria	19
Pseudoachondroplastic Form of Spondyloepiphyseal Dysplasia	90
Pyle's S.	101
Sanfilippo's S.	120
Schwartz's S.	33
Spondyloepiphyseal Dysplasia, X-linked	91
Stickler's Progressive Arthroophthalmopathy	24
Thoracic Asphyxiant Dystrophy	87

Occasional in

Basal Cell Nevus S. (fusions)	71
Conradi's S.	98
Diastrophic Nanism	89
Down's S.	1
Goldenhar's S.	40
Hallerman-Streiff S. (spina bifida)	18
Incontinentia Pigmenti S.	73
Larsen's S.	27
Marfan's S.	123
Nail-Patella S. (spina bifida)	110
Neurofibromatosis	67
Osteogenesis Imperfecta	126
Popliteal Web S. (spina bifida)	43
Radial Aplasia–Thrombocytopenia	50
Rubinstein-Taybi S.	14
Turner-like S.	12
13 Trisomy S.	4
18 Trisomy S.	3
No. 21 Long Arm Deletion S.	8

11. LIMBS

Arachnodactyly

Frequent in

Marfan's S.	123

Occasional in

Basal Cell Nevus S.	71
Homocystinuria	124

Short Limbs

Frequent in

Achondroplasia	85
Cartilage-Hair Hypoplasia	95
Conradi's S. (short femur and/or humerus)	98

Diastrophic Nanism	89
Dyschondrosteosis	111
Ellis-van Creveld S.	88
Metatrophic Dwarfism	86
Pseudoachondroplastic Form of Spondyloepiphyseal Dysplasia	90

Occasional in

Cornelia De Lange S.	13
Hypophosphatasia	99
Osteogenesis Imperfecta	126

Small Hands and Feet

Frequent in

Apert's S.	106
Brachydactyly Type E	113
Carpenter's S.	107
Cornelia De Lange S.	13
Down's S.	1
Mohr's S.	45
Prader-Willi S.	26
Stanesco's Dysostosis S.	105
Werner's S.	20
XXXXX S.	10

Occasional in

Rothmund S.	75

Fifth Finger Hypoplasia with Clinodactyly

Frequent in

Carpenter's S.	107
Cornelia De Lange S.	13
Down's S.	1
Mohr S.	45
Seckel's S.	17
Silver's S.	15
XXXXX S.	10
XXXXY S.	2

Occasional in

Cri-du-Chat S.	6
Fibrodysplasia Ossificans Congenita	127
Laurence-Moon-Biedl S.	25
Myotonic Dystrophy S.	31
Nail-Patella S.	110
Oral-Facial-Digital S.	44
Prader-Willi S.	26
Rubinstein-Taybi S.	14

Thumb Hypoplasia to Aplasia

Frequent in

Fanconi's S.	49
Holt-Oram S. (may be triphalangeal)	51
Radial Aplasia–Thrombocytopenia	50

Occasional in

Aminopterin-Induced S.	109
Cornelia De Lange S.	13
Fibrodysplasia Ossificans Congenita	127
18 Trisomy S.	3

Radius Hypoplasia to Aplasia

Frequent in

Holt-Oram S.	51
Radial Aplasia–Thrombocytopenia	50

Occasional in

Cornelia De Lange S.	13

Metacarpal Hypoplasia — Third, Fourth, and/or Fifth

Frequent in

Occasional in

Metacarpal Hypoplasia — First Metacarpal with Proximal Placement of Thumb

Frequent in

Occasional in

Polydactyly

Frequent in

Occasional in

Broad Thumb and/or Toe

Frequent in

Occasional in

Syndactyly, Cutaneous or Osseous

Frequent in

Occasional in

Elbow Dysplasia

Frequent in

Occasional in

Patella Dysplasia

Frequent in

Occasional in

12. LIMBS; NAILS, CREASES, DERMATOGLYPHICS

Nail Hypoplasia or Dysplasia

Frequent in

Clenched Hand; Index Finger Tending to Overlie the Third, and the Fifth Finger Tending to Overlie the Fourth

Frequent in

18 Trisomy S. 3

Occasional in

Smith-Lemli-Opitz S. 52
13 Trisomy S. 4

Joint Hypermotility

Frequent in

Cartilage-Hair Hypoplasia 95
Down's S. 1
Ehlers-Danlos S. 125
Marfan's S. 123
Morquio's S. 119
Oculo-Cerebro-Renal S. 29
Seckel's S. 17

Occasional in

Goltz's S. 72
Osteogenesis Imperfecta 126

Joint Dislocation

Frequent in

Larsen's S. (elbow, knee, hip) 27
Oto-Palato-Digital S. (elbow) 48

Occasional in

Aminopterin-Induced S. (hip) 109
Conradi's S. 98
Ehlers-Danlos S. 125
Mieten's S. (hip) 46
Neurofibromatosis 67
Oculodentodigital S. 47
Osteogenesis Imperfecta 126
Popliteal Web S. 43
Riley-Day S. 132
Seckel's S. (hip) 17
Silver's S. 15

14. SKIN AND HAIR

Skin Pigmentation, Melanomata

Frequent in

Basal Cell Nevus S. (nevi) 71
Berardinelli's S. (hyperpigmentation, especially axillae) 58
Chediak-Higashi S. (partial albinism) 135
Dyskeratosis Congenita S. (reticular) 74
Fanconi's S. (general increase) 49
Goltz's S. (poikiloderma) 72
Hypohidrotic Ectodermal Dysplasia (diminished pigment) 76
Incontinentia Pigmenti (spidery pigment) 73
Maffucci's S. (viteligo) 65
McCune-Albright S. (irregular) 68
Neurofibromatosis (café au lait spots) 67
Peutz-Jeghers S. (perioral spots) 69
Rothmund-Thomson S. (reticular) 75
Tuberosclerosis 66
Waardenburg's S. 55
XO S. 11

Occasional in

Ataxia-Telangiectasia (altered skin or hair pigmentation, café au lait spots) 36
Bloom's S. (café au lait spots) 16
Silver's S. (café au lait spots) 15

Hemangiomata and Telangiectases

Frequent in

Ataxia-Telangiectasia (telangiectases) 96
Bloom's S. (telangiectases) 16
Fabry's Disease (nodular lesions) 130
Goltz's S. 72
Maffucci's S. (hemangiomata) 65
Osler's S. (telangiectases) 131
Riley's S. (hemangiomata) 64
Rothmund S. (telangiectases) 75
Sturge-Weber S. 62
Tuberosclerosis (glioma-angioma lesions) 66
13 Trisomy S. (hemangiomata) 4

Occasional in

Dyskeratosis Congenita S. (telangiectases) 74
Rubinstein-Taybi S. 14
XO S. 11
18 Trisomy S. 3

Deep Sacral Dimple, Pilonidal Cyst

Frequent in

No. 4 Short Arm Deletion S. 5

Occasional in

Bloom's S. 16
Carpenter's S. 107
Cerebro-Hepato-Renal S. 28
Conradi's S. 98
Smith-Lemli-Opitz S. 52

Alopecia (Usually Sparse Hair)

Frequent in

Cartilage-Hair Hypoplasia 95
Clouson-type Ectodermal Dysplasia 81
Cockayne's S. 21
Dyskeratosis Congenita S. 74
Hallerman-Streiff S. 18
Homocystinuria 124
Hypohidrotic Ectodermal Dysplasia 76
Incontinentia Pigmenti 73
Menkes' S. 38
Oculodentodigital S. 47
Pili Torti–Deafness S. 80
Progeria 19
Werner's S. 20

Occasional in

Conradi's S. 98
Ellis-van Creveld S. 88
Goltz's S. 72
Oral-Facial-Digital S. 44
Popliteal Web S. 43
Rothmund S. 75
Seckel's S. 17

Hirsutism

Frequent in

Berardinelli's S. 58
Cornelia De Lange S. 13
Hunter's S. 118
Hurler's S. 116

Abnormal Form of Hair

15. CENTRAL NERVOUS SYSTEM

Hypotonicity

Hypertonicity

Ataxia

Seizures

16. DEAFNESS

17. CARDIAC ANOMALY

Congenital Heart Defect

18. ABDOMINAL ANOMALY

Inguinal and/or Umbilical Hernia

Hepatomegaly

Pyloric Stenosis

Incomplete Rotation of Colon

19. RENAL ANOMALIES

Kidney Malformation

Renal Insufficiency

20. GENITAL ANOMALIES

Hypospadias, or Ambiguous External Genitalia

22. HEMATOLOGY-ONCOLOGY

REFERENCES

1. Summitt, R. L.: Cytogenetics in mentally defective children with anomalies: a controlled study. J. Pediat., *74*:58, 1969.

MAJOR TEXTS FOR RECOGNITION OF PATTERNS OF MALFORMATION

General

1. Gorlin, R. J., and Pindborg, J. J.: Syndromes of the Head and Neck. New York, McGraw-Hill Book Co., 1964.
2. McKusick, V. A.: Mendelian Inheritance in Man: Catalogs of Autosomal Dominant, Autosomal Recessive, and X-linked Phenotypes. Baltimore, The Johns Hopkins Press, 1968.

Connective Tissue Disorders

1. McKusick, V. A.: Heritable Disorders of Connective Tissue. St. Louis, C. V. Mosby Co., 1966.

Chondrodystrophies

1. Rubin, P.: Dynamic Classification of Bone Dysplasias. Chicago, Year Book Medical Publishers, 1964.

Dermatological Disorders

1. Butterworth, T., and Strean, L.: Clinical Genodermatology. Baltimore, Williams and Wilkins Co., 1962.

Chapter Three

MORPHOGENESIS

Knowledge of normal morphogenesis may assist in the interpretation of malformations, and malformations may assist in the understanding of normal morphogenesis. Each anomaly must have a logical mode of development and cause. When interpreting a malformation the clinician is looking back to an early stage in development with which often he has had little acquaintance. This chapter sets forth some of the phenomena of morphogenesis and the normal stages in early human development, followed by the types of abnormal morphogenesis and the relative timing of particular malformations.

NORMAL MORPHOGENESIS

Phenomena of Morphogenesis

The genetic information that guides the morphogenesis and function of an individual is all contained within the zygote. After the first few cell divisions, differentiation begins to take place, presumably through activation or inactivation of particular genes, allowing cells to assume diverse roles. The entire process is programmed in a timely and sequential order with little allowance for error, especially in early morphogenesis.

Although little is known about the fundamental processes that control morphogenesis, it is worthwhile to mention some of the normal phenomena which occur and examples of each.

Cell Migration. The proper migration of cells to a predestined location is critical in the development of many structures. For example, the germ cells move from the yolk sac endoderm to the mesonephric ridge where they interact with other cells to form the gonad.

Control over Mitotic Rate. The size of particular structures, as well as their form, is to a large extent the consequence of control over the rates of cell division.

Interaction Between Adjacent Tissues. The optic cup induces the morphogenesis of the lens from the overlying ectoderm, the ureteral bud induces the development of the kidney from the adjacent metanephric tissue, the notochord is essential for normal development of the overlying neural tissue, and the prechordal mesoderm is essential for the normal morphogenesis of the overlying forebrain. These are but a few examples of the many interactions that are essential features in morphogenesis.

Adhesive Association of Like Cells. In the development of a structure such as a long bone the early cells tend to aggregate closely in condensations, a membrane comes to surround them, and only later do they resemble cartilage cells. The association of like cells is dramatically demonstrated by admixing trypsinized liver and kidney cells in vitro and observing them to reaggregate with their own kind.

Hormonal Influence over Morphogenesis. Androgen effect is one example of a hormonal influence over morphogenesis—in this case, that of the external genitalia. Normally the individual with a Y chromosome has testosterone from the fetal testicle which induces enlargement of the phallus, closure of the labia minoral folds to form a penile urethra, and fusion of the labioscrotal folds to form a scrotum. Prior to eight weeks the genitalia appear female in type and will remain so unless androgenic hormone is present.

Normal Stages in Morphogenesis

The general stages in normal morphogenesis as set forth here are illustrated in Figures 14 to 26. The first week is a period of cell division without much enlargement, the conceptus being dependent on the cytoplasm of the ova for most of its metabolic needs. By seven to eight days the zona pellucida is gone and the outlying trophoblast cells invade the endometrium and form

295

the early placenta which must function both to nourish the parasitic embryo and to maintain the pregnancy via its endocrine function. During this time a relatively small inner cell mass has become a bilaminar disc of ectoderm and endoderm, each with its own fluid-filled cavity, the amniotic sac and yolk sac respectively. By the end of the second week a small mound, Hensen's node, has developed in the ectoderm, and behind it a primitive streak forms. The embryo now has an axis to which further morphogenesis will relate. Cells migrate forward from Hensen's node between the ectoderm and endoderm to form an elastic cord, the notochord, which temporarily provides axial support for the embryo as well as influencing the adjacent morphogenesis. Ectodermal cells migrate through Hensen's node and the primitive streak to specific areas between the ectoderm and endoderm, becoming the mesoderm. One of the early mesodermal

derivatives is a circulatory system; during the third week the heart begins to develop, vascular channels form in situ, and blood cells are produced in the yolk sac. By the end of the third week the heart is pumping, a neural groove has formed anterior to Hensen's node, the para-axial mesoderm has begun to be segmented into somites, the anterior and posterior regions of the embryo have begun to curl under, and the foregut and hindgut pouches become distinct. The stage is now set for the period of major organogenesis which is best considered in relation to individual structures.

The morphogenesis of certain structures is set forth in Figures 27 to 48. As noted in the illustrations found on the inside front cover and inside back cover of this book, each stage of development represents a synchronous syndrome of characteristics.

General Morphogenesis

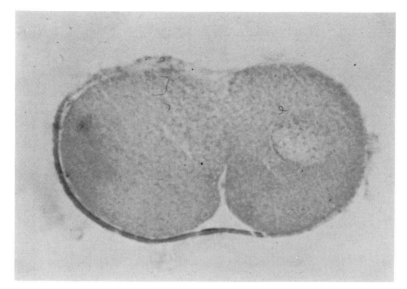

Figure 14. Two cell stage, within zona pellucida.

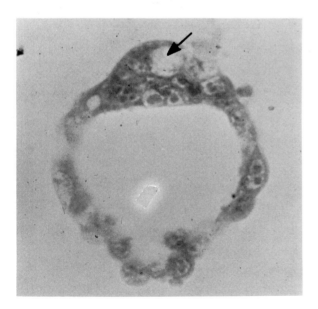

Figure 15. **Four to five day** blastula stage. The embryonic cell mass (top) shows the first indication toward an amniotic space (arrow).

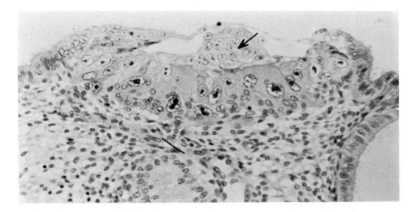

Figure 16. **Seven days.** The major part of the conceptus, the cytotrophoblast, has invaded the endometrium, and the embryo (arrow) is differentiating into two diverse cell layers, the ectoderm and endoderm.

Figure 17. **Fourteen to sixteen days.** The thicker ectoderm (arrow) has its continuous amniotic sac, whereas the underlying endoderm has its yolk sac. Major changes will now begin to take place.

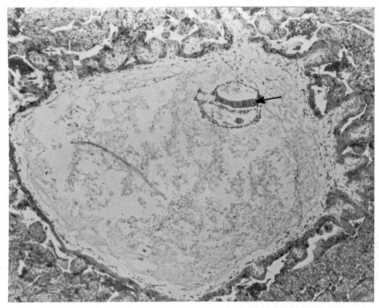

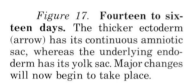

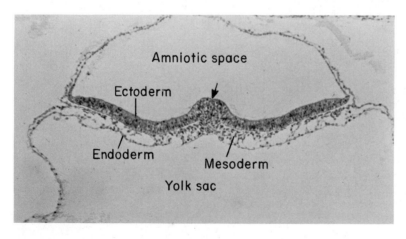

Figure 18. **Seventeen to eighteen days.** Mesioblast cells migrate from the ectoderm through Hensen's node (the hillock marked by the arrow) and the primitive streak to specific locations between the ectoderm and endoderm, there constituting the highly versatile mesoderm. Anterior to Hensen's node the notochord develops, providing axial support and influencing subsequent development such as that of the overlying neural plate.

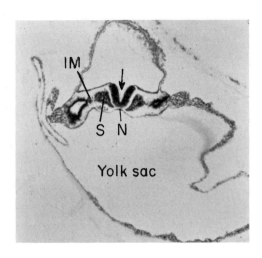

Figure 19. **Twenty-one to twenty-three days.** The mid-axial ectoderm has thickened and formed the neural groove (arrow), partially influenced by the underlying notochord (N). Lateral to it the mesoblast has now segmented into somites (S), intermediary mesoderm (IM), and somatopleura and splanchnopleura as intervening stages toward further differentiation. Vascular channels are developing in situ from mesoderm, blood cells are being produced in the yolk sac wall, and the early heart is beating. Henceforth development is extremely rapid with major changes each day.

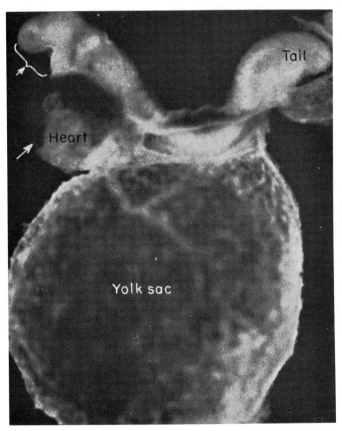

Figure 20. **Twenty-four days.** The fore part of the embryo is growing rapidly, especially the anterior neural plate. The cardiac tube, under the developing face (arrow), is functional.

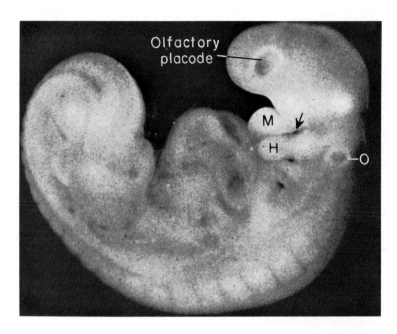

Figure 21. **Twenty-six days.** The olfactory placode has begun to invaginate. Between it and the mandibular process is the area of the future mouth, where the buccopharyngeal membrane, with no intervening mesoderm, is breaking down. Within the recess of the mandibular (M) and hyoid (H) processes the future external auditory canal will develop (arrow), and dorsal to it the otic placode (O) is invaginating to form the inner ear. The relatively huge heart must pump blood to the yolk sac and developing placenta as well as to the embryo proper. Foregut outpouchings and evaginations will now begin to form various glands and the lung and liver primordia. Foregut and hindgut are now clearly delineated from the yolk sac. The somites, which will differentiate into myotomes (musculature), dermotomes (subcutaneous tissue), and sclerotomes (vertebrae), are evident on into the tail, which will gradually regress.

Figure 22. **Thirty days.** The brain is rapidly growing and its early cleavage into bilateral future cerebral hemispheres is evident in the telencephalic outpouching of the forebrain (FB). To the right of this is the developing eye with the cleft optic cup (arrow) and the early invagination of the future lens from surface ectoderm. From the somatopleura the limb swellings (L) have developed. The loose mesenchyme of the limb bud, interacting with the thickened ectodermal cells at its tip, carries all the potential for the full development of the limb. The liver is now functional and will be a source of blood cells. The mesonephric ducts, formed in the mesonephric ridges, communicate to the cloaca which is beginning to become septated, and the yolk sac is regressing.

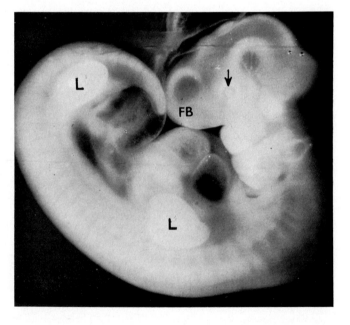

Figure 23. **Thirty-six days.**
The retina is now pigmented, still incompletely closed at its inferior medial margin. Closure of the lip is nearly complete. The hillocks of His are forming the early auricle (arrow) from the adjacent borders of the mandibular and hyoid swellings. The hand plate (H) has formed with condensation of mesenchyme into the five finger rays. The lower limb lags behind the upper limb in its development. The ventricular septum is partitioning the heart. The ureteral bud from the mesonephric duct has induced a kidney from the mesonephric ridge, which is also forming gonad and adrenal. Cloacal septation is nearly complete, the infraumbilical mesenchyme has filled in all the cloacal membrane except the urogenital area, and the genital tubercles are fused whereas the labioscrotal swellings are unfused. The gut is enlongating, and a loop of it may be seen projecting out into the body stalk.

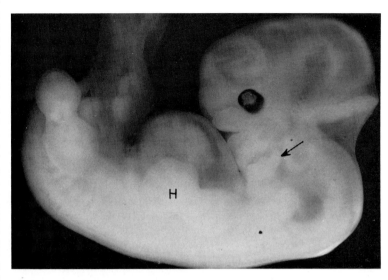

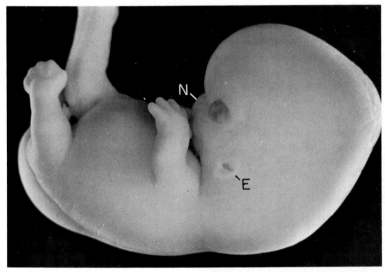

Figure 24. **Forty-one days.**
The nose (N) is relatively flat, and the external ear (E) is gradually shifting in relative position as it continues to grow and develop. A neck area is now evident, the anterior body wall has formed, and the thorax and abdomen are separated by the transverse septum (diaphragm). The fingers are now partially separated, and the elbow is evident. The major period of cardiac morphogenesis and septation is complete. The urogenital membrane has now broken down, yielding a urethral opening. The phallus and lateral labioscrotal folds are the same for both sexes at this age. This is the end of the so-called embryonic period and the beginning of the fetal era.

Figure 25. **Ten week male.** The eyelids have developed and fused, not to reopen until four or five months. Muscles are developed and functional, normal morphogenesis of joints is dependent on movement, and primary ossification is occurring in the centers of developing bones. In the male the testicle has produced androgen and masculinized the external genitalia with enlargement of the genital tubercle, fusion of the labioscrotal folds into a scrotum, and closure of the labia minoral folds to form a penile urethra, these structures being unchanged in the female. The testicle does not descend into the scrotum until eight or nine months.

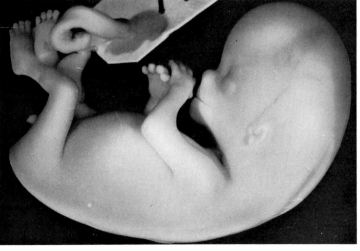

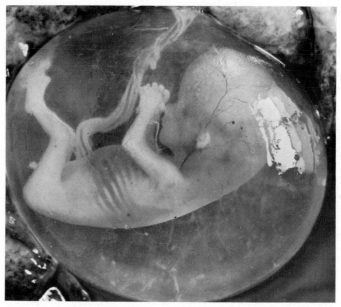

Figure 26.   **Three and one half month male.** The fetus is settling down for the latter two thirds of prenatal life. The morphogenesis of the lung, largely solid at this point in development, will not have progressed to the capacity for aerobic exchange for another three to four months. The skin is increasing in thickness, and its accessory structures are differentiating. The form of the volar surface of the hand and foot, especially the character of the prominent apical and other pads, will influence the patterning of parallel dermal ridges which form transversely to the relative lines of growth stress on the palms and soles between 16 and 19 weeks. Subcutaneous tissue is thin, and adipose tissue does not develop until seven to eight months.

Examples of Morphogenesis of Specific Structures

MORPHOGENESIS OF LENS AND EYE

An Example of Induction, Invagination, and Long-Term Differentiation

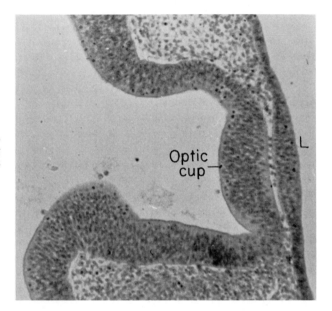

Figure 27. Twenty-seven days. Optic cup evagination from forebrain induces overlying ectoderm to thicken and begin development toward a lens (L).

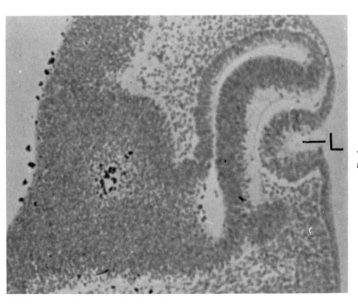

Figure 28. Twenty-nine days. Invagination of lens epithelium (L) into area of optic cup.

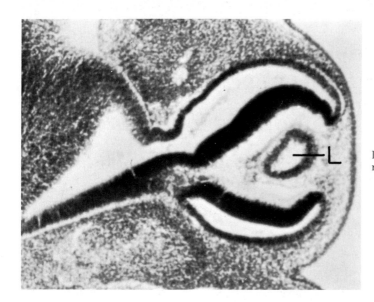

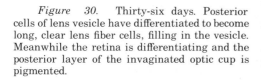

Figure 29. Thirty-two days. The lens epithelium (L) is now fully invaginated as a hollow vesicle.

Figure 30. Thirty-six days. Posterior cells of lens vesicle have differentiated to become long, clear lens fiber cells, filling in the vesicle. Meanwhile the retina is differentiating and the posterior layer of the invaginated optic cup is pigmented.

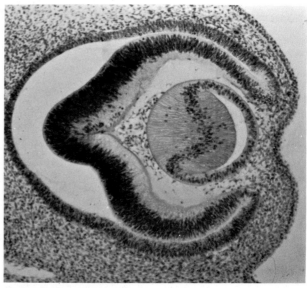

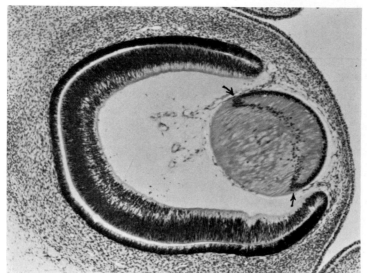

Figure 31. Thirty-eight days. Solid lens. New lens fiber cells (arrows) will continue to differentiate from the outer lens epithelial cells until adult life. Death of these early lens cells will yield a central cataract. Note the beginning neuromesodermal organization into an iris. Also note the hyaloid vessels behind the lens, which occasionally persist and lead to opacity behind the lens.

304

MORPHOGENESIS OF THE KIDNEY

An Example of Induction, Differentiation, Condensation, and Separation

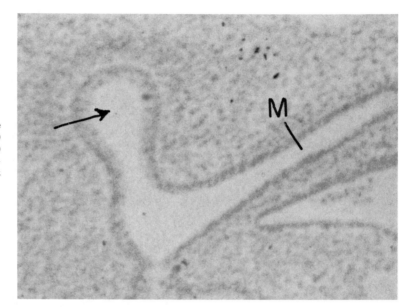

Figure 32. Thirty-one days. The ureteral bud (arrow) from the mesonephric duct (M) has induced a halo-like condensation of cells from the adjacent mesonephric ridge.

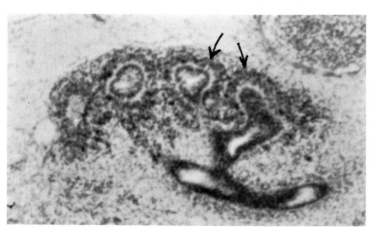

Figure 33. Thirty-six days. Successive branchings of the ureteral bud have led to a calyceal system, at the ends of which further condensations of early renal parenchyma have been induced (arrows). Note that the "kidney" has no limiting membrane from the surrounding tissue at this stage.

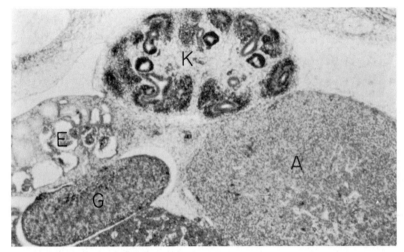

Figure 34. Thirty-eight days. The kidney (K) is now a separate organ structure, in close association with the other glands of mesonephric origin: the adrenal (A) and smaller gonad (G) with its associated mesonephros nephron-like units, the only residua of which will be parts of the epididymis (E).

Figure 35. Eleven weeks. Individual nephron units are more readily evident in this section. Each unit starts as an S-shaped hollow vesicle. Within one cup of the S a glomerulus develops and the other end elongates, connects with the arborizing collecting duct of ureteral origin, and then continues to elongate. The distal tubules are short at this stage and hence the urine is of relatively low osmolarity. New calyceal branches and nephron units develop until the latter period of fetal life.

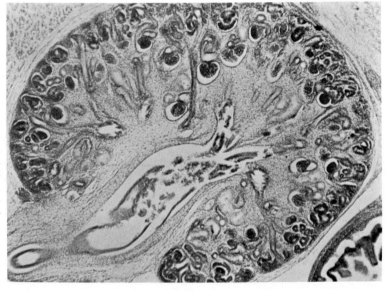

LIMB MORPHOGENESIS

An Example of in Situ Condensation, Differentiation, Separation, and Genetic Determination of Form

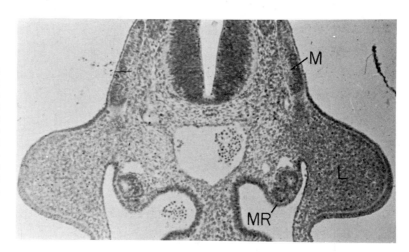

Figure 36. Twenty-eight days. Early limb buds (L) with loose, undifferentiated mesenchyme. Note the condensations of myotome cells (M) dorsal to the limb buds. These will form skeletal musculature other than that of the limb, which will differentiate in situ. Note also the mesonephric ridge (MR), with its transient nephron-like elements.

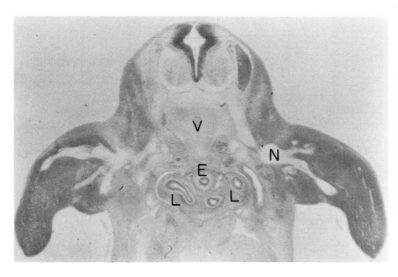

Figure 37. Thirty-one days. Nerve axon trunks (N) move out into condensing mesenchyme. Ectodermal cells at the tip of the limb bud are thickened. These cells exert an important interacting role with the mesenchyme in the guidance of morphogenesis of the limb. Note also (1) vertebral body (V) now formed, but as yet no spinous processes; (2) esophagus (E) in the center with main bronchi and undifferentiated early lung tissue (L).

307

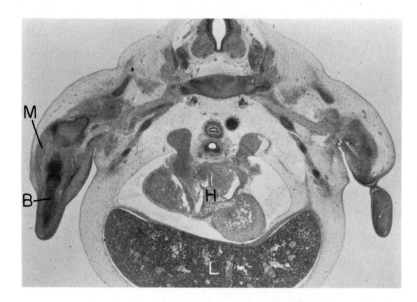

Figure 38. Thirty-six days. Mesenchyme has condensed into distinctive bones (B) and muscles (M). Note also the heart (H) and liver (L).

Figure 39. Thirty-eight days. Humerus (H) and scapula (S). Note how the general form of bone is set, that joint morphogenesis (arrow) occurs secondarily, and that as differentiation progresses the structures become more sharply delineated from surrounding tissues.

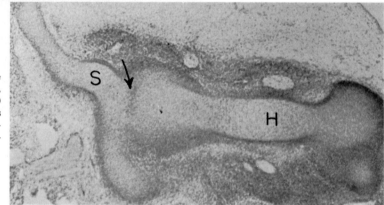

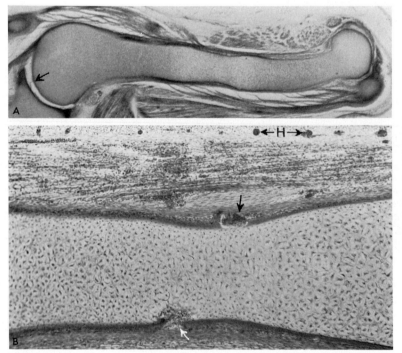

Figure 40. A, Forty-seven days. Humerus and shoulder. Solid cartilaginous humerus, clearly demarcated shoulder joint (arrow), and differentiated functional muscle. B, Fifty-one days. Invasion of bone from without (arrows) will develop marrow cavities for blood cell production. Primary ossification will be occurring in the near future. Note also the early developing hair follicles (H).

308

THYROID MORPHOGENESIS

*An Example of Outpouching, Migration of a Mass of Cells, and
Differentiation Toward Follicular Form*

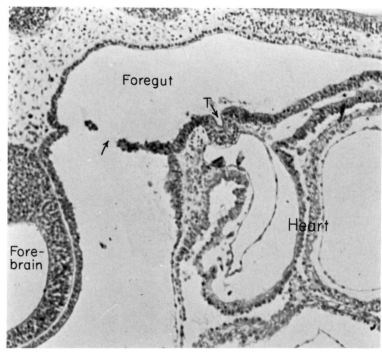

Figure 41. Twenty-six days. Thyroid invagination (T) from floor of foregut just at the time of breakdown of the buccopharyngeal membrane (arrow).

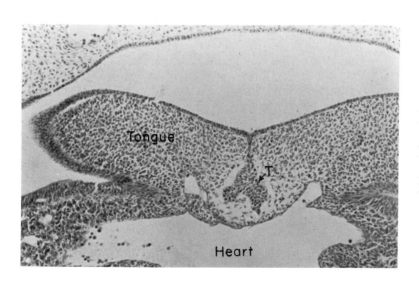

Figure 42. Twenty-nine days. The thyroid (T) has become an irregular solid structure, about to detach from its site of origin, which has now come to be the posterior tongue in this asymmetric coronal section. Note the immediate proximity to the underlying heart.

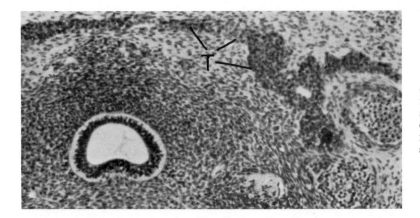

Figure 43. Thirty-six days. The thyroid (T) has now reached its usual locale at either side of the trachea with a straddling isthmus of thyroid anterior to the trachea. It is still a solid tissue.

Figure 44. Eleven weeks. Now a well developed gland, the thyroid cells have begun to organize as groups and develop follicles (arrows). The thyroid is functional from at least this age. Note the associated parathyroid glands.

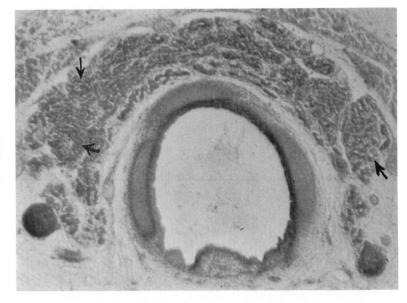

PITUITARY MORPHOGENESIS

An Example of Evagination from Endoderm and Neural Ectoderm, and Differentiation

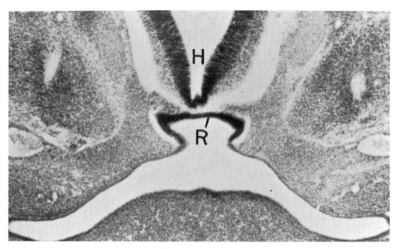

Figure 45. Thirty-two days. Rathke's pouch (R) evaginates from the roof of the pharynx to meet the base of the hypothalamus (H).

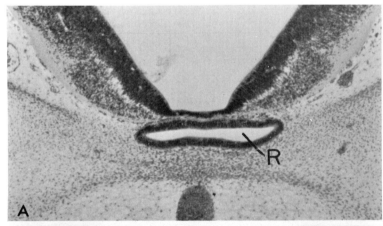

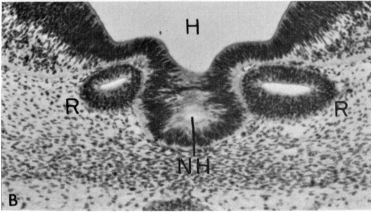

Figure 46. Thirty-six days. *A*, Rathke's pouch (R) becomes a vesicle. *B*, Slightly posterior, an outpouching occurs from the base of the hypothalamus (H) to become the neurohypophysis (NH), which indents Rathke's vesicle (R), this section being through the posterior margins of the indented vesicle. Note the early condensation of mesenchyme which will eventually form the base of the skull.

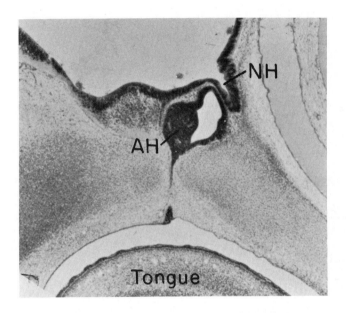

Figure 47. Thirty-eight days. Sagittal section showing obliterating tract of Rathke's outpouching with differentiation from the wall of Rathke's vesicle giving the early adenohypophysis (AH). The neurohypophysis (NH) is still represented by the simple outpouching from the floor of the hypothalamus. Note the progression in skeletal condensation of mesenchyme with a lack of clinoid processes at this time.

Incidentally, the pituitary marks the anterior level of extension of the notochord, and anterior to the hypophysis is the area into which the prechordal mesoderm has migrated.

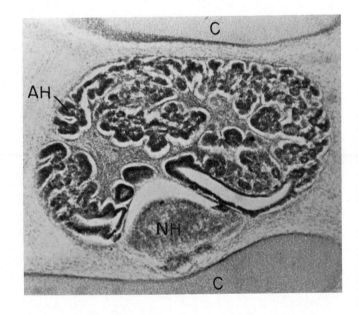

Figure 48. Eleven weeks. Cross section through the pituitary. The adenohypophysis (AH) has now organized into discrete groups of cells, the neurohypophysis (NH) may be noted posteriorly, and the clinoid processes (C) are now cartilaginous.

ABNORMAL MORPHOGENESIS

TYPES OF ABNORMAL MORPHOGENESIS

Structural anomalies can be divided crudely into several categories, each having somewhat different implications as to the type of error which occurred during morphogenesis.

Incomplete Morphogenesis. These are anomalies which represent incomplete stages in the development of a structure; they include the following subcategories, with one example listed for each:

Lack of development: renal agenesis secondary to failure of ureter formation.

Hypoplasia: micrognathia.

Incomplete separation: syndactyly (cutaneous).

Incomplete closure: cleft palate.

Incomplete septation: ventricular septal defect.

Incomplete migration of mesoderm: exstrophy of bladder.

Incomplete rotation: malrotation of the gut.

Incomplete resolution of early form: Meckel's diverticulum.

Persistence of earlier location: cryptorchidism.

Aberrant Form. An occasional anomaly may be interpreted as an aberrant form which never exists in any stage of normal morphogenesis. An example is the pelvic spur in the Nail-Patella syndrome. Such an anomaly may be more specific for a particular clinical syndrome entity than anomalies of incomplete morphogenesis.

Accessory Tissue. Accessory tissue — such as polydactyly, preauricular skin tags, and accessory spleens — all may be presumed to have been initiated around the same time as the normal tissue such as finger rays, auricular hillocks of His, and spleen, respectively.

Hamartomata. These anomalies represent an organizational defect leading to an abnormal admixture of tissues, often with a tumor-like excess of one or more tissues. Some have malignant potential. Examples of hamartomata are hemangiomata, melanomata, fibromata, lipomata, adenomata, and some strange admixtures that defy traditional classification.

Functional Defects. As an example, function is a necessary feature in joint development, and hence joint contractures such as club foot may result from functional deficit in use of the lower limb. Another potential clue toward defects of function of the limb may be derived from observing the creases of the hand. Creases on the palm or surface of the hand develop at planes of flexion of the early hand, and an anomaly such as early finger contracture (camptodactyly) will usually result in a lack of a crease at the nonfunctioning joint.

RELATIVE TIMING OF MALFORMATIONS

Malformations resulting from incomplete morphogenesis usually have their origin *prior to* the time when normal development would have proceeded beyond the form represented by the malformation. This type of developmental timing should not be construed as indicating that something happened *at* a particular time; all one can say is that a problem existed *prior to* a particular time.

Serious errors in early morphogenesis seldom allow for survival; hence only a few malformation problems are seen which can be said to have occurred prior to 23 days. Conjoined twins represent a partial to complete duplication of Hensen's node, the primitive streak, or both, and hence must have been initiated prior to 16 days. The cyclopia-cebocephaly type defect and the sirenomelia-sympodia type defect appear to be the consequence of defects in prechordal and postaxial mesoderm respectively, and presumably developed prior to 23 days. Aside from these examples, the vast majority of serious malformations represent errors that occur after three weeks of development.

Table 1 sets forth the relative timing as well as the presumed developmental error for some of the malformations which appear to represent incomplete stages in morphogenesis.

REFERENCES

1. Ebert, J. D.: Interacting Systems in Development. New York, Holt, Rinehart, and Winston, 1965.
2. Hamilton, W. J., Boyd, J. D., and Mossman, H. W.: Human Embryology. Baltimore, Williams and Wilkins Co., 1962.
3. Millen, J. W.: Timing of human congenital malformations. Develop. Med. Child. Neurol., 5:343, 1963.
4. Nilsson, L., Ingelman-Sundberg, A., and Wirsen, C.: A Child Is Born. New York, Delacorte Press, 1965.
5. Streeter, G. L.: Developmental Horizons in Human Embryos; Age Groups XI to XXIII. Washington, D.C., Carnegie Institute of Washington, 1951.
6. Willis, R. A.: The Borderland of Embryology and Pathology. Washington, Butterworth, 1962.
7. Longman, J.: Medical Embryology. Baltimore, Williams and Wilkins Co., 1963.

Table 1. Relative Timing and Developmental Pathology of Certain Malformations

TISSUES	MALFORMATION	DEFECT IN	CAUSE PRIOR TO	COMMENT
Central nervous system	Anencephaly	Closure of anterior neural tube	26 days	Subsequent degeneration of forebrain
	Meningomyelocele	Closure in a portion of the posterior neural tube	28 days	80% lumbosacral
Face	Cleft lip	Closure of lip	36 days	42% associated with cleft palate
	Cleft maxillary palate	Fusion of maxillary palatal shelves	8-9 weeks	
	Branchial sinus and/or cyst	Resolution of branchial cleft	8 weeks	Preauricular and along the line anterior to sternocleidomastoid
Gut	Esophageal atresia plus tracheoesophageal fistula	Lateral septation of foregut into trachea and foregut	30 days	
	Rectal atresia with fistula	Lateral septation of cloaca into rectum and urogenital sinus	6 weeks	
	Duodenal atresia	Recanalization of duodenum	7 to 8 weeks	
	Malrotation of gut	Rotation of intestinal loop so that cecum lies to right	10 weeks	Associated incomplete or aberrant mesenteric attachments
	Omphalocele	Return of midgut from yolk sac to abdomen	10 weeks	

	Malformation	Developmental process disturbed		Remarks
	Meckel's diverticulum	Obliteration of vitelline duct	10 weeks	May contain gastric and/or pancreatic tissue
	Diaphragmatic hernia	Closure of pleuroperitoneal canal	6 weeks	
Genitourinary system	Extroversion of bladder	Migration of infraumbilical mesenchyme	30 days	Associated müllerian and wolffian duct defects
	Bicornuate uterus	Fusion of lower portion of müllerian ducts	10 weeks	
	Hypospadias	Fusion of urethral folds (labia minora)	12 weeks	
	Cryptorchidism	Descent of testicle into scrotum	7 to 9 months	
Heart	Transposition of great vessels	Directional development of bulbus cordis septum	34 days	
	Ventricular septal defect	Closure of ventricular septum	6 weeks	
	Patent ductus arteriosus	Closure of ductus arteriosus	9 to 10 months	
Limb	Aplasia of radius	Genesis of radial bone	38 days	Often accompanied by other defects of radial side of distal limb
	Syndactyly, severe	Separation of digital rays	6 weeks	
Complex	Cyclopia, holoprosencephaly	Prechordal mesoderm development	23 days	Secondary defects of midface and forebrain
	Sirenomelia (sympodia)	Development of posterior axis	23 days	Associated defects of cloacal development

Chapter Four

GENETICS AND GENETIC COUNSELING

relative to single primary defects and dysmorphic syndromes of multiple primary defect

The basic process of morphogenesis is genetically controlled, being dependent on the environment for full expression of the genetic potential.

Judging from the malformation problems for which a mode of etiology has been strongly indicated, the major cause is genetic aberration. There are three general genetic modes of determination for abnormal morphogenesis: polygenic determination, mutant genes in single or double dose, and gross genetic imblance due to a chromosomal abnormality. These are considered separately as they relate to problems of malformation, especially multiple defect syndromes. Recommended genetic counsel is presented at the end of each section.

POLYGENIC INHERITANCE AS A MAJOR FACTOR IN THE ETIOLOGY OF COMMON SINGLE PRIMARY MALFORMATIONS

Much of the usual variability among individuals as well as many common disorders within a species may be ascribed to minor differences in a number of gene loci involved in the determination of a particular characteristic. A polygenically determined abnormality is herein defined as one that is predominantly the consequence of minor differences at many gene loci, no one of which may be held fully responsible for the abnormality. Obviously it is difficult to prove polygenic inheritance, but present evidence in the human indicates that this is the major mode in the etiology of many of the single localized defects in morphogenesis, namely, cleft lip and palate, cleft palate alone, pyloric stenosis, congenital dislocation of the hip, club foot, and the anencephaly-meningomyelocele type of anomaly (defects of neural tube closure). These anomalies account for about 47 per cent of the babies with obvious malformations in early infancy. The following indirect evidence for polygenic inheritance for the single common defects comes predominantly from the work of Carter[1] and has recently been summarized by Smith and Aase.[2]

Frequency of the Defect in Relatives

The frequency of *recurrence* for the same type of defect in offspring from unaffected parents ranges from 2 to 5 per cent (Table 2), 20 to 40 times the general frequency within that population group. The collected data are not compatible with autosomal dominant or recessive inheritance.

Concordance in Twins

The question asked in these surveys is the following: if one twin has a defect, with what frequency does the other twin have the same type of defect? If both twins have the defect, they are concordant for that anomaly; if one twin has the defect and the other does not, they are nonconcordant. These surveys include all the previously mentioned defects except those of neural tube closure. The incidence of concordance in nonidentical twins is of similar magnitude to that of siblings born of separate pregnancies and thereby gives no evidence toward a major environmental etiology for these defects. The frequency of concordance in identical twin sets is four to eight times the incidence in nonidentical twins, providing evidence for genetic factors in the etiology. Yet the highest concordance rate in identical twin sets, 40 per cent for cleft lip with or without cleft palate, amply demonstrates that given the same genetic background and similar intrauterine environment, the majority of identical twin sets are not concordant for these defects. This fact emphasizes the subtlety of the phenomena involved in the developmental pathology of these malformations.

Influence of Genetic Background

Sex. The difference between the XX and the XY genetic background is one major genetic difference that has an appreciable effect on the occurrence of these major malformations, no one of which has an equal sex incidence (Fig. 49). Considering a malformation such as pyloric stenosis for which genes on the X and/or Y chromosome play an especially large role, it is worthwhile to view recurrence risks in relation to the sex of the individual (Table 2).

These sex differences provide cogent evidence for polygenic inheritance. Taking the example of pyloric stenosis, Carter[1] reasoned as follows: if it takes more genetic factors to give rise to this anomaly in the female, then the affected female should pass on more of these genetic factors to her offspring, who would have a higher frequency of pyloric stenosis than would offspring of affected males. This is precisely what Carter found, the incidence of pyloric stenosis from affected mothers being four times as high as the incidence from affected fathers (24 per cent vs. 6 per cent). This is the type of quantitative effect that would be expected with polygenic inheritance.

Race. Numerous subtle genetic differences exist among racial groups. Persistent genetic isolation increases the differences between groups, and genetic admixture obviously lessens these differences.

The types of minor genetic differences hypothesized as being the predominant cause for the foregoing malformations would presumably differ among racial groups. Therefore the incidence of these anomalies would show racial variance. This is precisely what has been found, there being variability for the *types* of single malformation among racial groups (Fig. 50).[3]

Among particular racial groups or subgroups the incidence of a particular anomaly may be relatively high. For example, severe club foot is a more frequent anomaly among Polynesians than Chinese. The racial make-up in Hawaii provided Chung[4] the opportunity to determine the effects of racial admixture on the occurrence of this anomaly, as noted in Figure 51. These findings are compatible with a polygenic mode of determination for club foot in the Hawaiians, with dramatic reduction in the incidence of the defect following admixture with Chinese.

Another similar example is polydactyly as studied in Sao Paulo. The incidence of the defect was 0.7 per cent in Negroes, 0.24 per cent among the Caucasians, and 0.52 per cent among the mulatto racial admixture.[5]

Variation in Recurrence Risk in Relation to Severity of Malformation

In accordance with the hypothesis of polygenic inheritance for the foregoing anomalies, the more severe the degree of malformation, the greater the adverse genetic influences involved and thereby the greater the chance for recurrence from the same parentage. Carter[1] has obtained some preliminary data which support this hypothesis. The risk for recurrence in subsequent children when an offspring has a bilateral cleft lip and palate is 5.7 per cent, as contrasted to a 2.5 per cent recurrence risk when the offspring has only a unilateral cleft lip.

EVIDENCE FOR POLYGENIC MODE OF DETERMINATION FOR INDIVIDUALS WITH A SINGLE COMMON MALFORMATION

Recurrence risk data among relatives of an individual with a single common malformation are compatible with a polygenic mode of determination and not with usual mendelian dominant or recessive inheritance. The data from twin studies indicate a genetic etiology with a very subtle end point in the development of a single malformation, so subtle that unrecognized chance factors apparently are important. The genetic factors involved are apparently numerous and genes on the sex chromosomes

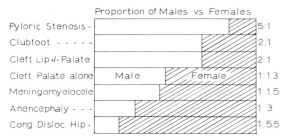

Figure 49. Relative sex incidence of single common malformations.

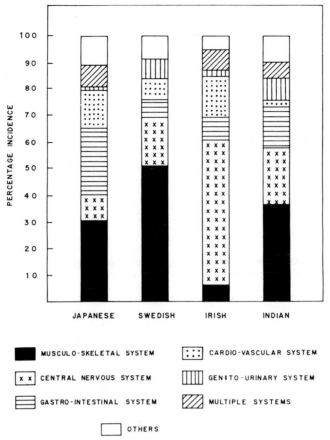

Figure 50. Racial differences in incidence of particular types of malformations. (From Kolah, P. J., Master, P. A., and Sanghvi, L. D.: Am. J. Obstet. & Gynec., *97*:400, 1967.)

play a role, no common malformation having an equal sex incidence. Racial differences also have a major influence on the incidence of a given common anomaly, with racial admixture altering the incidence of particular defects toward a median incidence between those for the respective racial groups. Further evidence of quantitative inheritance is derived from the observation that the risk for recurrence is greater when the degree of anomaly is more severe. Taken together and in context these data support polygenic inheritance as the most prevalent mode of determination of common single malformations. It is quite significant that the recurrence risk for

normal parents who have one affected child is so similar for each of these structural defects, in the range of one in 30 to one in 20.

It is not presently possible to transpose these data for common single malformations to the less common single defects, such as some of those presented in Chapter One. However, it is interesting to note that unequal sex occurrence is also a feature of these disorders, which are usually sporadic occurrences in a family with occasional instances of recurrence. Much more data are needed for each of these rare single defects before we can state recurrence risks or imply that they also appear to have a polygenic basis.

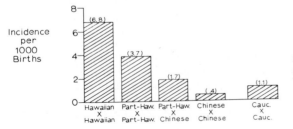

Figure 51. Relative incidence of severe club foot (talipes equinovarus) among various racial groups and combinations in Hawaii. (Courtesy of C. S. Chung, University of Hawaii.)

ENVIRONMENTAL FACTORS AND SINGLE MALFORMATIONS

Environmental influences can play a role in determination of these malformations. However, the fact that the concordance rate for nonidentical twins is of similar magnitude to the recurrence rate for siblings born of separate pregnancies gives little indication of environmental factors having the major role in etiology. This latter statement cannot be applied to the anencephaly-meningomyelocele type of anomaly, because adequate twin data are not yet available for this defect. Some indications of environmental effects have been observed in Scotland and England in studies of anencephaly-meningomyelocele families, namely, seasonal variability[6] and social class differences.[7] However, no significant seasonal variability was noted for these defects in Rhode Island,[8] and no social class differences were noted in Lebanon.[9] Birth order influences have also been noted, congenital dislocation of the hip and pyloric stenosis being more likely to occur in first born.[1]

The genetic background may have a profound influence on the likelihood of a given environmental teratogen causing malformation. For example, Fraser[10] could regularly produce cleft palate in mouse embryos of the A/Jax strain by giving the mothers a high dosage of cortisone during early gestation, but the same treatment in a different strain gave rise to only 17 per cent affected offspring.

The search for environmental factors that can allow for expression of a single malformation obviously should continue. However, it should be appreciated that present evidence indicates a subtle polygenic mode as the predominant basis for the more common single defects. Furthermore, just as the polygenic mode implies multiple minor genetic differences that are difficult to individualize, so environmental factors are likely to be multiple and subtle in character. The total factors combine to approach the subtle threshold for a particular defect in morphogenesis, a threshold predominantly set by the genetic makeup of the individual.

Counsel for Single Primary Defects for Which Polygenic Inheritance Has Been Indicated

1. Explain the developmental pathology of the defect so that the parents can appreciate that there was only a single localized defect in the early development of their child. Then discuss the management and prognosis for the child. When the single defect is of the type which—with repair—need not interfere with the social acceptance or function of the child, it is often helpful to tell the parents that the *child* is normal. For example, given a child with isolated cleft lip, the parents may be told, "Your *child* is normal; the *lip* did not close completely, and therefore we shall have a plastic surgeon bring about the closure." The purpose of this approach is to assist in the parental acceptance of the child by not branding the whole child as malformed, but localizing the defect to what it actually represents in an anatomical and functional sense.

2. Explain that the localized problem in development must have occurred *prior to* a particular time in gestation, and reassure the parents that it was not related to any factor after that time.

3. Ask the parents if they have any ideas concerning the cause of the malformation. Most of the parental concerns relative to etiology can be dispelled.

4. Explain that morphogenesis is a genetically determined process in which numerous genes play a role, as a team, in the development of a given structure. Then indicate that the "set of genes" derived from *both* parents did not allow for full normal development of the particular structure leading to the malformation. Indicate

Table 2. Empiric Recurrence Risk Data for Some Common Single Malformations[2]

	GIVEN—UNAFFECTED PARENTS WITH ONE AFFECTED OFFSPRING		GIVEN—AFFECTED ADULT
	RISK FOR SUBSEQUENT OFFSPRING:		RISK OF AFFECTED OFFSPRING:
Cleft lip with or without cleft palate	4.9%		4.3%
Cleft palate alone	2.0%		6.0%
Club foot	2-8%		?
Anencephaly*	3.4%		
Meningomyelocele*	4.8%		
Dislocation of hip	3.5%	Brothers—0.5% Sisters—6.3%	?
Pyloric stenosis	3.2%	Brothers—4.0% Sisters—2.4%	Affected father—4.6% Affected mother—16.2%

*The recurrence risk for anencephaly and for meningomyelocele includes about an equal risk for either defect, because these anomalies seem linked etiologically as defects in neural tube closure.

how subtle the end point is, toward normal or malformation, for such single defects.

5. Indicate to the parents that the likelihood of a subsequent offspring having a similar set of genes allowing for a similar malformation is of low magnitude, 5 per cent or less for the single common defects. In giving this counsel the risk figures may be mildly increased when the defect is severe in degree and decreased when the anomaly is mild in degree. The risk figures may be separately stated for the sex of the offspring, especially for pyloric stenosis and congenital dislocation of the hip. If two offspring are affected, the risk for subsequent offspring being affected is two- to threefold greater than the previously mentioned figure, around 10 to 15 per cent. The risk of an affected individual having affected offspring is of similar magnitude to that of the sibling recurrence risk, around five per cent.

Note: This counsel is obviously crude, being based on indirect evidence and empiric data. However, to the author it seems the most appropriate at our present state of knowledge and is thereby preferable to not giving the parents any perspective on etiology and recurrence risk. Hopefully future knowledge will allow for more precise counseling relative to individuals with a single localized malformation.

MENDELIAN TYPE INHERITANCE OF MUTANT GENES

The genes are contained as a part of the chromosomes. Those genes located in the X chromosome are referred to as X-linked genes and those on the autosomes (the non-sex chromosomes) as autosomal-linked genes.

Man is a diploid organism with two sets of chromosomes, one set being derived from each parent. Each pair of chromosomes will have comparable gene determinants located at the same position on each chromosome of the pair. The pair of genes may be referred to as *alleles,* or partners, which normally work together. Thus, with the exception of the genes of the X and Y chromosomes in the male, each genetic determinant is present in *two doses,* one from each parent. A *mutant* gene indicates a *changed* gene. A major mutant gene is herein defined as a genetic determinant which has been changed in such a way that it can give rise to an abnormal characteristic. If a mutant gene in single dose gives rise to an abnormal characteristic despite the presence of a normal allele (partner), then it may be referred to as *dominant* because it causes abnormality even when counterbalanced by a normal gene partner. A mutant gene which only causes an abnormal characteristic when present in double dosage (or single dosage without a normal partner, as for an X-linked mutant gene in the male) is referred to as recessive. There are gradations from a mutant gene that always causes an abnormal characteristic in single dosage (dominant), to one that occasionally causes some abnormality in single dosage (semidominant), and one that never causes an evident alteration except when present in double dosage (recessive).

Expression is a term used to indicate the extent of abnormality that is due to a genetic aberration. The expression may be stated as severe, usual, mild, or no expression, the latter being synonymous with lack of penetrance in an individual who has the genetic aberration. Individuals with the same genetic aberration frequently show variance in expression, especially with respect to malformations.

Traditionally, the mutant gene disorders have been categorized into those due to genes located on the autosomes—autosomal dominant and autosomal recessive—and disorders due to genes on the X-chromosome—X-linked recessive and X-linked dominant.

AUTOSOMAL DOMINANT—SINGLE DOSE AUTOSOMAL MUTANT GENE DISORDERS

Autosomal dominant disorders often show wide variation in expression among affected individuals, presumably because of minor differences in the normal allele (partner) of the mutant gene as well as other differences in the genetic or environmental background of the affected individual. Figure 52 demonstrates the variance in expression for an autosomal dominant disorder, ectrodactyly. The risk of the single mutant gene being passed to a given offspring is 50 per cent, yet the risk of a severe defect of hand development is less than 50 per cent because of variance in expression. To utilize the example of Waardenburg's syndrome, the risk of inheritance of the mutant gene from an affected individual is 50 per cent, yet only about 20 per cent of affected individuals have deafness, the most disturbing expression of the syndrome. Hence the risk for deafness in offspring of a parent with Waardenburg's syndrome is the risk of receiving the mutant gene (50 per cent) times the likelihood of expression for deafness in the disorder (20 per cent), or 10 per cent. This dichotomy between the risk of receiving the gene and the risk of a particular expression of the disorder in individuals with the mutant gene must be utilized in counseling, especially for autosomal dominant disorders.

The first question to ask oneself after making the clinical diagnosis of an autosomal single mutant gene disorder is: "When did the gene mutation occur?" If the disorder is one which always shows some expression and the parents are quite normal, then this may be presumed to be a *fresh gene mutation* which happened in one of the germ cells that went to form the conceptus and thereby is present in all the cells of the resulting individual. The parents of a child who represents a fresh gene mutation therefore have a negligible risk for recurrence. Actually a high proportion of individuals with autosomal domi-

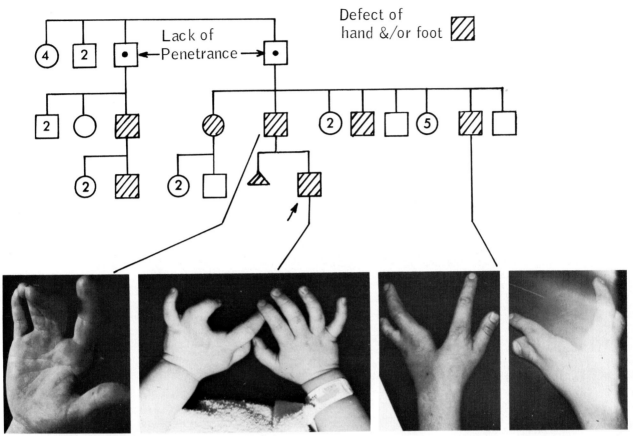

Figure 52. Variation in expression for autosomal dominant ectrodactyly among various related individuals. Note also the *intra-individual* asymmetry of expression in the propositus (arrow). (From Smith, D. W.: J. Pediat., *69*:1150, 1966.)

nant patterns of malformation represent fresh gene mutations. Since the affected individuals often have limited capability of reproduction, the majority of cases seen are fresh mutations. For some conditions such as Apert's syndrome there have been only a few reported cases of offspring from affected individuals, but these demonstrated the autosomal dominant inheritance. Some of the sporadic syndromes of unknown etiology may also be single gene mutations, but lack of reproduction prevents a testing of the hypothesis. Fresh gene mutation appears to be more likely at *older paternal age*. Hence paternal age should always be noted in the evaluation of disorders which may be the consequence of a single mutant gene.

Counseling in Autosomal Dominant Disorders (Utilize Fig. 53)

1. Examine the parents and siblings and occasionally other relatives to determine whether any of them show features of the disorder in question. If neither parent shows any expression of an autosomal dominant disorder, which always shows some effect on the individual, the parents may be told, "A single gene was altered in one of the germ cells prior to the development of the child. This event is extremely unlikely to happen again, and therefore your risk for further affected children is negligible." They should also be reassured that relatives need have no concern of having affected children.

2. The risk for an *affected* individual having an affected child is 50 per cent for each offspring. When possible, be acquainted with the frequency of various features in affected individuals so as to relate not only the risk of a given offspring receiving the mutant gene but also the likelihood of any particular defect occurring.

3. Explain, when feasible, the developmental pathology and how all the aspects of altered development are secondary to the effects of the single altered gene. Outline the natural history of the condition and the management for the child.

AUTOSOMAL RECESSIVE – DOUBLE DOSE (PAIR) AUTOSOMAL MUTANT GENE DISORDERS

Autosomal recessive disorders generally have less variation in expression than do autosomal dominant syndromes. Possibly this is because both genes of a pair are mutant, and therefore there is *no* normal partner gene to carry on the function of that particular gene. The inheritance is from clinically normal parents who both have the *same* recessive mutant gene in *single dose,* the risk of which is obviously enhanced if the parents are related. Hence consanguinity should always be asked about in disorders known to be autosomal recessive as well as when evaluating unknown syndromes of questionable cause.

The recurrence risk from the same parentage is 25 per cent for each subsequent offspring. The genes involved in the autosomal recessive patterns of malformation are relatively rare in the population, and therefore the parents may be reassured that there is little risk of other relatives or their normal children having affected offspring. This would not hold true for an inbred population group.

Counsel for Autosomal Recessive Disorders (Utilize Fig. 54)

1. Explain that the child has one pair of altered genes and that the disturbance in development is caused by that pair of altered genes. Outline the natural history and management for the child.

2. Explain to the parents that most individuals have several altered genes that cause no problem because each is counterbalanced by its normal gene partner. They happen to have one altered gene in common, and the chance of any given offspring receiving both of these altered genes and being affected is 25 per cent for each pregnancy.

3. Explain that the chance of their normal children having a single altered gene (carrier) is two out of three, but since the chance of randomly marrying another carrier is very small their risk of having affected children should be very small. The general risk of any unaffected relative having an affected child may be calculated, as set forth in Figure 54.

X-LINKED RECESSIVE—SINGLE DOSE X-LINKED MUTANT GENE, EXPRESSED IN THE MALE

The X-linked genes in the XY male are present in but a single dose with no allele in the male, and hence the full recessive disorder is expressed with but a single mutant gene. The frequency of X-linked recessive disease in the male is thereby a direct reflection of the frequency of X-linked recessive genes per X chromosomes in the population. The chance of an XX female having a pair of such X-linked recessive genes and expressing the same disorder as the male is very small. Hence the following precepts are the important ones in detecting X-linked recessive inheritance:

1. With rare exception only males are affected and the transmission is through unaffected heterozygous (carrier) females.

2. There is no male to male transmission.

X-linked recessive disorders in the male, especially the more severe ones, may represent a fresh gene mutation. These disorders present a problem in trying to determine at what level the gene mutation arose, for it could be in the patient alone, or in the mother, or even back one or two generations and silently passed through carrier females. For some X-linked disorders this dilemma can be solved by demonstrating the presence or absence of a heterozygous (carrier) subclinical expression in the females in question. Such observations can also be of value in determining whether any related female at risk is a carrier or not.

Counsel for X-Linked Recessive Disorders (Utilize Fig. 55)

1. First, try to determine by family pedigree evaluation, or observation of heterozygous expression, whether the mother is a carrier or not.

2. Explain the X-linked single mutant gene and how it caused trouble because the male has no normal partner gene to counter the mutant gene. Then relate the natural history and management for the boy.

3. If the mother is a carrier she may be told that there is a 50 per cent risk of any future male being affected; that all daughters will be normal with a 50 per cent risk of being a carrier; that normal sons cannot transmit the disorder; and that affected sons would have normal sons who cannot transmit the disease, and all their daughters would be unaffected carriers.

4. If the mother is *not* a carrier, then the risk for recurrence from the mother is negligible and the affected boy's risk is as listed above.

X-LINKED DOMINANT

X-linked single gene *dominant* disorders show expression in the XX female, usually with a more severe effect in the XY male. This type of inheritance is most commonly confused with autosomal dominant inheritance from which it may be discriminated in the following ways:

1. There is usually a more severe expression in affected males.

2. Affected males have normal sons (no male to male transmission) and all their daughters are affected.

The counseling is the same as for X-linked recessive except that all carrier females are affected (utilize Fig. 56).

SINGLE MUTANT GENE WITH SEX LIMITATION

Several disorders, such as the oral-facial-digital syndrome, are found almost exclusively in females and apparently cause early lethality in the affected male because there is a 50 per cent deficiency in sons as compared to daughters from affected females, with about 50 per cent of the daughters and none of the sons being affected. At present it has not been possible to determine whether this disorder is an X-linked dominant with early lethality in the male or an autosomal dominant which has a lethal effect in the male.

Genetic Counseling for a Single Mutant Gene Defect with Presumed Early Lethality in the Affected Male (Utilize Fig. 57)

1. Explain that this is due to a single altered gene and discuss the natural history and management.
2. Examine the parents, especially the mother. If they are quite normal, assume a fresh gene mutation with a negligible recurrence risk.
3. If the mother is affected, then her risk would be one in three for a normal male, one in three for an affected female, and one in three for a normal female. The same risks would apply for any affected female.

CHARTS FOR GENETIC COUNSEL REGARDING MUTANT GENE DISORDERS

Figures 53 to 57 are designed to be of assistance in providing genetic counsel. The following chart summarizes the genetic aberrations and sets forth the system utilized in the ensuing figures. The pair of genes under consideration are depicted in their usual situation, as loci on a pair of chromosomes, only one of which will go to a given offspring. The normal gene is a *dot,* the mutant dominant gene is a full *bar,* and the mutant recessive gene is depicted as a triangular *wedge.* The male is the large square, the female is a circle, and the affected individual is marked by diagonal lines. The dashed lines lead to the risk figures for future offspring. These charts have been designed for use in genetic counseling.

MENDELIAN INHERITANCE, WITH DESIGNATIONS TO BE UTILIZED IN THE FOLLOWING FIGURES

Normal		Except for the XY, there is a pair of genes for each function, located at the same loci on sister chromosomes. One pair of normal genes is represented as dots on a homologous pair of chromosomes.
Dominant		A single mutant (changed) gene is dominant if it causes an evident abnormality. The chance of inheritance of the mutant gene (■) is the same as the chance of inheriting a particular chromosome of the pair: 50 per cent.
Heterozygous Recessive		A single mutant gene is recessive (▶) if it causes no evident abnormality, the function being well covered by the normal partner gene (allele). Such an individual may be referred to as a *heterozygous* carrier.
Homozygous Recessive		When both genes are a recessive mutant (▶), the abnormal effect is expressed. The parents are generally carriers, and their risk of having another affected offspring is the chance of receiving the mutant from one parent (50 per cent) times the chance from the other parent (50 per cent), or 25 per cent for each offspring.
X-linked Recessive	X Y	An X-linked recessive will be expressed in the male because he has no normal partner gene. His daughters, receiving the X, will all be carriers, and his sons, receiving the Y, will all be normal.
	X X	An X-linked recessive will not show overt expression in the female because at least part of her "active" X's will contain the normal gene. The risk for affected sons and carrier daughters will each be 50 per cent.

(*Text continues on page 329*)

AUTOSOMAL DOMINANT
For Single Altered Gene Which
Always Shows Some Expression

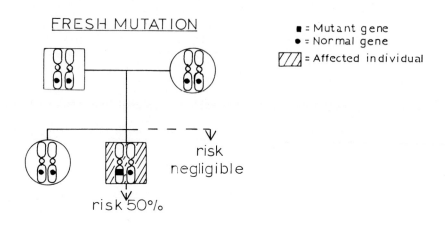

FRESH MUTATION

■ = Mutant gene
● = Normal gene
▨ = Affected individual

risk
negligible

risk 50%

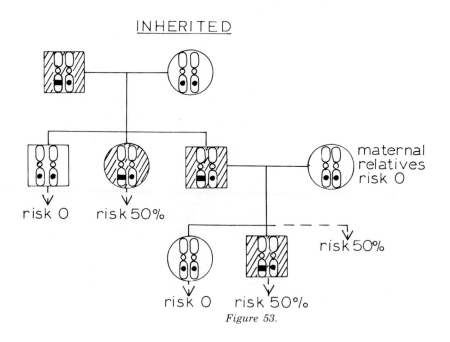

INHERITED

risk 0   risk 50%

maternal
relatives
risk 0

risk 50%

risk 0   risk 50%

Figure 53.

AUTOSOMAL RECESSIVE
The Affected Individual has
a <u>Pair</u> of Altered Genes

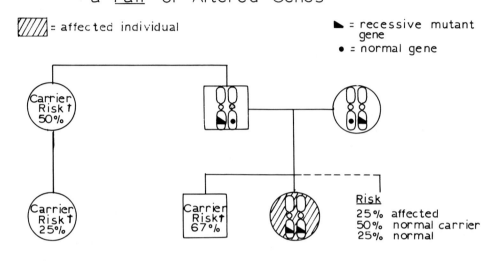

Risk of Unaffected Relative — Carrier × Gene ×25%
having Affected Child   = Risk   Frequency
                                    in Population

For example, ┐ ─ ─ ─ ─ Siblings: 67%   X   1%   X   25%=1 in 600
Gene Frequency │
1 in 100, with ├─Aunts and Uncles: 50%   X   1%   X   25%=1 in 800
Random Marriage┘─ ─ First Cousins: 25%   X   1%   X   25%=1 in1600

†Probability of this individual having the mutant gene.

Figure 54.

X-LINKED RECESSIVE
Single Altered Gene Expressed in Male

🔸 = X chromosome

🔸 = Y chromosome

◣ = recessive gene

• = normal gene

▨ = affected individual

INHERITED

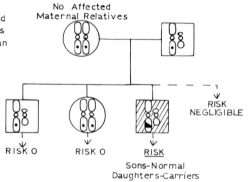

carrier risk † 50%

carrier risk † 25%

Paternal Relatives No Risk

RISK
Sons-50% affected
Daughters-50%carriers

RISK O

carrier risk † 50%

RISK
Sons-Normal
Daughters-Carriers

FRESH MUTATION

This can only be ascertained with assurance for conditions in which the carrier state can be __ruled out__ in the mother.

No Affected Maternal Relatives

RISK NEGLIGIBLE

RISK O   RISK O   RISK
Sons-Normal
Daughters-Carriers

† Probability of individual having the mutant gene.

Figure 55.

X-LINKED DOMINANT

Single Altered Dominant X-Linked Gene; Usually More Severe Expression in Male

////// = affected individual

= X chromosome

= Y chromosome

■ = mutant gene

● = normal allele

<u>INHERITED</u>

Paternal Relatives, No Risk

<u>RISK</u>
Sons 50%
Daughters 50%

<u>RISK</u>
Sons-Normal
Daughters-Affected

FRESH MUTATION

This can only be determined with assurance for X-linked dominant disorders which <u>always</u> show expression in both the male and female.

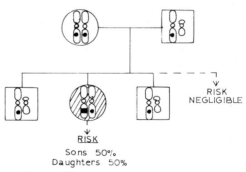

RISK
NEGLIGIBLE

<u>RISK</u>
Sons 50%
Daughters 50%

Figure 56.

SEX LIMITED
Single Altered Gene[†]
apparently an early lethal in affected males

▨ = affected individual

■ = Mutant gene, dominant
• = Normal gene

INHERITED

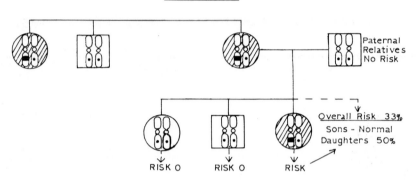

Paternal Relatives No Risk

Overall Risk 33%
Sons - Normal
Daughters 50%

RISK 0   RISK 0   RISK

FRESH MUTATION

Can only be stated with assurance for disorders in which the affected female always shows expression.

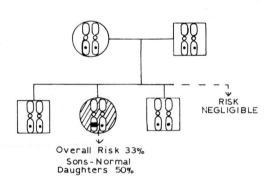

RISK NEGLIGIBLE

Overall Risk 33%
Sons-Normal
Daughters 50%

[†] The localization to the X chromosomes or an autosome has not been determined. Here it is depicted as an autosome.

Figure 57.

GENETIC IMBALANCE DUE TO GROSS CHROMOSOMAL ABNORMALITIES

The 46 normal chromosomes consist of 22 homologous pairs of autosomes plus the XX pair of sex chromosomes in the female and the XY in the male. Normal development is not only dependent on the genic content of these chromosomes, but on the gene balance as well. The genetic balance of cells is dependent on the integrity of the chromosomes and on their proper distribution at the time of cell division. During meiotic reduction division (Fig. 58) one of each pair of autosomes and one of the sex chromosomes are distributed randomly to each daughter cell, whereas during mitosis (Fig. 59) each replicated chromosome is separated longitudinally at the centromere such that each daughter cell receives an identical complement of genetic material.

Figure 60 shows the natural appearance of stained chromosomes at early, mid, and late stages of mitosis. It would obviously be difficult to count these chromosomes or to distinguish their individual structure from such preparations. In order to obtain adequate preparations for the study of chromosome number and morphology the cultured cells are treated with a toxic agent such as colchicine which blocks the spindle formation and thus leads to the accumulation of cells at the metaphase of mitosis. These cells are then exposed to a hypotonic solution that spreads the unattached chromosomes, allowing for such preparations as that shown in Figure 61.

Abnormal morphogenesis may result from genetic imbalance. Figure 62 illustrates some of the types of chromosomal abnormalities which can lead to gross genetic imbalance.

Chromosomal maldistribution at cell division is the most common type; in fact it appears to be the most prevalent serious genetic event occurring in man. At least 3 per cent of conceptuses have an altered number of chromosomes, principally one too many or one too few, collectively referred to as aneuploidy. The majority of these genetic imbalances do not allow for normal morphogenesis and result in early demise of the conceptus. For example, about 25 per cent of embryos spontaneously aborted have an abnormal number of chromosomes. Only a few of the gross genetic imbalances allow for prenatal survival, the frequency in the newborn being about 0.5 per cent. These are generally aneuploidy with one chromosome too many. An extra sex chromosome is the most common aneuploidy, at least partially because these aneuploidies give rise to the least disturbance in morphogenesis. The XYY, XXY, or XXX individual usually appears quite normal at the time of birth. The XYY individual may become relatively tall and may have aberrant aggressive behavior; the XXY male may be mentally dull, may have aberrant behavior, and usually has primary hypogonadism with infertility and inadequate androgen production; the XXX female seldom shows any apparent expression.

Only three autosomal trisomies have been discovered which allow for prenatal survival. Each results in a recognizable pattern of multiple malformations, demonstrating that unrelated individuals with the same type of genetic imbalance tend to have a similar disturbance in morphogenesis. The least affected of these are those with an extra 21 chromosome which gives rise to Down's syndrome, the most frequent mal-

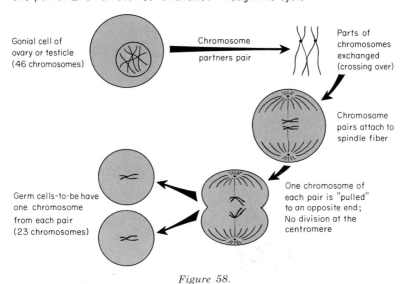

MEIOTIC REDUCTION DIVISION in development of gametes (sex cells) One pair of 21 chromosomes is followed through the cycle

Gonial cell of ovary or testicle (46 chromosomes)

Chromosome partners pair

Parts of chromosomes exchanged (crossing over)

Chromosome pairs attach to spindle fiber

One chromosome of each pair is "pulled" to an opposite end; No division at the centromere

Germ cells-to-be have one chromosome from each pair (23 chromosomes)

Figure 58.

USUAL CELL CYCLE
One chromosome 21 is followed through the cycle

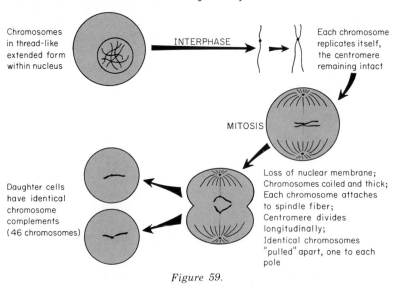

Figure 59.

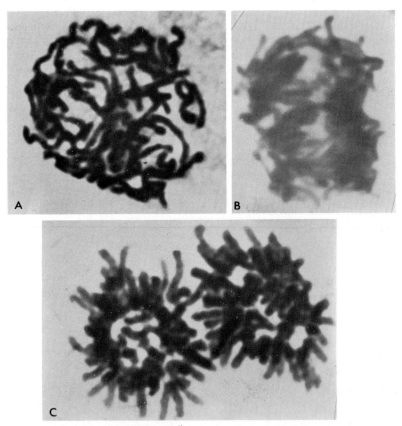

Figure 60. Chromosomes of untreated mitotic cells. *A,* Prophase cell. *B,* Metaphase cell with chromosomes attached to the spindle fibers and beginning to separate. *C,* Anaphase cell, with identical chromosomal complements having been "pulled apart" toward the development of two daughter cells.

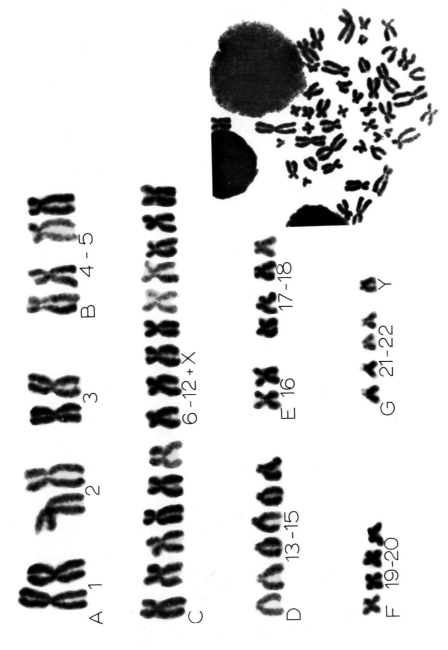

Figure 61. Chromosomes of a cultured normal human male cell, treated with Colcemid and then a hypotonic solution, are shown at the lower right. These have been cut out and arranged in the karyotype on the basis of length and position of the centromere.

TYPES OF CHROMOSOMAL ABNORMALITIES
LEADING TO GENETIC IMBALANCE

Chromosomal Maldistribution:

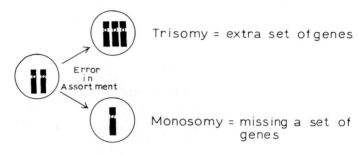

Trisomy = extra set of genes

Monosomy = missing a set of genes

Chromosomal Breakage:

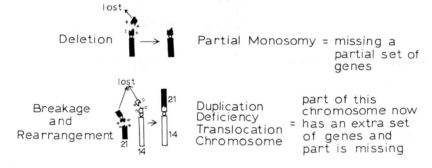

Deletion → Partial Monosomy = missing a partial set of genes

Breakage and Rearrangement → Duplication Deficiency Translocation Chromosome = part of this chromosome now has an extra set of genes and part is missing

Maldivision at Centromere:

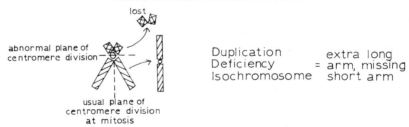

Duplication Deficiency Isochromosome = extra long arm, missing short arm

Figure 62.

formation problem in the human with an incidence of about one in 650 newborn infants. Judging from findings in the products of spontaneous abortion, the majority of 18 trisomy and 13 trisomy individuals do not survive the prenatal period. Those who do survive are born with multiple malformations and are seldom capable of extrauterine existence for very long. The only potentially viable monosomy is the XO imbalance, and studies of spontaneous abortuses indicate that the majority of these do not survive prenatal life. Those who are born have a pattern of malformations which usually allows for clinical recognition.

Though little is known about the etiology of faulty chromosomal distribution, one recognized factor is the increased likelihood of such errors at older maternal age. This applies especially to the autosomal trisomy syndromes and to a lesser extent to some of the sex chromosome aneuploidies. Figure 63 shows the progressive increase in the frequency of Down's syndrome during the latter period of a woman's reproductive life.

The timing of the error in chromosome distribution seldom can be stated with assurance, for it could occur prior to meiosis, during the first or second divisions of meiosis, or even during the first division of the zygote and still result in an aneuploid individual (see Fig. 64).

Errors in the assortment of chromosomes that occur during postzygotic cell division can give rise to mosaic individuals having at least two different cell populations from the stand-

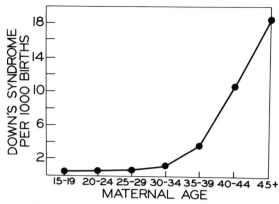

Figure 63. Increasing incidence of Down's syndrome during the latter period of a woman's reproductive period. (From Smith, D. W.: Am. J. Obstet. & Gynec., *90*:1055, 1964.)

point of chromosomal number (see Fig. 64). Those who are mosaics for XO/XX often have less abnormality than the wholly XO individual, and in similar fashion 21 trisomy–normal mosaic individuals show every gradation from Down's syndrome to near-normal appearance and function.

Less commonly, genetic imbalance can result from chromosomal breakage (Fig. 62). A broken piece of a chromosome may be lost. With more than one break, rearrangement of chromosomal pieces may take place between the broken chromosomes, a phenomenon referred to as translocation. An individual can have a translocation chromosome with no evident problem as long as he still has a balanced set of genes. However, a balanced carrier of a translocation chromosome is likely to produce unbalanced germ cells during meiotic reduction division (Fig. 65). Should a germ cell receive a translocation chromosome containing a large part of a 21 chromosome and also receive the normal 21 chromosome from that same parent, the resulting zygote would have partial trisomy 21. Such individuals generally have Down's syndrome. About 6 per cent of Down's syndrome patients have 46 chromosomes, with the extra dose of 21 chromosome being attached to another chromosome. Similarly, a small proportion of patients with the 18 trisomy syndrome or the 13 trisomy syndrome have the extra set of genes attached as part of a translocation chromosome.

The major reason for doing chromosome studies on individuals with autosomal trisomy syndromes, beyond confirmation of the clinical diagnosis, is to determine whether the patient has a translocation chromosome rather than the more usual full trisomy. This applies predominantly to younger mothers, because the vast majority of such babies born to older mothers have full trisomy. If it is a translocation case, then both parents should be studied to determine whether either of them is a balanced translocation carrier with a consequent high risk of having

affected offspring. Fortunately only about one third of the patients with partial translocation trisomy will be found to have a translocation carrier parent, because most of them represent fresh occurrences for which there is a negligible recurrence risk.

Chromosomal breakage with or without rearrangement allows for a wide variety of individually rare genetic imbalances with extra or missing segments of chromosomes. Many of these do not survive prenatal life. Of those who are born there are a wide variety of partial trisomies (mostly with a question as to the source of the extra piece of chromosome), and we have come to recognize certain specific autosomal deletion (missing piece) syndromes. Summitt,[11] evaluating undiagnosed multiple defect children, found 8 per cent with chromosomal abnormalities. Obviously, with our present techniques many small chromosomal exchanges or deletions will be missed. Chromosomal studies should be carried out on the parents of any child with structural chromosome aberration in an effort to determine whether either parent is a balanced carrier of the chromosome abnormality.

Another type of chromosomal abnormality that can lead to genetic imbalance is misdivision or breakage at the centromere during mitosis leading to the formation of an isochromosome, as depicted in Figure 62. The daughter cell receiving the isochromosome has an extra dose of the long arm of the altered chromosome and is missing the set of genes on the short arm of that chromosome. Occasional cases of the autosomal trisomy syndromes may be found to have a presumed isochromosome of the long arm of 21, 13, or 18 chromosome causing the genetic imbalance. X-isochromosome X has not been infrequent in individuals who have partial expression of the XO syndrome.

COUNSELING FOR CHROMOSOMAL ABNORMALITIES

Autosomal Trisomy Syndromes

1. If there is any question as to diagnosis, if the mother is young (generally less than 30 years), or if there are other cases of the same syndrome in the family pedigree, then chromosomal studies should be carried out on the patient in order to determine whether it is a full trisomy or a translocation case. If it is a full trisomy, then the future risk for younger mothers is less than 1 per cent, and for older mothers it is about the same as for any mother of that age (see Fig. 63). Should it be a translocation case, both parents should be studied to determine whether either parent is a balanced translocation carrier, a finding in about one third of such cases. The recurrence risk from chromosomally normal parents is apparently very small, certainly less than 1 per cent. The risk from a translocation carrier parent is often of major concern, particularly

FAULTY CHROMOSOME DISTRIBUTION
#21 chromosome as an example

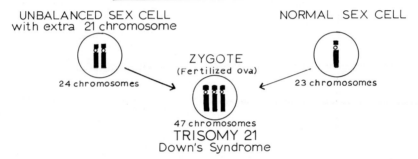

PRIOR TO FERTILIZATION

UNBALANCED SEX CELL
with extra 21 chromosome

NORMAL SEX CELL

ZYGOTE
(Fertilized ova)

24 chromosomes

23 chromosomes

47 chromosomes
TRISOMY 21
Down's Syndrome

AFTER FERTILIZATION

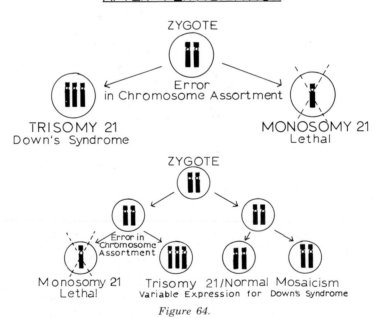

ZYGOTE

Error
in Chromosome Assortment

TRISOMY 21
Down's Syndrome

MONOSOMY 21
Lethal

ZYGOTE

Error in
Chromosome
Assortment

Monosomy 21
Lethal

Trisomy 21/Normal Mosaicism
Variable Expression for Down's Syndrome

Figure 64.

POTENTIAL INHERITANCE FROM 'BALANCED' TRANSLOCATION CARRIER

21/"14" translocation carrier example [t]
showing only the 21 and "14" chromosomes

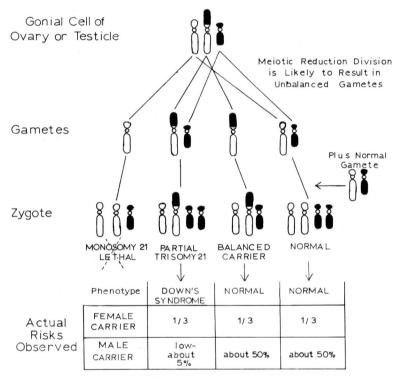

	Phenotype	DOWN'S SYNDROME	NORMAL	NORMAL
	FEMALE CARRIER	1/3	1/3	1/3
	MALE CARRIER	low-about 5%	about 50%	about 50%

The lower risk of Down's Syndrome from the carrier male may be due to reduced likelihood of an unbalanced sperm reaching the ova first! This is a good example of how it is difficult to predict the actual outcome in offspring of translocation carriers.

[t] The translocation could be a fresh occurrence in the development of this gonial cell. The above example occurred in a past generation and this individual is a balanced translocation carrier.

Figure 65.

when the risk of having translocation carrier normal children is added to that of having a child with the respective trisomy syndrome (see Fig. 65).

2. Inform the parents that the chromosome abnormality amounts to a gross genetic imbalance that upsets the pattern of development. Then explain what is *usual* for this genetic imbalance—the natural history for the syndrome.

3. For the 18 or 13 trisomy syndromes the parents may be told that most affected individuals with these trisomies are so seriously altered that they do not survive the first few months of pregnancy and that the parents "must have a good genetic background" and/or the mother "must be very good at carrying babies" in order to allow for prenatal survival of a baby with this genetic imbalance. This sets the stage for informing them of the limited capacity for postnatal survival, the outcome if the baby should survive early infancy, and the indications for providing comfort without medical intervention if they are in agreement with this approach. Whether the parents take the baby home or have the baby taken care of elsewhere is their decision; they simply should be reassured that survival will be limited no matter where the baby is being cared for.

Other Chromosomal Disorders

XO Syndrome. Suspicion of XO syndrome should lead to both buccal smear for sex chromatin *and* a chromosome study. An appreciable proportion of cases with partial expression of the full XO syndrome are found to be XO/XX mosaic, X iso-X, XX/X iso-X mosaic, or X deleted-X. The recurrence risk for these conditions is apparently very low to negligible, and older maternal age has not been a significant factor. In fact, X-linkage studies have more commonly indicated a lack of paternal than maternal sex chromosome in the XO cases.

Any Case with Deletion or a Translocation Chromosome. Both parents should have chromosomal studies. The majority of them will be found to be normal, and their recurrence risk is

negligible. If a parent is a balanced translocation carrier, then there is a significant recurrence risk. This may be figured out on a theoretical basis in terms of the possible meiotic products. However, the theoretical and the actual risks may not coincide, as is evident in Figure 65 for translocation carrier males.

REFERENCES

1. Carter, C. O.: The inheritance of common congenital malformations. Prog. Med. Genet., *4*:59, 1965.
2. Smith, D. W., and Aase, J. M.: Polygenic inheritance of certain common malformations. J. Pediat., in press, 1969.
3. Kolah, P. J., Master, P. A., and Sanghvi, L. D.: Congenital malformations and perinatal mortality in Bombay. Am. J. Obstet. Gynec., *97*:400, 1967.
4. Chung, C. S., University of Hawaii School of Public Health: Personal communication.
5. Saldanha, P. H., Cavalcanti, A. A., and Lemos, M. S.: Incidencia de defeitos congenitos na populacao de Sao Paulo. Rev. Paul. Med., *63*:211, 1963.
6. McKeown, T., and Record, R. G.: Seasonal incidence of congenital malformation of the central nervous system. Lancet, *1*:192, 1951.
7. Edwards, J. H.: Congenital malformations of the central nervous system in Scotland. Brit. J. Soc. Med., *12*:115, 1958.
8. MacMahon, B., Pugh, T. F., and Ingalls, T. H.: Anencephalus, spina bifida and hydrocephalus. Incidence related to sex, age, race, and season of birth and incidence in siblings. Brit. J. Prev. Soc. Med., *7*:211, 1953.
9. Abou-Daoud, K. T.: Congenital malformations observed in 12,146 births at the American University Hospital in Beirut. J. Med. Liban., *19*:113, 1966.
10. Fraser, F. C.: The Use of Teratogens in the Analysis of Abnormal Developmental Mechanisms. First International Conference on Congenital Malformations. Philadelphia, J. B. Lippincott Co., 1961.
11. Summitt, R.: Cytogenetics in mentally retarded children with anomalies: a controlled study. J. Pediat., *74*:58, 1969.

Chapter Five

MINOR MALFORMATIONS
as clues to more serious problems and toward the recognition of malformation syndromes

Minor anomalies are herein defined as unusual morphological features that are of no serious medical or cosmetic consequence to the patient. The value of their recognition is that they may serve as indicators of altered morphogenesis in a general sense or may constitute valuable clues in the diagnosis of a specific pattern of malformations.

Regarding the general occurrence of minor anomalies detectable by surface examination (except for dermatoglyphics), Marden, Smith, and McDonald[1] found that 14 per cent of newborn babies had a single minor anomaly. This was of little concern because the frequency of major defects in this group was not appreciably increased. However, only 0.8 per cent of the babies had two minor defects, and in this subgroup the frequency of a major defect was five times that of the general group. Of special importance were the findings in babies with three or more minor anomalies. This was found in only 0.5 per cent of babies (20), and 90 per cent of them had one or more major defects as well. In summary, the finding of several minor anomalies in the same individual is unusual and often indicates that a more serious problem in morphogenesis has occurred.

These minor external malformations are most common in areas of complex and variable features such as the face, auricles, hands, and

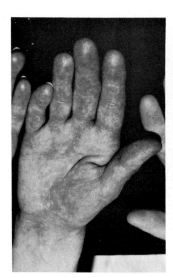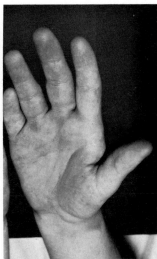

Figure 66. An otherwise normal mother (left) and daughter with clinodactyly of the fifth finger. A family history should be obtained before ascribing significance to a given minor anomaly.

feet. Before acribing significance to a given minor anomaly in a patient it is well to note whether it is found in other family members. Almost any minor defect may occasionally be found as a usual feature in a particular family, as noted in Figure 66.

The following figures illustrate certain minor anomalies, including dermatoglyphic features. Also depicted, for perspective, are some minor variants found in the newborn individual with sufficient frequency that they should not be classed as anomalies.

1. OCULAR REGION

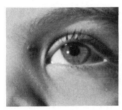 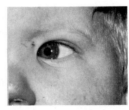 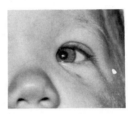

Varying degrees of inner epicanthic folds

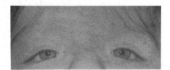 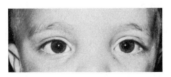 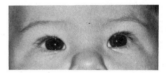

Lateral displacement of inner canthi and downslanting palpebral fissures

True ocular hypertelorism (see Appendix for normal measurements)

Mild lateral displacement of inner canthi and upslanting palpebral fissures

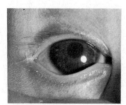 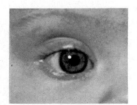 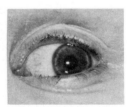

Brushfield spots: speckled ring about 2/3 of distance to periphery of iris with relative lack of patterning beyond it; Found in about 20% of individuals vs. 80% and more striking in Down's syndrome

Figure 67.

2. AURICULAR AREA

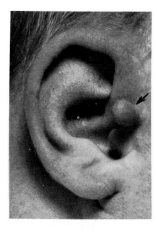

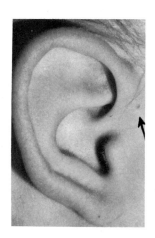

Cutaneous tags
or
pits

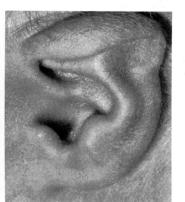

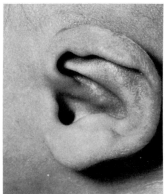

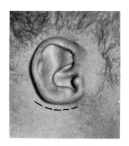

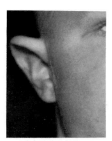

Lack of lobulus   Prominent ear

Incomplete scapha helix development (minor degrees not unusual in infants)

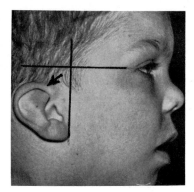

Ears low set: when the helix meets the cranium (arrow) at a level below that of a horizontal plane with the corner of the orbit

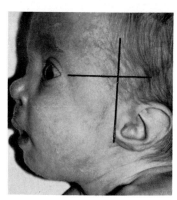

Ears slanted: when the angle of slope of the auricle exceeds 10 degrees from the perpendicular, a value which may be too low for prematures

Figure 68.

3. HAND—CREASES

(CLINODACTYLY, SYNDACTYLY)

The creases appear to reflect the early plane of flexion of the fingers and palm; mild alterations of form, function or both can alter the crease patterns

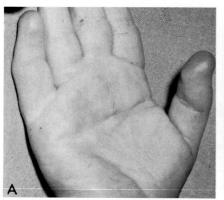
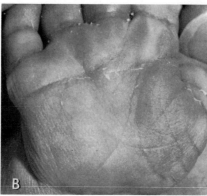
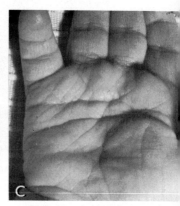

Single upper palmar*   Bridged palmar crease   Unusual crease pattern
simian crease

A and *B*, Single crease on short inturned fifth finger (clinodactyly)†
A, Partial syndactyly of third and fourth fingers (most common syndactyly of hand)

NAILS

(CAMPODACTYLY, ASYMMETRY)

The nails often reflect the form of the underlying distal phalanges

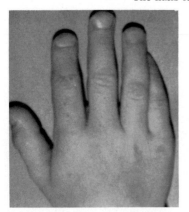
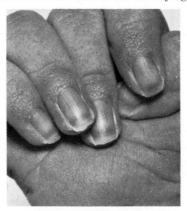
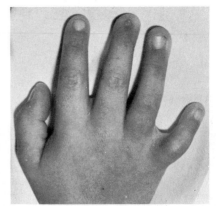

Short and broad nails   Narrow, hyperconvex   Hypoplasia of nail
nails,   and
especially fifth   camptodactyly of fifth finger;
asymmetry of short third finger

*About 4% unilateral in Caucasians, less than 1% bilateral
†Eight degrees or less inturning of the distal fifth finger is within normal limits

Figure 69.

4. DERMAL RIDGE PATTERNS

(DERMATOGLYPHICS)

The parallel dermal ridges on the palms and soles form between the thirteenth and nineteenth fetal weeks. Their patterning appears to be dependent on the surface contours at that time, and the parallel dermal ridges tend to develop transversely to the planes of growth stress.[2] Curvilinear arrangements occur where there was a surface mound, as over the fetal pads which are prominently present during early fetal life on the fingertips, on the palm between each pair of fingers, and occasionally in the hypothenar area. Indirect evidence suggests that a high fetal fingertip pad tends to give rise to a whorl pattern, a low pad yields an arch pattern, and an intermediate pad produces a loop, as illustrated in Figure 70B.

The dermal ridge patterning thereby provides an indelible historical record that indicates the form of the early fetal hand (or foot). Mild to severe alterations in hand morphology occur in a variety of syndromes, and hence it is not surprising that dermatoglyphic alterations have been noted in numerous dysmorphic syndromes. These alterations have seldom been pathognomonic for a particular condition. Rather, they simply provide additional data which, viewed in relation to the total pattern of malformation, may enhance the clinician's capacity to arrive at a specific overall diagnosis.

Dermal ridge patterning may be evaluated utilizing a seven-power illuminated magnifying device such as an otoscope, or a stamp-collector's flashlight which has a wider field of vision. Permanent records may be obtained by a variety of techniques listed in Appendix H.

There are two general categories of dermatoglyphic alterations: an *aberrant pattern* and an *unusual frequency* and/or *distribution of a particular pattern on the fingertips*.

Aberrant Patterning

Distal Axial Palmar Triradius (Fig. 70A). Triradii occur at the juncture of three sets of converging ridges. There are usually no triradii between the base of the palm and the interdigital areas of the upper palm. However, patterning in the hypothenar area often gives rise to a distal axial triradius located, by definition, greater than 35 per cent of the distance from the wrist crease to the crease at the base of the third finger.

This alteration, found in about 4 per cent of Caucasians, is a frequent feature in a number of patterns of malformation.

Open Field in Hallucal Area (Arch Tibial) (Fig. 70A). Open field simply means a relative lack of complexity in patterning and thereby implies a low surface contour in that area at the time ridges developed. The hallucal area of the sole usually has a loop or whorl pattern and a lack of such pattern is unusual in the normal but is found in about 50 per cent of patients with Down's syndrome and as an occasional feature in other syndromes.

Lack of Ridges. Failure of development of ridges in an area, most commonly the hypothenar area of the palm, is an occasional but nonspecific feature in the Cornelia de Lange syndrome.

Other Patterns. There are a number of other unusual patterns, especially in the upper palmar, hypothenar, and thenar areas, which may be of clinical significance, but these are so rarely of value in an individual case that they will not be discussed.

Unusual Frequency or Distribution of Patterns on the Fingertips

A quantitation of the overall extent of patterning on the ten fingertips may be achieved by obtaining fingerprints and recording the total fingertip ridge count, as illustrated in Figure 70C.

High Frequency of Low Arch Configurations. It is unusual to find a normal person with more than six of ten fingertips having a low arch configuration; however, this is a frequent feature in the 18 trisomy syndrome and the XXXXY syndrome, presumably reflecting hypoplasia of the fetal fingertip pads in these disorders. High frequency of low arches is nonspecific, being an occasional finding in certain other syndromes and in about 0.9 per cent of normal individuals.

High Frequency of Whorl Patterning. It is unusual to find nine or more fingertip whorls in an individual (3.1 per cent in normals). Excessive patterning, presumably reflecting prominent fetal pads, is more likely to be found in the XO syndrome, the Smith-Lemli-Opitz syndrome, occasionally in other patterns of malformation, and in some normal individuals.

Unusual Distribution, Especially of Radial Loop Patterns. Loops opening to the radial side of the hand are unusual on the fourth and fifth fingers. Radial loop pattern on these fingers is more common in Down's syndrome (12.4 per cent) than in the normal (1.5 per cent).

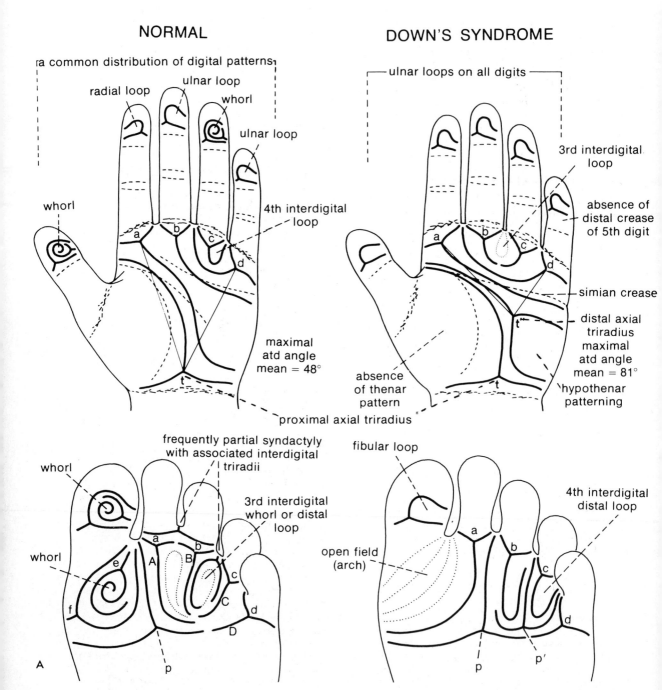

Figure 70. *A,* The solid lines and dotted lines denote the dermal ridge configurations, and the dashes within the palm represent the creases. (Courtesy of Dr. M. Bat-Miriam; prepared by Mr. R. Lee of the Kennedy-Galton Center near St. Albans, England.)

(Illustration continues on opposite page)

Ridge Count

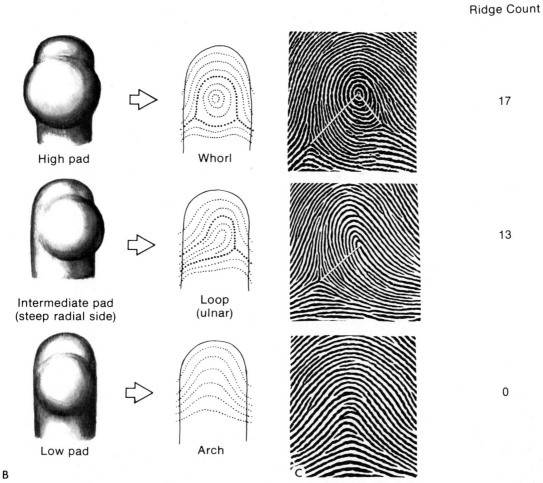

High pad → Whorl   17

Intermediate pad
(steep radial side) → Loop
(ulnar)   13

Low pad → Arch   0

B

Figure 70 (Continued). *B,* Presumed relationship between fetal fingertip pads at 16 to 19 weeks of fetal life and the fingertip dermal ridge pattern, which develops at that time. *C,* Technique for dermal ridge counting. A line is drawn between the center of the pattern and the more distal triradius, and the number of ridges which touch this line is the fingertip ridge count. The sum of the ten fingertip ridge counts is the total ridge count; this averages 144 in the male and 127 in the female. (From Holt, S.: Brit. Med. Bull., *17:*247, 1961.)

5. FEET

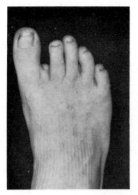
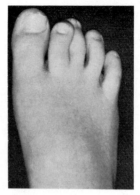
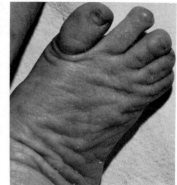

Asymmetrical   Clinodactyly   Short first metatarsal
length of toes   of second toe   with dorsiflexion of hallux
                      with overlapping

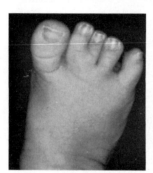
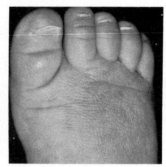
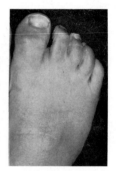

Syndactyly,   Hypoplasia of nails   Short, broad
most common 2-3   (2½ year old)   toenail

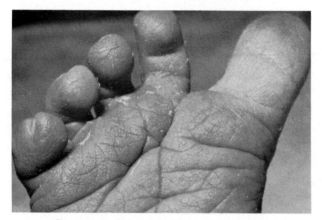
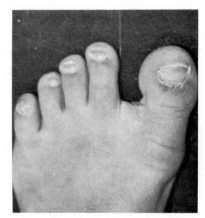

Deep crease between hallux and second toe   Wide gap between hallux
                                                   and second toe

Figure 71.

6. SKIN AND HAIR

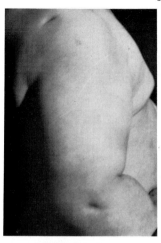

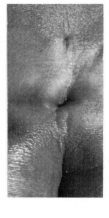

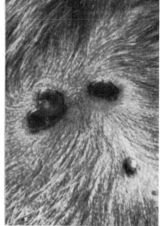

Deep dimples,
usually at bony
promentories

Deep sacral
dimple, often with
subsidiary creases
or pits

"Punched out"
ulceration,
posterior scalp

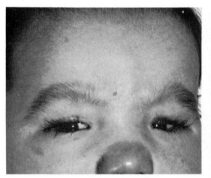

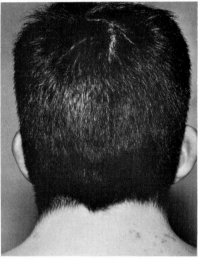

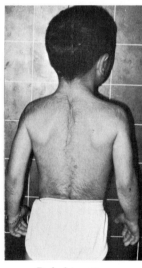

Abnormal eyebrows

Low posterior hairline,
especially at lateral
borders

Body hirsutism,
not secondary to
failure to thrive

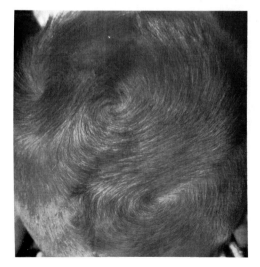

Multiple hair whorls

Figure 72.

7. MOUTH, THORAX AND GENITALIA

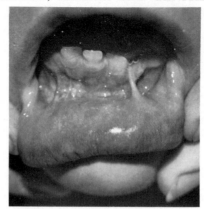

Aberrant frenula

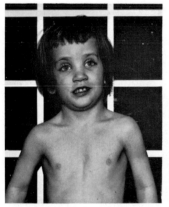

Mild pectus excavatum

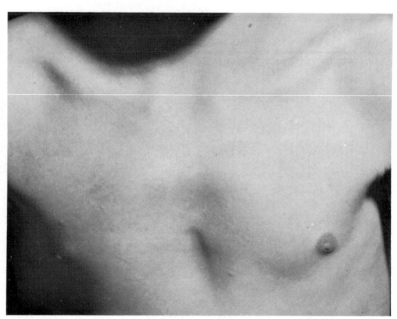

Short sternum

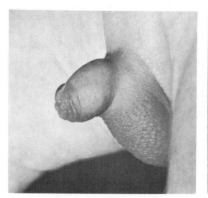

Scrotum extends distally
on phallus

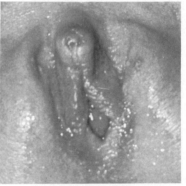

Hypoplasia of labia majora such
that clitoris *appears* prominent

Figure 73.

8. MINOR VARIANTS IN THE NEWBORN
WHICH SHOULD *NOT* BE CLASSED
AS ANOMALIES

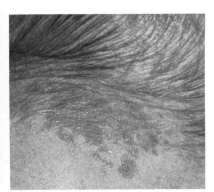 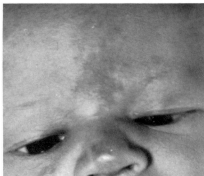 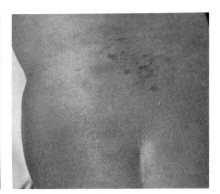

Fine nonelevated pink to red capillary hemangiomata (left to right) at nape of neck,
over central forehead and eyelids, and in lumbosacral area

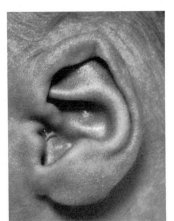 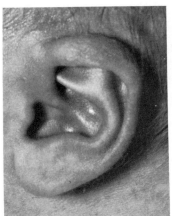 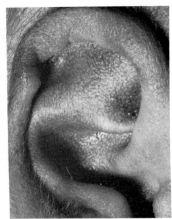

Incompletely outfolded scapha helix   Darwinian tubercle

Figure 74.

9. MINOR VARIANTS IN THE NEWBORN WHICH SHOULD *NOT* BE CLASSED AS MINOR ANOMALIES

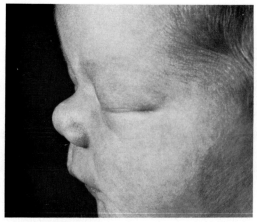

"Saddle" nose, mildly upturned nares

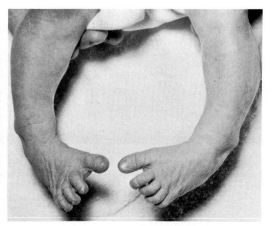

Mild to moderate inbowing of lower leg with tibial torsion

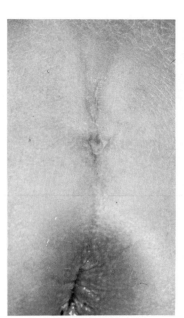

Sacral dimple, not deep

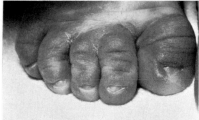

Mild syndactyly of second and third toes; also toenail hypoplasia in newborn

Figure 75.

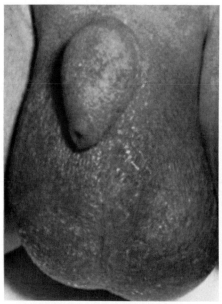

Hydrocele of testicle

REFERENCES

1. Marden, P. M., Smith, D. W., and McDonald, M. J.: Congenital anomalies in the newborn infant, in-cluding minor variations. J. Pediat., *64*:357, 1964.

2. Mulvihill, J., and Smith, D. W.: Genesis of dermal ridge patterning. J. Pediat., *75*:579, 1969.

APPENDICES

APPENDIX A

OUTLINE OF HISTORY AND PHYSICAL EVALUATION
FOR PATIENTS WITH MALFORMATIONS

PEDIGREE:

GESTATION: Duration_____ weeks; weight gain_____lb.; fetal activity began_____mo.

Vigor:_____

Possible illness, teratogens, or problems during pregnancy:_____

_____

BIRTH: Mode:_____ Birth weight:_____ Length:_____

Placenta and cord:_____ Amniotic fluid:_____

Problems:_____

_____

POSTNATAL: Growth:_____

_____

Developmental progress:_____

_____

OTHER HISTORY:

350

PHYSICAL EXAMINATION: Age_____ Height_____, _____%

Weight_____, _____% Head circumference_____

Developmental age or IQ_____

(Borderline findings in parenthesis)

CNS:_____

Neurological:_____

Cranium:_____

Ears:_____

Eyes:_____

Nose:_____

Mandible and mouth: _____

Face (other):_____

Neck:_____

Thorax:_____

Heart:_____

Abdomen:_____

Back:_____

Pelvis, hip, anus: _____

Genitalia:_____

Arms:_____

Hands: General:_____

         Creases:_____

         Dermal patterns:_____

Legs:_____

Feet:_____

Skin:_____

Hair:_____

Other:_____

COMMENT ON SPECIFIC ANOMALIES:

APPENDIX B

PERCENTILE CHARTS FOR MEASUREMENTS OF CHILDREN

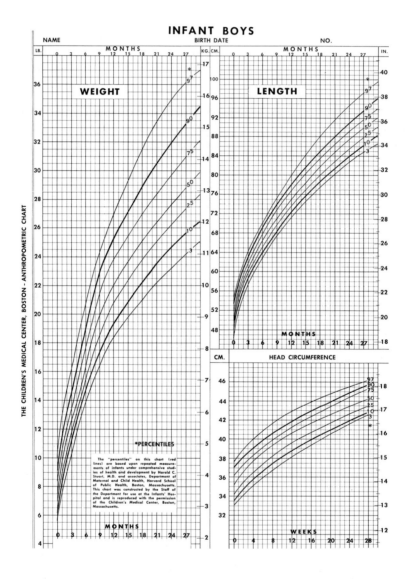

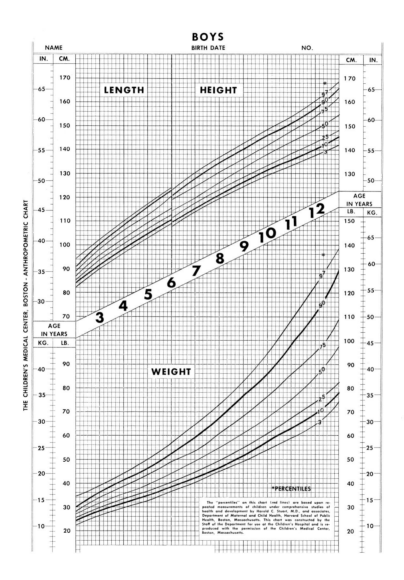

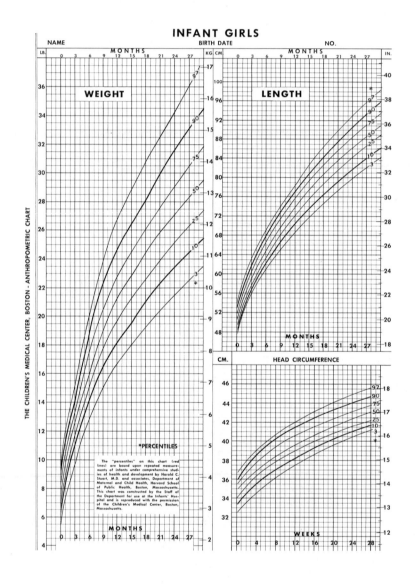

INFANT GIRLS

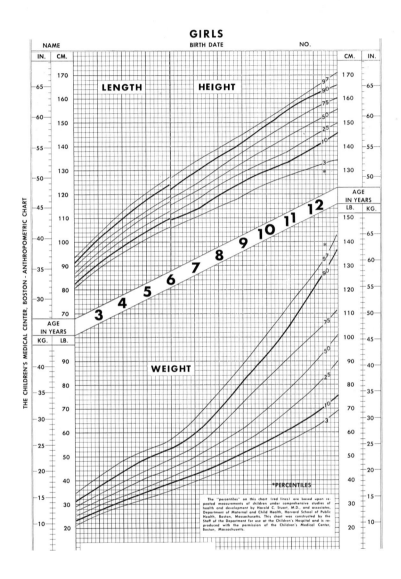

APPENDIX C

HEAD CIRCUMFERENCES

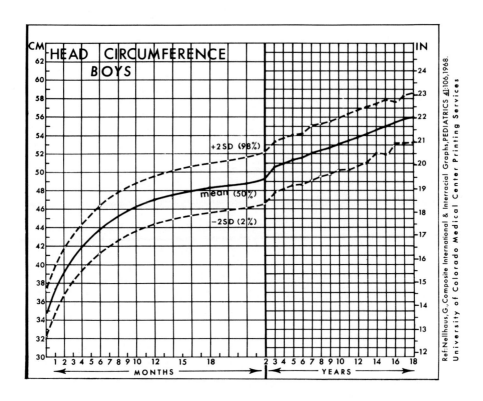

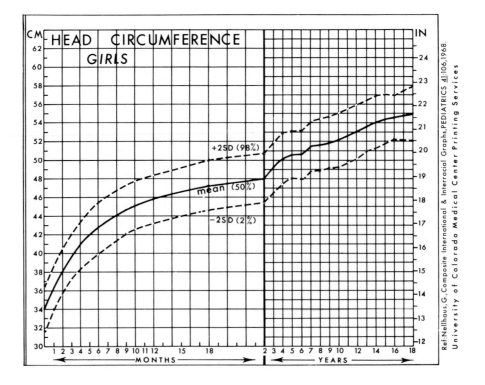

APPENDIX D

PRENATAL MEASUREMENTS

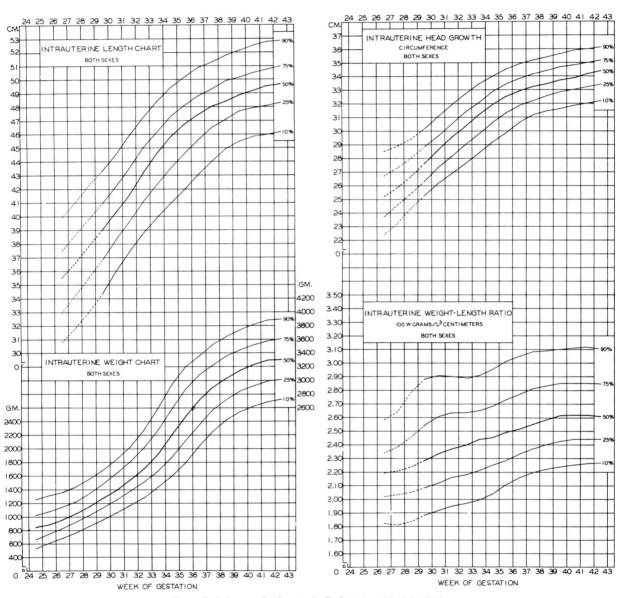

(From Lubchenco, L. O., et al.: Pediatrics, *37*:403, 1966.)

APPENDIX E

TABLES OF INNER CANTHAL AND OUTER ORBITAL DIMENSIONS

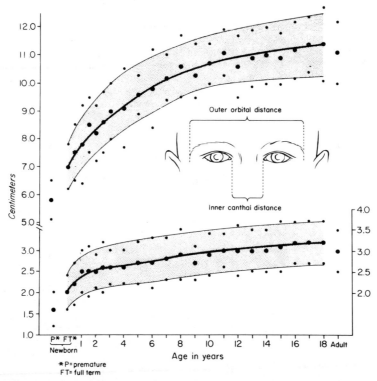

The large dots represent the mean value, and the small dots represent two standard deviations above (ninety-seventh percentile) and below (third percentile) the mean. Note that 70 per cent of the adult inner canthal distance is achieved by two years of age. (From Laestadius, N., et al.: J. Pediat., 74:465, 1969.)

APPENDIX F

Interpupillary and Palpebral Width Measurements

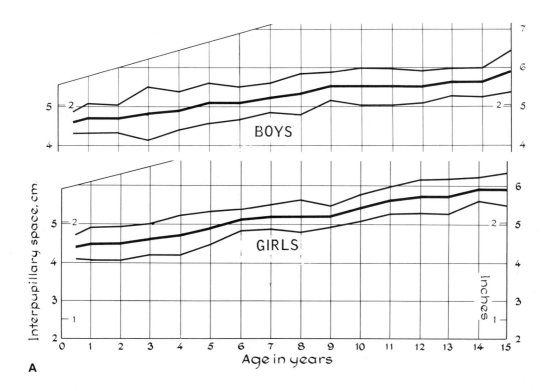

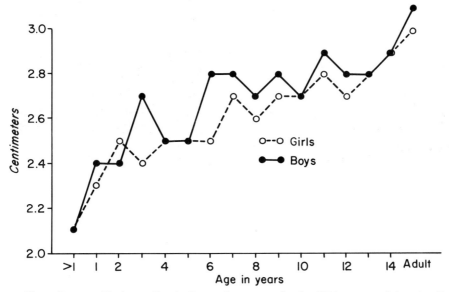

A, Interpupillary distance. The heavy line indicates the mean value for 6000 cases, and the other lines indicate one standard deviation above and below the mean (eighty-fourth and sixteenth percentiles respectively). (From Pryor, H. B.: J. Pediat., *68*:615, 1966.) *B*, Palpebral width measurement. (From data of Chouke, K. S.: Am. J. Phys. Anthropol., *13*:255, 1929.)

APPENDIX G

AURICULAR LENGTH AND ANATOMY OF AURICLE

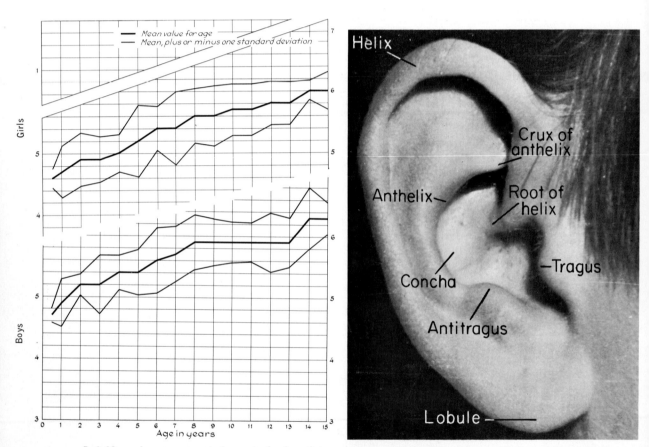

Left, Normal measurements for auricular length in centimeters. (From data of Lucas, W. P., and Pryor, H. B.: J. Pediat., *6*:533, 1935.) *Right,* Nomenclature for anatomical features of the normal auricle.

APPENDIX H

METHODS OF RECORDING DERMATOGLYPHICS

Faurot's Inkless Method

Materials. Special fluid (available in bulk or in individual packets) and paper from Faurot, Inc., 299 Broadway, New York, New York 10007. Soft thin sponge.

Technique. Wash and dry hands; sparingly and evenly rub fluid onto entire surface; lightly press hand to paper over sponge; reapply fluid to fingertips and roll them individually on paper; label impressions and repeat if incomplete.

Use. A good, general method for cooperative patients, not messy or cumbersome; but the correct amounts of fluid and of pressure on the paper are difficult to master.

Reference

Ford-Walker, N.: Inkless methods of finger, palm and sole printing. J. Pediat., *50*:27, 1957.

Hollister Printer Set

Materials. Hollister printing set with special inking pad and glossy paper, from Hollister, 211 East Chicago Avenue, Chicago, Illinois 60611. Soft thin sponge.

Technique. Wash and dry hands; apply ink evenly from pad to hand; firmly press hand to paper over sponge; label impressions and repeat if incomplete.

Use. Fairly good for younger children and infants, but untidy to handle and smudges easily.

Reference

Uchida, I. A., and Soltan, H. C.: Evaluation of dermatoglyphics in medical genetics. Pediat. Clin. North America, *10*:409, 1963.

Dry Pigment and Adhesive Transparent Tape

Materials. Clear adhesive tape in bulk roll, 5 inches wide (2VEF, Minnesota Mining and Manufacturing); tape cut in 6 inch lengths and applied to peel-off backing paper; thin carbon paper; clear acetate plastic sheet.

Technique. Wash and thoroughly dry hands; evenly coat hand with carbon from paper; cut tape to hand size and apply the tape at wrist, then distally to outspread fingers and into the central palm, the interdigital areas, and around fingers; peel off the tape from wrist distally and apply it smoothly to clear acetate; label impressions and repeat if incomplete.

Use. Very good for uncooperative individuals; good clarity, even of sweat pores; not cumbersome; one print includes palm and fingertips. The materials are difficult to obtain presently, and carbon paper can be somewhat messy.

Reference

Aase, J. M., and Lyons, R. B.: A new technique for recording dermatoglyphics. (In manuscript form.)

Photography by Internal Reflection

Materials. Norelco Inkless Fingerprint Instrument from North American Philips Company, Inc., 100 East 42nd St., New York, New York 10017. Price: $1500. Polaroid film.

Technique. Lightly press hand onto glass prism surface; expose and develop film.

Use. Quick, with unmatched detail and clarity, especially with infants. Disadvantages: initial high cost; small viewing surface such that multiple exposures are necessary to cover entire hand of older children and adults; instrument is nonportable; fingertip cannot be rolled to include necessary lateral margins.

Reference

Harrick, N. J.: Fingerprinting via total internal reflection. Philips Tech. Rev., *24*:271, 1962, 1963.

Plastic Mold

Materials. Silican latex (Silastic RTV 882, Dow Corning Corporation) and catalyst. Small cup and tongue blades.

Technique. Prepare mixture as directed; wash hands in soap and water, then rinse in alcohol and dry with acetone; with tongue blade, apply mixture sparingly to entire hand with close attention to interdigital palmar areas; let set for five to 15 minutes; gently peel off; label with ball-point pen; repeat if incomplete.

Use. Only way to record prints in three dimensions; gives clear detail with cooperative individuals; readily photographed after inking the mold. Tedious and time consuming because mixture must be prepared separately for each person; difficult to store mold; possible contact dermatitis.

Reference

Tips, R. L., Shininger, F. S., and Perkins, A. L.: Plastic mold method for recording dermatoglyphics. Human Bio., *36*:1, 1964.

Printer's Ink

Materials. Fingerprint ink; rubber roller; glass plate; heavy paper; soft thin sponge.

Technique. Wash and dry hands; apply a small amount of ink to glass plate and roll to a fine film; touch entire hand to plate; press hand onto paper over sponge; roll fingertips on inked plate and then on paper; label impressions, and repeat if incomplete.

Use. Standard method of police and federal agents; good dark prints with cooperative individuals; but messy, time consuming, and requires much equipment.

Reference

Cummins, H., and Midlo, C.: Finger Prints, Palms and Soles, New York, Dover Publications, 1961, pp. 45-52.

For Fetal Prints

Materials. 25× power binocular microscope; depilatory cream; talcum powder.

Technique. View hand directly under microscope. If patterns are unclear in the younger fetuses, apply talcum power to reduce glare; if still unclear, rub skin with depilatory cream and dry with tissue.

Use. For fetuses greater than 70 mm. crown-rump length.

Reference

Miller, J. R.: Dermal ridge patterns. Technique for their study in human fetuses. J. Pediat., *73*:614, 1968.

Index

NOTE: Page numbers in *italic* type refer to illustrations. Entries that begin with numbers (e.g., 13 Trisomy syndrome) are listed at the end of this Index.

Mouth. See also *Oral*.
  anomalies of, 284
  downturning corners of, syndromes featuring, 283
  minor malformations of, *346*
Mucopolysaccharidoses, 242-257
  I, 244, *245*
  II, 248, *249*
  III, 252, *253*
  IV, 250, *251*
  V, 254, *255*
  VI, 246, *247*
Multiple epiphyseal dysplasia, 200, *201*
Multiple exostoses, 208, *209*
Muscular disorders, with associated defects, 88-101
Mutant gene(s), mendelian inheritance of, 320-322
  single, with sex limitation, 322-323
    counseling for, 323, *328*
Myopia, syndromes featuring, 280
Myositis ossificans congenita, 266, *267*
Myotonic dystrophy, 96, *97*

Nail-patella syndrome, 234, *235*
Nails, hypoplasia or dysplasia of, syndromes featuring, 287
  minor malformations of, *340*
Nanism, diastrophic, 194, *195*
Neck, anomalies of, 285-286
  web, syndromes featuring, 285
Nervous system, central, anomalies of, 290
Neural tube closure, primary defect in, meningomyelocele and anencephaly resulting from, 3, *4, 9*
Neurofibromatosis, 162-163, *163*
Neurological disorders other than mental deficiency, with associated defects, 102-109
Neurovisceral lipidosis, familial, 242, *243*
Newborn, minor variants in, *347-348*
Nipple anomaly, syndromes featuring, 285
Noonan's syndrome, 60, *61*
Nose, anomalies of, 281-282
Nostrils, anteverted, small nose with, syndromes featuring, 281-282
Nystagmus, brachydactyly, cerebellar ataxia, and, 103
  syndromes featuring, 280

Obesity, syndromes featuring, 293
Occiput, flat or prominent, syndromes featuring, 278
Ocular. See also *Eye(s)*.
Ocular region, anomalies of, 279-280
  minor malformations of, *338*
Oculo-auriculo-vertebral syndrome, 112, *113*
Oculo-cerebro-renal syndrome of Lowe, 94
Oculodentodigital syndrome, 126, *127*
Oculomandibulodyscephaly with hypotrichosis, 72, *73*
OFD syndrome, 120, *121*
Opacity(ies), of cornea, syndromes featuring, 281
  penticular, syndromes featuring, 281
Opitz syndrome, 140, *141*
Oral. See also *Mouth*.
Oral frenula, syndromes featuring, 284
Oral region, anomalies of, 283
Oral-facial-digital associations of defects, 120-129
Oral-facial-digital syndrome, 120, *121*
Orbital dimensions, outer, measurement of, *358*
Orbital ridges, shallow, syndromes featuring, 279
Osler's hemorrhagic telangiectasia, 274
Osseous syndactyly, syndromes featuring, 287
Osteitis fibrosa cystica, 164, *165*
Osteochondrodysplasias, 186-215

Osteodystrophy, hereditary, Albright's, 238, *239*
Osteogenesis imperfecta, 264, *265*
Osteo-onychodysplasia, hereditary, 234, *235*
Osteopetroses, 216-225
  severe, 218, *219*
Oto-palato-digital syndrome, 128, *129*

Pachyonychia congenita, 184, *185*
Palate, cleft, cleft lip and, 2, *3*
    syndromes featuring, 283, 284
  narrow, maxillary hypoplasia and, syndromes featuring, 283
Palm, upper, single crease of, syndromes featuring, 288
Palpebral fissure, short or slanted, syndromes featuring, 279
Palpebral width measurements, *359*
Pancytopenia, Fanconi's syndrome of, 130, *131*
Patella, dysplasia of, syndromes featuring, 287
Pectus carinatum, syndromes featuring, 285
Pectus excavatum, syndromes featuring, 285
Penis, small, syndromes featuring, 292
Penta-X syndrome, 56, *56*
Peutz-Jeghers syndrome, 166, *167*
Philtrum, abnormal, syndromes featuring, 283
Photography by internal reflection, for recording dermatoglyphics, 361
Physical evaluation, outline of, for patients with malformations, *350-351*
Pierre Robin anomaly, 2, *8*
Pigmentation, of retina, syndromes featuring, 281
  of skin, abnormal, syndromes featuring, 289
Pili torti, deafness and, 181
Pilonidal cyst, syndromes featuring, 289
Pituitary, morphogenesis of, *311-312*
Pleonosteosis, Leri's, 82, *83*
Poikiloderma congenita, 176, *177*
Poland's anomaly, 6, *6*
Polygenic inheritance, in etiology of single primary malformations, 316-320
Polyposes, 166-168, *167*
Popliteal web syndrome, 118, *119*
Potter's syndrome, 5, *12*
Prader-Willi syndrome, 88, *89*
Prechordal mesoderm, primary defect in, defects resulting from, 3, *10*
Prenatal measurements, *357*
Prints. See *Dermatoglyphics*.
Progeria, 74-76, *75*
Prognathism, syndromes featuring, 283
Progressive arthro-ophthalmopathy of Stickler, 84, *85*
Pseudoachondroplastic form of spondyloepiphyseal dysplasia, 196, *197*
Pseudo-Hurler's syndrome, Caffey's, 242, *243*
Pseudohypoparathyroidism, 238, *239*
Pseudopseudohypoparathyroidism, 238, *239*
Pseudoxanthoma elasticum, 268, *269*
Ptosis, of eyelid, syndromes featuring, 280
Pyknodysostosis of Maroteaux and Lamy, 220, *221*
Pyle's disease, 216, *217*
Pyloric stenosis, syndromes featuring, 291

Racial groups, differences in incidence of malformations in, 317, *318*
Radial aplasia or hypoplasia, syndromes featuring, 286
Radial aplasia–thrombocytopenia, 132, *133*

FETAL DEVELOPMENT

AGE weeks	LENGTH cm. C-R	LENGTH cm. Tot.	WT. gm.	GROSS APPEARANCE	CNS	EYE, EAR	FACE, MOUTH	CARDIO-VASCULAR	LUNG
7	2.8				Cerebral hemisphere / Infundibulum, Rathke's	Lens nearing final shape	Palatal swellings / Dental lamina, Epithel.	Pulmonary vein into left atrium	
8	3.7				Primitive cereb. cortex / Olfactory lobes / Dura and pia mater	Eyelid / Ear canals	Nares plugged / Rathke's pouch detach. / Sublingual gland	A-V bundle / Sinus venosus absorbed into right auricle	Pleuroperitoneal canals close / Bronchioles
10	6.0				Spinal cord histology / Cerebellum	Iris / Ciliary body / Eyelids fuse / Lacrimal glands / Spiral gland different	Lips, Nasal cartilage / Palate		Laryngeal cavity reopened
12	8.8				Cord-cervical & lumbar enlarged, Cauda equina	Retina layered / Eye axis forward / Scala tympani	Tonsillar crypts / Cheeks / Dental papilla	Accessory coats, blood vessels	Elastic fibers
16	14				Corpora quadrigemina / Cerebellum prominent / Myelination begins	Scala vestibuli / Cochlear duct	Palate complete / Enamel and dentine	Cardiac muscle condensed	Segmentation of bronchi complete
20						Inner ear ossified	Ossification of nose		Decrease in mesenchyme / Capillaries penetrate linings of tubules
24		32	800		Typical layers in cerebral cortex / Cauda equina at first sacral level		Nares reopen / Calcification of tooth primordia		Change from cuboidal to flattened epithelium / Alveoli
28		38.5	1100		Cerebral fissures and convolutions	Eyelids reopen / Retinal layers complete / Perceive light			Vascular components adequate for respiration
32		43.5	1600	Accumulation of fat		Auricular cartilage	Taste sense		Number of alveoli still incomplete
36		47.5	2600						
38		50	3200		Cauda equina, at L-3 / Myelination within brain	Lacrimal duct canalized	Rudimentary frontal maxillary sinuses	Closure of: foramen ovale ductus arteriosus umbilical vessels ductus venosus	
First postnatal year +					Continuing organization of axonal networks / Cerebrocortical function, motor coordination / Myelination continues until 2-3 years	Iris pigmented, 5 months / Mastoid air cells / Coordinate vision, 3-5 months / Maximal vision by 5 years	Salivary gland ducts become canalized / Teeth begin to erupt 5-7 months / Relatively rapid growth of mandible and nose	Relative hypertrophy left ventricle	Continue adding new alveoli